The Cheater's Diet

The Cheater's Diet

The Sneaky Secrets
to Losing Up to
20 Pounds in 8 Weeks
Eating (and Drinking)
Everything You Love

MARISSA LIPPERT

DUTTON

DUTTON
Published by Penguin Group (USA) Inc.
375 Hudson Street, New York, New York 10014, U.S.A.
Penguin Group (Canada), 90 Eglinton Avenue East, Suite 700, Toronto, Ontario M4P 2Y3,
Canada (a division of Pearson Penguin Canada Inc.); Penguin Books Ltd, 80 Strand,
London WC2R 0RL, England; Penguin Ireland, 25 St Stephen's Green, Dublin 2, Ireland
(a division of Penguin Books Ltd); Penguin Group (Australia), 250 Camberwell Road,
Camberwell, Victoria 3124, Australia (a division of Pearson Australia Group Pty Ltd);
Penguin Books India Pvt Ltd, 11 Community Centre, Panchsheel Park, New Delhi – 110 017,
India; Penguin Group (NZ), 67 Apollo Drive, Rosedale, North Shore 0632, New Zealand
(a division of Pearson New Zealand Ltd); Penguin Books (South Africa) (Pty) Ltd,
24 Sturdee Avenue, Rosebank, Johannesburg 2196, South Africa

Penguin Books Ltd, Registered Offices: 80 Strand, London WC2R 0RL, England

Published by Dutton, a member of Penguin Group (USA) Inc.

First printing, April 2010
10 9 8 7 6 5 4 3 2 1

 REGISTERED TRADEMARK—MARCA REGISTRADA

LIBRARY OF CONGRESS CATALOGING-IN-PUBLICATION DATA

Lippert, Marissa.
   The cheater's diet : the sneaky secrets to losing up to 20 pounds in 8 weeks eating (and
drinking) everything you love / Marissa Lippert.
         p. cm.
   Includes bibliographical references and index.
   ISBN 978-0-525-95152-0 (hardcover : alk. paper)   1. Reducing diets.   2. Weight loss.
I. Title.
   RM222.2.L5356 2010
   613.2'5—dc22
                                                                2009050456

Printed in the United States of America
Set in Stempel Garamond • Designed by Victoria Hartman

For Zayde
Even in your absence,
you provide daily inspiration.

CONTENTS

ACKNOWLEDGMENTS

In true Cheaters style, this book came to life over countless Sunday brunches, mimosas included, with Alexandra Machinist, my literary agent and good friend. Al, thank you for being a constant source of inspiration and support.

Thanks to my mom, Sharon, and my grandmothers for instilling in me a love and appreciation for the kitchen and fresh, home-cooked food. Thanks to my dad, Ed, for his determination, stubbornness, and energy—all of which I've inherited. And thanks to my brother, Monte, for challenging me in and out of the kitchen.

A big thank-you to my publicist, Carla Nikitadis, for understanding me right from the get-go and making the next steps of this project so fun and infused with life.

Many thanks to Amy Abrams and Adelaide Lancaster for listening and pushing me forward and simply being the incredible women they are.

Thanks to my intern, Sarah Russell, for all her help and the excitement she oozes about nutrition, healthy eating, and cooking.

Thanks to Angelica Glass, Jeanine Donofrio, and Pryce McDowell for their talent.

Thanks to Barbara, Kim C., Margarita, Sunny, and Kim T., for giving me an avenue to reach so many people and help them think about food a little differently.

Thanks to my editor, Amy Hertz, and everyone at Dutton for seeing potential in this book.

And finally, a very grateful thank-you to all of my clients and my close-knit group of girlfriends (you know who you are). You all made this book, period.

INTRODUCTION

Cheaters Always Win . . .

Here's one of the best pieces of advice you'll ever receive: Cheaters always win. Sounds nothing like what your mother taught you, but when it comes to what you eat, it's the best-kept secret to smart, sustainable weight loss and a style of eating that is actually enjoyable, healthful, *and* rich with indulgence. Bottom line, this is a book about cheating and eating. Get excited. You'll not find any deprivation within these pages, so you can breathe a little easier. The word's finally out: Diets don't work, plain and simple. You know this, I know this, and the millions of other women and men, nearly 60 percent of Americans, attempting to shed a few pounds know this. But here's what so many of us still don't know—how to eat. And I'm not talking about proper fork and knife etiquette. I mean the basic building blocks of a healthy, balanced, sane diet, one that actually includes chocolate, cheese, and wine. It always amazes me to think about the countless clients, family, friends, and acquaintances who plead, "I just want to know how to eat . . . normally, wholesomely, and healthfully without being restricted to bland, boring diet food. And learning how to cook a simple chicken breast that doesn't resemble a burnt hockey puck would be nice, too. Can you please, for the love of God, help me?"

The Definition of Cheating

Before we get ahead of ourselves, what really defines cheating? It's a word with a pretty naughty connotation. Isn't "cheating" what always kills our valiant efforts to lose a few pounds? We're so fearful of it, yet it feels so damn good. Who doesn't like being a little "naughty" once in a while, honestly? This book erases the dividing line between "good" and "bad" food and turns the notion of cheating upside down, making it more acceptable in hopes of making food—really amazing, mouthwatering food—something you can actually enjoy. Relishing in cheating, or indulging in good quality food, allows you to love everything that you bite into.

The following chapters will help you *cheat* the system. It's a no-frills but extremely fun and tasty guide that halts the vicious cycle of "good food versus bad food" dieting and roller-coaster weight loss—and weight gain. Instead, you and your rear end will reap the benefits of utterly delicious food—and understand how to fit it easily into your life, shop for it, and cook it. You'll begin to see healthy, delicious food in a fresh, new light, and those extra pounds will start to fall off and stay off. You'll be able to bring balance between the "cheat" foods you love and a solid foundation of healthy basics.

You'll master how to navigate the grocery store and plan for the week ahead—snacks, simple lunches and breakfasts, and quick, healthy weeknight dinners. You'll lose weight wisely (without fear or loathing), you'll connect with your food, your hunger, and your cravings, and you'll understand how to keep off those damn pounds for good, once and for all! And you'll be ready and able to accomplish all of this, even with the inevitable slips and falls, because you're planning ahead, thinking more strategically. You'll have an outline of goals—each and every week. You want to live well, eat well, and lose weight all at once. Who doesn't? It's all at your fingertips, and the tip of your tongue. You'll be playing the game smarter, not harder, in no time, and cheating it up all the way.

Before we go further, who am I really to be writing about all this stuff? I'm a registered dietitian (so I'd better know what I'm talking about). Thinking, talking, and writing about great food and good health is what I do, and I'm passionate about it. It's a love affair that was sparked by the long line of masterful cooks and bakers in my family and that was solidified by the sights and smells of my mother's and grandmothers' kitchens. My mom started me young in the kitchen and without realizing it, my family helped shape me into the cheating nutritionista-foodie I am today. Healthful, home-cooked meals, fresh fruit on the counter for snacking, and not a sugary cereal in sight were the focus, while ice cream and homemade brownies in the freezer and chips in the pantry served as understated but unrestricted treats. I was pretty lucky, looking back. I unconsciously grew up understanding good food, great cooking, and healthful balance.

From all that, I emerged as an avid home cook and a restaurant lover who now lives and works in New York City. I'm in my early thirties, am forced to make do with the tiny kitchen in my apartment, am typically on the go, or rather five minutes behind, and am always finding fresh, simple ways to cook for just one—or for a group of ten. I'm known as "the organizer" among my friends, scouting out new local restaurants to try and hosting impromptu dinners. I come from a close-knit group of friends who love to go out and party just as much as we love to stay in and get completely wrapped up in solid conversation. I will rarely pass up a good glass of wine or four (hey, we all have those nights). Some of my favorite foods are ice cream (the real stuff), french fries, and a salty piece of sharp Pecorino Romano cheese—right up there with summer cherries, peppery arugula, and my mother's roasted carrots. And over the years, I've worked with hundreds and hundreds of individuals, helping them to improve their eating habits, lose weight, increase energy, figure out when and why to fit in grocery shopping and cooking, and to do it all without going nuts. In other words, I've heard it all (or at least a whole lot of what your needs and frustrations are) and I'm actually a lot like you—just a fun-loving, regular gal trying to do right for herself and her body.

My hope is that this book will serve as a road map, helping to make your life and the way you view food easier, healthier, greener, and hell of a lot more indulgent and appetizing. So get in the driver's seat—the following pages praise real food, real women, and real life. Visions of your skinny jeans are on the horizon! See, told ya cheaters always win. Let's get this party started.

Cheater's Basics: Learning to Plan Ahead for Pitfalls

"It's amazing what some great food, a couple of liters of water, and a forty-five-minute session on the elliptical will do for a girl."

—Margo

WEEK I GOALS

- Eat 2 fruits and at least 2 different vegetables per day. Fill up on more nutrients, fewer calories.
- Boost your water intake. Drink at least 1 ½ liters.
- Revise portion sizes by 15 to 25 percent. This chapter details all you'll need to know about servings sizes of all your basic food groups and favorite items.
- Work in one to two *cheat meals* and one to two *cheat treats* throughout the week . . . love them and don't dare feel guilty!
- Don't skip meals! Eating is too good to pass up. You've got to eat to lose those pounds.
- Get to the gym or get exercising. Add one or two more days of physical activity than you're already doing. If you already have a strong fitness routine of five to six days a week, up your intensity level or increase the length of your workouts by five to fifteen minutes.
- Decrease your alcohol intake by 25 percent of what you're currently drinking each week. If you average eight drinks a week, cut it back to six . . . or less.
- Start keeping a food journal. It's the only way you'll know what you've eaten.

All right, ladies, lock the door, turn off the cell phone, and take a deep, calming breath. Ready or not, open your fridge and kitchen cabinets and take a good, long look. If you're still standing and haven't passed out from sheer shock or horror, you might be facing one of the following scenarios:

a) **The social-butterfly party girl**—Who needs food when you've got martinis—don't the olives count? Your social calendar is packed tighter than your closet. You come home basically to sleep and shower, so it's no surprise that your fridge is completely barren aside from a few bottles of forgotten Chanel nail polish, some Gatorade (for Sunday morning hangovers), two bottles of champagne circa New Year's 2005, and what appears to be a block of cheese.

b) **The perpetual roller-coaster dieter**—Your cabinets are chock-full of every sugar-free, low-carb, non-fat cracker, cookie, and canned soup known to humankind. The fridge follows a close second with "lite" artificially sweetened yogurt, fat-free cheese (aka plastic orange squares), frozen diet dinners, some baby carrots, and a half-eaten jar of salsa. And you wonder why your meals taste like cardboard.

c) **The workaholic jetsetter**—Your fridge has a few apples, some gourmet Brie and smoked Gouda, last night's leftover Chinese (steamed chicken and broccoli), last week's leftover Italian (eggplant parm and penne alla vodka); the freezer boasts a few pints of your favorite boys Ben & Jerry (a lovely "welcome home" ritual after those extra-grueling workdays). And right on cue, that high-powered professional inner voice of yours scoffs, "I mean, come on now, let's be realistic here . . . who honestly has time to grocery shop or cook?"

d) **The green goddess wannabe**—You know who you are. Subscribing to the organic, environmentally conscious mantra, you've got some great stuff, like organic oatmeal and cage-free eggs, standing right alongside organic chocolate chip cookies, organic double fudge caramel brownie ice cream, organic ranch dressing, and organic mac 'n cheese. And damn, why are you still struggling to fit into that horrid bridesmaid's dress? Your sister's wedding is only three weeks away!

Okay, investigation of the crime scene's over, you can shut the fridge and the cabinets. Time to be realistic. Take a step back and think for a second; what's your real intention and goal in this whole "eating-food" game? You obviously picked up this book for a reason, and my guess is that it wasn't just to look pretty on your coffee table. I will repeat myself: This is *not* another diet book (you can let out a second huge sigh of relief), and it won't restrict you to beets and grapefruit all day or ban pasta or ice cream or bananas for the rest of your life. What it *will* do is inform and empower you, helping you make your relationship with food, your kitchen, and the grocery store a little easier and a lot more comfortable (with the added bonus that you'll see the scale drop a number of pounds in the process).

Welcome to Week 1, the first week of the rest of your healthier, tastier, greener, shiftier, and oh-so-slimmer life. We're starting anew and are rolling out the red carpet to build a fresh foundation and a tactical plan for the week ahead, baby step by baby step. Equate this week to reorganizing your closet with the essential staples that comprise a fantastic wardrobe: the little black dress, a killer pair of pumps, a couple of warm cashmere sweaters, a lovely lacey camisole or two. What you eat is just like what you wear. Would you ever consider donning something that's not of great quality or is itchy or unflattering or makes your boobs sag or your bum look larger than life? Probably not. The same goes for what you're putting in your mouth. Our bodies don't understand junk foods that are too processed, packaged, or prodded. Shop the good stuff—real fresh food—and your body will respond. So let's build the groundwork for your healthy eating wardrobe.

The Plan

We're starting with the bare-bones basics. This week's goals are going to help you jump-start the shedding of excess baggage and reinforce daily habits to keep the weight off. Let's reiterate your first week's plan of attack.

A Look at the Week Ahead:

Revise Portion Sizes
Cut your current portions by 15 to 25 percent. Read on in this chapter for precise portions of all your essential food groups. Why curb portions? Because the majority of Americans eat far more than is necessary. By no means is tackling serving sizes an easy task, but it's absolutely your best weapon for slimming down, staying that way, and eating things you actually enjoy. You'll learn specific details about what real-woman portions are as you read through this chapter. I don't eat like a peckish bird and I definitely don't expect you to, either. When in doubt about exact amounts, ounces, or cups, DO NOT overstress. This is not rocket science. Shave portions down by 15 to 25 percent and your body will do the rest.

Eat 2 Fruits and 2 Vegetables per Day
Fruits and vegetables fill you up fast, boost your health and immune system, and are quite calorie-friendly. Work them into the picture fast and furiously—we're aiming for two a day of each at a bare minimum.

Drink 1 ½ to 2 Liters or More of Water per Day
Better skin, better digestion, better energy, better waistline.

Don't Skip Meals
We want to maximize your ability to burn up calories, not hinder it. Once you've read through this chapter, you'll be eating smaller meals and satisfying snacks like it's your job. You paid good money for this book—give it a chance and you'll start building trust just like you would in a new relationship.

Have One or Two Cheat Meals and Treats Each Week
Because it stinks feeling deprived, like you're on a "diet." Clearly that's not what this book is about, so we're starting with the good stuff from day one. A cheat meal is defined as something fun, something "naughty," if you will. Things you love, like mac 'n cheese and pizza, but thought you weren't "allowed" to have. You're still moderating portions and ideally balancing out the meal with vegetables,

but go ahead and eat and don't feel bad about it. A cheat treat is defined as 200 to 300 calories of pure, unadulterated indulgence. Such as sharing a decadent dessert at a restaurant, a single scoop of real-deal ice cream, a cupcake, half of a gigantic chocolate chip cookie, or a small serving of french fries. The options are endless.

Hit the Gym or Get Active

If exercise or physical activity was an afterthought before this book, get off the couch, please! Increase exercise by at least one to two days (at least thirty minutes a clip). And if you're already a gym rat, try increasing your intensity level or tacking on an extra five to fifteen minutes to your workout. Though diet is the large majority, usually 60 to 70 percent or more, of the weight loss equation, a weekly fitness routine is extremely beneficial and speeds this whole weight loss process up. Walking, running, biking, dancing, skiing, even golfing . . . just get moving!

If You're a Boozer, Cut the Number of Drinks You Consume

Excess alcohol will put extra weight on in a heartbeat. Consider cutting back at least 25 percent of your intake per week. Don't fret, you'll get your alcohol in this book, and plenty of it.

Start Keeping a Food Journal

I saved this goal for last for good reason. It's *muy importante*! Writing down your meals, snacks, alcohol intake, and gym time means accountability, and it works wonders. It ensures that you're on track and are hitting this week's goals (as well as every week to follow). On the very next page you'll find a blank week's calendar to start using. Go ahead and rip it out to make copies if you wish—I don't care if you deface my book.

The Food Journal: Instructions on Use

Jot down each day's food, exercise, beverages, and "oops" moments. Oopses are for situations like: "Oh crap, I had one too many cocktails at happy hour and found myself knee deep in nachos and cheese fries at 2 a.m." Obviously, situations like that are few and far between now that you're on a mission to lose those pounds for

Week 1: Your Weekly Food Journal

Week 1:	Monday	Tuesday	Wednesday
BREAKFAST *300-400 calories* *(Note your hunger level on a scale of 1 to 10 after each meal)*			
SNACK *less than 100 calories* *(If you're not hungry, skip it!)*			
LUNCH *400-550 calories*			
SNACK *100-200 calories*			
DINNER *400-600 calories*			
SNACK *100-150 calories* *(Work in desserts and treats when you really want them and they're damn worth it!)*			
WATER			
ALCOHOL/ OOPS!			
EXERCISE			

Thursday	Friday	Saturday	Sunday

good, but being realistic and writing EVERYTHING down will help you reach your goals that much faster. I encourage you to take note of your hunger level on a scale from 1 to 10, 1 being famished and 10 being stuffed. This can be a helpful way of gauging what meals and snacks really fill you up and satisfy you and which ones don't. You may have been eating cereal for breakfast the past ten years but never realized that it doesn't fill you up and you're consistently starving soon after. Journaling and assessing your hunger levels tells you what works best for your particular body. It also tells you when you've gone overboard on portion sizes and are too full.

Tally up your workouts, your cheat treats and meals, and your alcohol intake each week. If the scale is stuck, that's a quick indicator to kick up your workouts and take down the cheats, oopses, and alcohol a notch or two. Take time to look back at what you've written down each week and assess what worked well and what kinks in your schedule or your meals still need to be adjusted. Help yourself by resetting your own personal goals in addition to those laid out in each chapter.

> *Cheater's Secret:* If hand-writing your journal is too old school for you, or simply not practical because you're constantly on the move, try keeping it on your computer or get the super-convenient Cheater's Diet Food Journal, which you can easily download at www.cheatersdietbook.com.

The Plan, Part Deux

I've taken the liberty of completing a sample week's food and exercise map for you for Week 1, and every other week to follow. The meals and snacks laid out are by no means set in stone—there's always room to play around and swap ingredients or change days around to fit your schedule and food preferences. Each sample calendar depicts how I myself might set a week up, taking into account work commitments, social engagements, gym time, travel, grocery shopping, and more. Week after week, you'll build upon the goals and lessons from the prior chapter.

So take a good look, let it sink in, and gather whatever questions you have swimming in your head. Each chapter bears a straight-forward plan and a sample food calendar for the week ahead. Each calendar incorporates a few recipes from the little cooking lessons you'll get at the end of each chapter. Cooking better helps you eat better, which all helps bust those extra pounds. Assess each week's plan first, then read the remainder of the chapter to see how easily you'll be able to simulate and implement it.

Week 1—Cheater's Shopping List:

- ❑ Vegetables: 3 to 5 (or more) for the week: spinach, asparagus, red bell peppers, snow/snap peas, carrots
- ❑ Fruit: 2 to 4 types (or more), your pick (enough to get you through 5 to 7 days, 2 servings a day): apples, bananas, grapefruit, strawberries, pears
- ❑ Protein: eggs, 1 pound chicken breasts, 8 ounces flank steak or tofu, 1 pound shrimp, 1 whole roasted chicken from the grocery store *grab on the way home the night you're eating it
- ❑ Healthy carbs: 1 sweet potato, whole grain cereal (more than 5 grams fiber, less than 7 grams sugar), whole grain bread
- ❑ Dairy/calcium: string cheese, shredded mozzarella cheese, feta cheese, 3 to 4 low-fat plain yogurts or cottage cheese, skim or soy milk
- ❑ Other: 2 28-ounce cans of whole plum tomatoes, honey, pine nuts, currants/raisins
- ❑ Fresh herbs and spices: chives, parsley, garlic, ginger
- ❑ Seasonings and oils: bottle of balsamic vinegar, olive oil and canola oil, low-sodium soy sauce and low-sodium chicken or vegetable broth, 2 lemons
- ❑ Snack stuff and staples (for work/home): all-natural peanut or almond butter, hummus (any flavor), all-natural granola bars (more than 3 grams fiber)
- ❑ Dessert/treat: dark chocolate (more than 70% cacao), all-natural/organic frozen yogurt

Week 1: Sample—Starting Simple
based on 1400-1600 calories

Week 1:	Monday	Tuesday	Wednesday
BREAKFAST 300-400 calories 7-9:30 a.m.	6 ounces plain low-fat yogurt with 1 cup fresh fruit (e.g., mixed berries or banana—your choice) For an extra boost: Toss in 1 to 2 tablespoons chopped almonds or pecans, or ½ cup whole grain cereal such as Kashi Heart to Heart, bran flakes, or good ol' Shredded Wheat	1 slice seven grain bread (or 1 whole wheat English muffin) with 1 ½ tablespoons natural peanut butter and banana slices (1 medium banana)	HIT THE GYM Post-gym recharge: 2 hard-boiled eggs and 1 slice whole wheat toast with ½ grapefruit (or a serving of fruit) (Don't know how to hard-boil an egg? Check out page 41 for the recipe.)
SNACK About 100 calories 10-11 a.m. (If you're not hungry, SKIP IT!)	1 serving of fruit	1 part-skim string cheese or 1 ounce cheddar cheese and a small apple or handful of grapes	4 ounces (½ cup) cottage cheese or a quick swig of skim milk or soy milk (snag it from the office fridge)
LUNCH 400-550 calories 12-2 p.m.	At the corner deli—open-face turkey sandwich (take the top half of that sucker off—the bread, that is) with 1 slice seven grain bread, 3 to 4 slices all-natural turkey breast (such as Applegate Farms, or freshly roasted if you can get it), Dijon mustard, lettuce, tomato, and 2 to 3 thin avocado slices or 1 slice light Swiss or cheddar cheese	Make-your-own-salad 1. mixed greens, spinach, or arugula 2. some type of protein, such as grilled chicken, salmon, plain tuna, hard-boiled egg, beans, tofu 3. whatever veggies or fresh fruits you wish to add 4. a sprinkle (about 2 tablespoons) of 1 or 2 of the following: cheese, dried fruit, nuts, olives, and avocado 5. 1-2 tablespoons dressing: olive oil and vinegar or lemon juice; balsamic, red wine, Dijon vinaigrette, to name a few	The office cafeteria (make the best of it)—1 to 1 ½ cups veggie or turkey chili with a sprinkle of shredded cheddar cheese and side of steamed broccoli
SNACK 100-200 calories 3-5 p.m.	1 piece of fruit and handful of trail mix from office vending machine (½ bag) HIT THE GYM and go GROCERY SHOPPING early this week to get things rolling!	All-natural granola bar (such as Kashi TLC Bars, Nature Valley, or Gnu Flavor and Fiber Bars)	Apple and 1 tablespoon all-natural peanut butter or almond butter
DINNER 400-600 calories 7-8:30 p.m.	Got home late, unpack groceries and do up a quick dinner—Eggs with Fresh Chives and Mozzarella (page 61), with 1 slice whole grain toast	2 cups Ginger-Soy Stir-fry (page 52) and ¾ cup brown rice or soba noodles	4 ounces roast chicken (pick up a preroasted chicken from the grocery store) and spinach sautéed with 2 teaspoons olive oil and garlic and 1 small baked sweet potato (to save on time, microwave it for 4 to 5 minutes)

Thursday	Friday	Saturday	Sunday
1 cup whole grain cereal (such as Kashi Golean— look for anything with more than 5 grams of fiber) with 1 cup strawberries (or a serving of fruit) with ¾ cup skim or low-fat soy milk	6 ounces plain low-fat yogurt with fresh fruit (such as mixed berries or banana—your choice) and ¼ cup granola (go for the brand lowest in sugar, such as Bear Naked or Feed)	HIT THE GYM Banana before the gym No-brainer breakfast: 1 cup whole grain cereal with 1 cup strawberries and ¾ cup low-fat soy milk	SLEEP LATE
1 serving of fruit	1 handful of roasted, unsalted almonds or cashews	Skip it, you slept in.	Skip it, you're heading to brunch instead!
Favorite salad joint— 3 to 4 ounces grilled chicken breast (or 3 ounces flank steak strips) over 3 cups mixed greens with 2 tablespoons blue cheese, ½ cup sliced red pears, 2 teaspoons dried cranberries, 1 tablespoon chopped pecans, with 1 tablespoon balsamic vinaigrette	PB&J from home (who doesn't love it?) and an apple	Veggie wrap: 1 grilled portobello mushroom, 2 tablespoons goat cheese, romaine lettuce or mixed greens, ⅓ cup jarred roasted red peppers, in an 8-inch multigrain wrap (such as Ezekiel or Aladdin)	Brunch out—omelet with spinach, tomato, and goat cheese, 2 slices turkey bacon (if you can get it), and fruit salad
12 ounces skim latte with cinnamon	1 cup fresh cut vegetables and ¼ cup hummus	4 cups low-fat popcorn (like Smart Pop or Newman's Own)	CHEAT TREAT—You're dying for a chocolate chip cookie from the best bakery in town. It's enormous, so split it with your friend. Iced coffee with a dash of milk
CHEAT MEAL #1 dinner out with the girls	1 ½ cups Baked Shrimp with Feta and Tomatoes (page 56), ¾ cup whole wheat penne, and 2 cups arugula salad with 2 teaspoons olive oil and 1 teaspoon balsamic vinegar	CHEAT MEAL #2 dinner date Split tuna tartare to start, share 8-ounce filet mignon and mushroom risotto	4 ounces Balsamic-Glazed Steak or Chicken Breast (page 47) and 6 or 7 steamed asparagus spears with lemon zest

Continued

Week I:	Monday	Tuesday	Wednesday
SNACK 100-150 calories 8:30-9:30 p.m. (Again, if you're not hungry, SKIP IT!—work in desserts and treats when you really want them and they're damn worth it!)	2 small squares dark chocolate (look for 70% cacao content or more, like Green & Blacks, Ghirardelli, or Dagoba)	Fresh fruit (e.g., I cup strawberries, 2 clementines, or I cup watermelon chunks)	
WATER	I ½ liters and an unsweetened iced tea	2 liters	I ½ liters and a glass of seltzer with lime
ALCOHOL/ OOPS!			I glass wine or skip it!
EXERCISE	45 to 60 minutes		60 minutes

Map It Out

First things first—in order to kick up the slim-down process, it's unbelievably helpful to map out your week ahead. Rock out your type-A tendencies (we all have them, whether they're blatant or latent) and take a quick glance at your week's schedule, noting major work meetings and deadlines, social events, dinners . . . you get the idea. Now take a second look and start plugging in your healthy foundation—when exactly you're hitting the gym for forty-five minutes, when you're going to the grocery store, and when you'll have thirty minutes to cook at home. This is called "you time," and I swear it'll make you a more sane, refreshed person, and it *should* be what you eventually build the rest of your week around, obviously barring things out of your control, like that bout of strep throat that wiped you out for over a week last winter or your friend's birthday party during the last week of your monthly cycle when you just couldn't resist eating three cupcakes. When you map out

Thursday	Friday	Saturday	Sunday
½ cup frozen yogurt, like Stonyfield Farms, with berries on top			Fresh fruit or skip it!
1 ½ liters	2 liters	2 liters	1 liter (Water on weekends can be tough sometimes—try carrying a bottle with you or remembering to drink at mealtimes)
	1 vodka-soda, glass of wine, or light beer	2 glasses wine and 2 vodka/sodas and 1 slice late-night pizza	
		60 to 90 minutes—it's the weekend, enjoy a good long workout when you can!	

your schedule and specific healthy eating goals (you'll do this each week in your trusty food journal), those goals become set in stone, and soon enough they become habitual. You wouldn't think not to do them. Personally, I tend to go the old-school route and employ a basic date book/scheduler that details each week out, but choose whatever weapon works best for you, whether it's your Outlook calendar, your BlackBerry or iPhone, or the ever-economical piece of scrap paper lying around on your desk.

The point is, mapping it out allows you to see what the week has in store for you. You're playing smart, avoiding being ambushed and planning out healthy cheating habits according to what your week's like. For instance, say you've got a massively important meeting on Wednesday at 10 a.m. Your standard day prior to this book might have looked like this:

9 a.m.—Rushing, late for work. Grab coffee on your way into the office. Sneak into 10 a.m. meeting with seconds to spare.

11:30 a.m.—Finish meeting and frantically run back to your desk to tackle a boatload of e-mails.

2:30 p.m.—The thought of eating something finally occurs to you and you're so hungry you're ready to eat whatever's in sight . . . times two.

Let's rework that scenario a bit. Thinking ahead and planning to grab a banana and a low-fat yogurt WITH your coffee in the a.m. gets your metabolism rolling, fuels you up to be a standout in the meeting, and helps cue your hunger after the meeting for your next meal, often called lunch. You might inhale the yogurt and banana five minutes before heading into the conference room, but at least we're onto something here. You're simply looking at your day from a slightly different perspective and making it more efficient.

Here's how a revamped Cheater's Diet day, up through lunch, would look:

9 a.m.—Rushing, late for work. Thankfully, you stock the office fridge each Monday with enough yogurt to last you through the week. You're prepared, and you're proud of it.

9:45 a.m.—Grab coffee and a banana from the deli next to your office. Snatch your trusty yogurt from the fridge and have just enough time to eat before heading to your 10 a.m. meeting.

11:30 a.m.—Finish meeting and sit down at your desk to respond to a flood of morning e-mails. A quick handful of some roasted cashews stashed in your desk drawer helps you plow through e-mail after e-mail like a fine-tuned machine. Small, simple midmorning snacks are excellent "energy bridges" to get you to lunch, even if you're eating later than you'd like.

Cheater's Secret: Have 10 to 20 nuts per serving and be done. Nuts pack in protein and healthy fat to hold you over, boosting satiety and energy so you're alert and efficient throughout the morning or in general between mealtimes. They can, unfortunately, also pack in the calories, so keep a portion to a handful, 10 to 20

(100 to 200 calories).We usually have the shortest gap between breakfast and lunch, so for a mini morning snack, you're likely good to go with the lower end, about 8 to 12. If nuts aren't your thing or you're allergic, just remember to keep the morning snack simple, around 80 to 150 calories—like a 1-ounce piece of cheese or a piece of fresh fruit. For more on snacks, see page 94.

2:30 p.m.—Lunchtime, finally. Those cashews did the trick and you were able to make it to lunch without turning into your evil, ravenous twin and ordering double the amount or opting for the most outrageous thing on the menu . . . with a side of fries.

While we're on the topic of time, let's take a moment to tackle the basics of when to have meals throughout the day.

Well Timed

- **Breakfast—Eat It!** Mom was right—breakfast is the most important meal of the day. Eating something within about ninety minutes after waking revs up your metabolism to effectively burn calories throughout the day. Imagine your metabolism is like a fire—you want to get those flames roaring as soon as you can early in the morning and keep them burning throughout the day. A common rebuttal against breakfast I hear is, "But if I eat breakfast, I'm starving a few hours later." My response, "Thank goodness! That means your body is cranked up and is working as it should be." It's a fact—you've got to eat to lose. You want to set the tone of your day from the get-go. A healthful, kickass day starts with a healthful, kickass breakfast. Research notes that eating the majority of your calories earlier in the day helps aid weight loss, keeps metabolism moving, and helps decrease the total amount of calories you take in throughout the day—not to mention it'll likely save you from getting tripped up by sneak-attack sugar cravings.
- **Skipping Meals Stinks!**—So do your best not to do it. The same theory applies here as with breakfast. If you snooze on

the food, you lose out on max calorie-burn potential (and not to mention, isn't it more fun and appealing to eat more frequently throughout the day rather than starve yourself until 5 p.m.?). It's not a pretty picture—your blood sugar's all out of whack, you've got a headache, feel light-headed, and are so cranky you could rip someone a new one if they look at you wrong. Skipping meals makes you ready to eat everything in sight and causes your metabolism to lag. Skipping may even cause you to gain weight if you tend to overeat at meals later in the day because you're so damn hungry. There's too much risk of blowing your calorie bank way out of the water, so don't cheat yourself out of multiple meals throughout the day.

CHEAT SHEET: It's All About Timing—A Sample Day of Meals and Snacks

8:30 a.m.—Breakfast
11 a.m.—Mini morning snack (if you're hungry)
1 p.m.—Lunch
4:30 p.m.—Afternoon snack
6:30 p.m.—Gym/exercise
8 p.m.—Dinner
9:30 p.m.—Small dessert/evening snack three or four times a week (try to leave at least 1 ½ to 2 hours between your last meal or snack and when you hit the sack)
11:30 p.m.—Lights out

- **Every Three to Four Hours**—That's about the amount of time in between meals and snacks you should be aiming for. Eating every few hours will help sensitize and stabilize your blood sugar and metabolism. Some days during the month you might be ravenous all day long and need to grab something small every two to three hours; other days you might be fine holding out for five hours. Just try to get in three balanced meals during the day (more on what "balanced" actually means to come) and at least one snack to keep you energized and fired up. When it comes to weekends, I realize that two full meals tend to be the standard, and that's just fine if you're sleeping late. After all, brunch is one of the best things ever invented.

- **Listen to Your Body**—This concept is completely foreign to many of us, particularly those of us tortured by every fad diet and food marketing claim that's surfaced in recent memory. You know, it's the mind game of "Well, the box says this sugar-free oatmeal will help me kick extra weight, so I *have* to buy it—even if I don't really like the taste and I'm ready to eat my hand an hour later." Read: That "diet-designed" oatmeal might *not* be your best breakfast option. Use this first week and the next few weeks to do a little detective work and try out something else that actually satisfies and sustains you. It's not easy distinguishing among hunger, satiety, and cravings (more on this in Chapter 4), but I promise your body won't let you down when you can read acute messages like "Waiting too long to eat gives me a headache" or "I'm really full and if I eat a second helping my stomach might explode." Start simple this week and just begin paying a bit more attention to your body's hunger and satiety signals—you might surprise yourself. Keep a handy list of what foods fill you up best on less.
- **Slow and Steady**—Slow down when you're eating. Eating shouldn't be something you race through. It takes fifteen to twenty minutes for your stomach to tell your brain it's full and well-fed. Slowing down your pace of eating allows you to actually *taste* your food and discover the wondrous flavors and textures that abound on your plate. You'll fill up faster, which, in turn, translates to you eating less. If you've traveled to Europe (or even if you haven't), you likely find that eating really is a pleasurable, often memorable experience that's meant to be enjoyed and appreciated. So take your time.

Portion Perfection

Portion size is not something that comes easy to the vast majority of Americans. With the double- or triple-size portions we receive at many restaurants, bagels and burgers that are as big as our heads, the allure of super-sizing (if you have yet to watch Morgan Spurlock's documentary *Super Size Me*, please do so), and average dinner plates that are more than 30 percent larger than they were forty years ago. All of this translates to increased consumption. Today, the average adult female consumes 335 more calories per day than she did in 1971, the average male, 168 more calories. Just twenty years ago, the bane of every fad dieter's existence, the bagel, was a mere 140 calories. Now bagels are nearly blimp-size, weighing in at 350 to upward of 500 calories. No wonder they tend to make you bloated—you just consumed the equivalent of four or five pieces of bread! When it comes to proper portions, I always find it interesting that when I visit my parents, my dad refuses to eat on a regular-size dinner plate (stubbornness is one of his finer qualities). He prefers to use a perfectly satisfying salad plate. It's not about being dainty or watching his waistline—he just knows what his body requires.

Bottom line, if you get portions down pat, you'll be loving life, your favorite foods, and how you feel in your clothing. Eat too much of anything, even if it's deemed healthy, and your body will store that excess as fat, like it's shoving it into a mini storage unit. And we've all seen how that scary scenario can play out in a tight black minidress. That's why having small portions of pleasurable food is a cheater's golden key. Portions aren't easy to tackle and refine, but your taste buds, your mind, and your stomach (and if a dish is *that* good, maybe even your loins sometimes)—will all be happy campers.

Here's a basic breakdown for mastering your own portion sizes:

- First, start with your plate. Use a salad plate if it's the easiest way for you to portion things. Otherwise, definitely whip out the gorgeous set of standard-size plates you purchased from Crate and Barrel and carefully consider the following appropriate portions.
- Divide your plate up into four equal parts, like we've done here, and take a second look next time you sit down to a meal. Time to test your knowledge of fractions back from fourth-

grade math class. Your plate proportions should typically look like this: ½ vegetables and/or fruit (two parts), ¼ lean protein, ¼ healthy complex carbohydrates/whole grains. Notice how the emphasis here is on fruits and vegetables. Unfortunately, a staggering 89 percent of the American public doesn't get its fill of fruits and veggies on a given day. It's obvious that this plays a part in our country's major health and obesity crisis. Packed with vitamins, minerals, disease- and wrinkle-fighting antioxidants, and filling fiber, fruits and veggies generally should be the primary focus at *every* meal. Your body likes color, and produce is a great way to get it. Your plate should be a rainbow of colors.

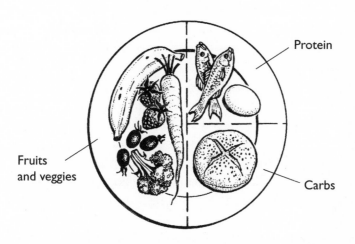

Protein

Fruits and veggies

Carbs

Cheater's Secret: Work fruit and vegetables into every meal, and oftentimes snacks. We're talking berries with your cereal; lettuce, tomato, onion, and sprouts on your sandwich; asparagus and mushrooms with your pasta. If you can conquer this little secret, you'll hit the daunting recommendation of "5 to 9 servings" without even thinking about it and you'll keep dropping pounds effortlessly. Fruits and vegetables are low in calories, so you're stockpiling your plate with water-rich and fiber-full food without a ton of calories. A cup of baby spinach has 7 calories, tomatoes 27, and strawberries 60. You can spare it.

- **Fruit**—A standard serving of fruit is a piece of whole, fresh fruit, such as a medium-size banana, apple, orange, peach, plum, etc. Or a cup of cut fruit, such as melon or pineapple, or a cup of berries or grapes. Despite what you've read in the past, there's no such thing as forbidden fruit. Some are slightly higher in sugar than others, but no one ever gained weight from eating a handful of grapes. So yes, bananas, mango, and pineapple are delicious and crazy healthful—eat up and don't be scared. Aim for 2 to 3 servings of low-cal, high-fiber fruit each day, and both your waistline and digestive tract will love you for it.

  Cheater's Secret: Be thoughtful when it comes to dried fruit and max out at a handful per serving. It's darn tasty, but it can also pack in calories and sugar quickly. Think about it—three dried peaches are essentially three entire fresh peaches. A serving of ¼ cup dried fruit contains about 130 calories. That's barely a handful. Three handfuls later, we're talking the amount of calories that go into a small meal. So be mindful if you're munching on dried fruit, or use it to toss into cereal, salads, or side dishes, or pair it with a tiny handful of nuts for a fast, energizing snack. Think of dried fruit more as a condiment if that helps. Also, beware of behemoth bananas—grab small to medium-size ones or use ½ banana to stay on track with portions.

- **Vegetables**—Love them or hate them, they're good for you, and hopefully you'll discover a few new veggies you like after reading this book and experimenting a little. Short and sweet, ½ cup of cooked vegetables is a serving and 1 cup of raw vegetables is a serving. Don't drive yourself crazy measuring stuff out—that would be insanity, and you might end up hating me and putting this book down right here and now. Your daily veggie goal is about 5 to 6 servings. I guarantee you'll achieve this if you work vegetables in somehow twice a day at meals or snacks. I think focusing on veggies at lunch and dinner is a no-brainer. Does that mean you're stuck eating salads every meal? Of course not. Vegetables can take the form of greens and salads, a raw or cooked side dish, soup along with your sandwich or as a light meal, crudité with some hummus or low-fat dip for a snack, one-pot stews, and so on. Do keep in mind, however, that some foods commonly defined as vegetables really fit best in the healthy carbohydrate category. Foods like corn, potatoes, sweet potatoes and other root vegetables, and butternut and acorn squash are more starchy (yet still fantastic for us) than most other vegetables, like spinach, green beans, and red bell peppers. Get the good, fresh stuff rather than tagging french fries and ketchup as "vegetables," and you'll never go wrong.

If you serve up some sautéed broccoli with your dinner, you're likely already getting 3 or more servings (1 ½ cups). Don't make eating well harder than it has to be—eating shouldn't be painful.

Cheater's Secret: Fresh or frozen? If you've ever questioned purchasing frozen vegetables, don't. Frozen vegetables are packed at peak nutrient value and can be a huge time-, flavor- and calorie-saver in the winter months when options are limited. Stash a few bags of frozen spinach or broccoli in your freezer for emergencies. Make cold-weather meals a little more tasty by freezing summer vegetables and fruits, like blueberries and corn kernels shaved off the cob at the end of the season in August or September. You'll have that farm-fresh taste saved all year long.

- **Protein**—Contrary to popular belief, we don't require mass quantities of protein. In fact, our bodies can't really handle too much of it all that well; it's pretty taxing for our kidneys to break it all down and it backs up our digestive systems if we're not careful. Your fist makes a great protein portion estimator; all you really need is about two fists total per day to cover your bases, around 50 to 60 grams or so. When was the last time you went to dinner and had a piece of steak or salmon the size of your fist? That's laughable. Your fist is probably about the size of 3 to 5 ounces, a bit larger than the size of an iPhone or BlackBerry. You're typically getting 6 to 12 ounces when you dine out. Cut it in half and bring it home. Your fist is a great eyeball trick at lunch and dinner, when we're most likely to consume meat. But protein is easy to sneak in at breakfast, too, with eggs, yogurt, oatmeal topped with some nuts, or even a good swig of skim, low-fat, or soy milk. Because small, normal servings of protein fill us up fast, that's why it's important to incorporate it at most meals. Don't stress yourself trying to calculate the number of grams; just make sure you've got a little protein in your meal somewhere.

A few quick points worth noting:

◆ If you're training for a marathon or an intense exercise regimen, bump up your portions just slightly, about another half fist or so—you'll need a little extra for muscle repair and endurance.

◆ To all you vegetarian and vegan readers, there are lots of vegetarian sources of protein, like tofu, edamame, nuts, quinoa, beans, and legumes, so don't feel left in the dark. If your meals tend to be carb- or pasta-heavy, make sure you toss some protein in there to fill you up faster. My theory on eating meat versus not: It's wherever your preference and personal philosophy lies. I'm not here to preach about the virtues or vices of animal protein, I just want you to understand the basics so you can take the information and run with it. I will, however, delve more into what you should be looking for when purchasing meat, fish, eggs, and poultry, the whole organic, wild, free-range conversation, but that's down the line in Chapter 7. Keep reading. If you're a meat-loving carnivore, work it in just one or two times a week to ensure you're getting a balance of other foods and are keeping calories and cholesterol levels at bay.

• **Carbs and Your New Best Friend, Mr. Fiber**—Carbohydrates are not the enemy, they are your friends. Where we often get tripped up is in the type and amount of carbs we're consuming. There's no such thing as a "good" or "bad" carb. We're

CHEAT SHEET: Protein

Here's a quick rundown of your basic lean sources of protein and their serving sizes:

- Skinless chicken breast or thigh, lean red meat, like flank steak, filet, 97% lean ground beef, white meat and ground turkey, pork, fish, and seafood (3 to 4 ounces)
- Beans, chickpeas, and legumes (½ cup)
- Eggs (1 to 2 whole eggs or 1 egg plus 1 to 2 whites per meal)
- Nuts (1 ounce or 1 handful, about 20, is a 200-calorie serving), nut butters (1 to 2 tablespoons)
- Tofu (3 to 4 ounces), edamame (1 cup), quinoa (½ cup)
- Cheese/soy cheese (4 to 5 dice or 1 ounce, about the size of a dental floss container—yikes, that's not a lot!)
- Low-fat or skim milk or soy milk (1 cup), low-fat yogurt or soy yogurt (your basic 4- or 6-ounce container), cottage cheese (4 ounces—a mini-size container, like Breakstone's or Light n' Lively)

(For more on the leanest cuts of meat and poultry, see page 225.)

just distinguishing among those that are less refined, higher in fiber, and more nutrient-rich. When eaten in normal amounts, your more refined comfort carbs, like pasta, white rice, and white bread, can absolutely have a place in your life. But we like variety and we also like good nutrients from complex carbs and whole grains. Complex carbs serve as our brain's best fuel source, our body's ideal energy source known as glucose, and they pack in countless vitamins, minerals, and antioxidants to increase energy, lower disease risk, and keep your skin and hair glowing. So essentially, more refined carbohydrates like white bread, flour, and sugar lack nutritional value, while complex, whole grain carbs are loaded with it. Complex carbs also are full of fiber, and fiber is any cheater's ultimate secret weapon when it comes to satiety and getting and maintaining a weight you want. Foods rich in fiber serve up a triple punch: a) They take longer for our bodies to digest and break down—like a gift that's underneath extra layers of wrapping—so they keep our blood sugar and energy levels much more steady and smooth-running and keep us fuller for a longer period of time. This in turn aids weight loss and weight maintenance because you don't get as hungry as quickly. Ever had a huge stack of pancakes with maple syrup and been hungry and tired an hour later? A straight shot of refined carbs and simple sugar will do that to anyone. Swap

---

CHEAT SHEET: The Dish on Dietary Fiber

What it is: An undigestable substance found in plant foods

- Insoluble fiber—absorbs water and speeds up digestion
- Soluble fiber—binds to cholesterol and helps remove it from the body

Benefits: Promotes bowel health and regularity, alleviates constipation, helps lower cholesterol levels, prevents heart disease and types of cancer, stabilizes blood sugar levels, increases satiety, and aids in weight loss and maintenance efforts

Daily recommendations: 25 to 35 grams (high-fiber foods have more than 3 to 5 grams of fiber per serving)

Where to find fiber: Complex carbohydrates; whole, unprocessed foods; bran and whole grains, like oatmeal, whole wheat pasta, barley, brown rice, quinoa, and millet; legumes and beans; fresh vegetables and fruits; root vegetables, like sweet potatoes, beets, and potatoes; dried fruit; nuts and seeds

A few fiber-rich examples:
Blueberries (½ cup)—4 to 5 grams
Bran cereal (1 cup)—5 to 10 grams
Broccoli (½ cup)—5 grams
Dried figs (3)—10 grams
Lentils (½ cup cooked)—6 grams
Oatmeal (½ cup dry)—4 grams
Sweet potato (½ cup)—5 grams

it for a small stack of silver-dollar multigrain pancakes and a side of yogurt and berries and you'll feel a hell of a lot better; b) Fiber-rich foods speed up digestion, which helps banish a bloated stomach, naturally sends toxins on their way out the door, and keeps your metabolism kicking. Your grandmother, who's trim and feisty at ninety, loves her morning prune juice and bran cereal—now you know why. Both are loaded with fiber; c) Foods high in fiber also help lower cholesterol levels by driving cholesterol out of the body. The claim on the Quaker Oatmeal canister is right!

Now that you've had a quick crash course on carbs, on to their portion sizes. The surprising truth: A single serving of cooked carbohydrates, like pasta, rice, beans, and whole grains such as couscous and brown rice, is a meager ½ cup, about 100 calories. If you own measuring cups, take a peek. Most restaurants serve up at least 3 whole cups of pasta, which is 6 servings. For the average female, ½ cup seems incredibly small. And for the average male, forget it. Here's the trick: At a given meal, aim for a ¾ to 1 cup serving, or 1 to 2 pieces of bread, or a combo, like a small ear of corn and 2 to 3 baby potatoes. Ideally you're having a healthy carb at most meals and snacks. Work with 1 to 2 servings at each meal, which actually adds up to a lot. And remember, you've got other stuff on your plate—vegetables or fruits and protein. So think of pasta (or rice or potatoes and the like) as a plate liner—it's the added bonus to the meal, not the starring feature. The feature should be the sauce glittering with veggies and grilled chicken, shrimp, beans, meatballs, or whatever lean protein you have in mind—obviously, all of those things can go on the side if you're a pasta purist. Do it like the Italians—they serve pasta in appetizer-size portions, as a small starter. Think about that next time you sit down to a massive plate of spaghetti.

Your head is likely swirling by now, but it will all come together—I promise.

CHEAT SHEET: Carb Portions

- Cooked rice, pasta, polenta, whole grains, like couscous, bulgur, quinoa, and barley (½ to 1 cup)
- Potatoes and sweet potatoes (1 small, about fist-size; otherwise, cut it in half)
- Starchy root vegetables and squash, like parsnips, beets, acorn and butternut squash, and pumpkin (½ to 1 cup, about fist-size)
- 1 ear of corn; 4 cups all-natural popcorn
- Cereal (1 cup, or the serving size as indicated on the label)—you'll be able to choose a solid cereal by looking for just two things on the nutrition label—aim for about 5 grams of fiber or more per serving and 7 grams of sugar or less
- Granola (¼ cup)—it packs in calories, so beware—½ cup can be up to 250 calories! Think of it as a condiment (just like dried fruit) to sprinkle in yogurt or mix with another lower-calorie cereal.
- Hot cereal and oatmeal (½ cup dry; if you're using steel-cut oats, it's ¼ cup dry)—skip the sugary, flavored stuff
- Bread, English muffins, and pita (1 slice/muffin/pita = 1 serving)— shoot for 100% whole wheat, multigrain, pumpernickel, dark rye, and the white stuff when it's worth it—like a phenomenal piece of baguette or artisan sourdough
- 1 all-natural granola bar (like Kashi TLC, 18 Rabbits, Clif Nectar, Larabar)

Cheater's Secret: Be confident in good carbohydrates. As stated above, carbs are not the enemy, but some are better than others, like whole grain and complex carbs (more fiber and nutrients). When beginning to build out your weekly Cheater's routine, take comfort in the following healthy, delicious carbohydrates (1 piece, ½ to 1 cup, or a fist-size portion at a time!): sweet potatoes, regular potatoes, brown and wild rice, whole wheat pasta, beans and lentils, butternut and acorn squash, quinoa, barley, wheatberries, bulgur/cracked wheat, millet, whole wheat couscous, spelt, rolled oats and steel-cut or old-fashioned oatmeal, whole grain breads, wraps, and crackers (with more than 3 grams of fiber per serving), whole grain cereal (with more than 5 grams of fiber per serving).

Cheater's Secret: Swap white rice and regular pasta for brown rice and whole wheat/multigrain pasta when you can for an extra dose of filling fiber. That said, having a nice aromatic white rice, like jasmine or basmati, or a great regular white pasta here and there during the week is definitely worth it—just watch those portions. Personally, I have a tough time cozying up to the idea of whole wheat pasta. My answer: I do the real deal but less frequently and experiment with interesting pasta shapes to keep things exciting.

Cheater's Secret: Keep the skin on potatoes for extra fiber. Sweet potatoes are loaded with antioxidants and beta-carotene (vitamin A), which is great for your eyes and skin and helps lower risk of heart disease and cancer. One small sweet potato contains well over your daily recommended value of vitamin A. And despite what low-carb diets taught us, regular potatoes aren't off-limits—they're packed with nutrients and are a great source of quick energy. A small potato contains 45 percent of your daily vitamin C and about as much potassium as a banana! Keep eating piles of butter-drenched mashed potatoes, however, and your hips will surely pay a price.

Cheater's Secret: Reach for whole grain and whole wheat bread with at least 3 grams of fiber per slice when you can. Look for bread that's not "squishable" in your hand, which often means it'll be more easily digested and won't be super-satisfying. Opt for a denser, heartier, firmer, and possibly seedier, nuttier bread—way more filling and nutrient rich. When it comes to picking out a quality bread, if it looks like an Amish farmer baked it, you're in good shape. Sandwiches can make a great meal option. What causes their downfall is often their size and what's in them. If a sandwich is bigger than your head, wrap half of it up. If it has a stack of turkey a foot tall and four slices of cheese, knock the turkey down to two to four slices and the cheese to one to two.

- **Fats**—Fat is a necessary, healthful part of your diet. That statement does not open the floodgates for a tidal wave of fried, creamy, butter-dripping goodness (granted, a small wave is too good to pass up sometimes). Feast your eyes and focus your attention on the "healthy fats" you hear so much talk about. Fat is essential in our diet, as we need it to act as a cushion for our organs and to aid the digestion and absorption of certain vitamins (A, D, E, and K) and phytochemicals (a type of antioxidants) found in plant foods—fruits and vegetables like lettuce, carrots, grapes, onions, and garlic, to name just a few. Fat also helps the whole digestion process and provides some serious energy stores. And finally, fat can be glorious when used well. Fat provides something called mouthfeel, that sense of comfort, texture, overall goodness, and satiety. Fat is calorie- and energy-dense, so a little goes a long way and actually helps us stay fuller and satisfied for longer. Recall the days of fat-free SnackWells. You could eat the entire box without guilt because they were fat-free, but you were always left hungry. Because fat-free doesn't mean calorie-free; if you'd eaten just one real chocolate chip cookie, you'd probably be much happier and you'd have saved a couple hundred calories. Aside from skim milk, I usually suggest going low-fat or full-fledged fat for most things and aiming to have smaller amounts of them. However, if you eat too much fat, you have too much to store and you can no longer zip your jeans up. This is exactly why it's so important to consider what type of fats you're consuming and how much. A fast and furious breakdown of fats:

◆ **Saturated**—The not-so-good, artery-clogging kind of fat. Whole milk dairy products, butter, cream, heavily marbled fatty cuts of red meat, fried and processed foods. Aim for a max of 20 grams total of saturated fat per day. When checking out nutrition labels, the saturated fat number falls right beneath total fat. Saturated fat should be low. Total fat in the item might seem high, but don't stress it, as there's good, healthy fat mixed in there, too. Here's what I'm talking about: 2 tablespoons (a single serving) of peanut butter contains 16 grams of total fat but only 2.5 grams of saturated fat. That's a big winner on the fat front, and that's why we call peanut butter healthy. When in doubt, use foods high in saturated fat, like butter and heavy cream, sparingly, keep fried foods to a minimum, and eat red meat one to two times a week.

◆ **Super-Saturated Trans Fats**—Also known as hydrogenated, or partially hydrogenated. These words are a major red flag if you spot them on an ingredients list. Trans fats are artificially produced to help extend a food's shelf life and may increase "bad," LDL cholesterol and decrease "good," HDL cholesterol. Many food companies have removed or limited trans fats in products, and a number of places, including New York City and the state of California, have banned restaurants from using trans fats altogether. Here's where you might find them: premade and packaged cookies, baked goods, pastries and chips, packaged and frozen meals, fast food, margarine, vegetable shortening.

◆ **The Good Stuff: Monounsaturated and Polyunsaturated Fats**—Awesome heart-healthy fats that help protect against heart disease and increase "good," HDL cholesterol and decrease "bad," LDL cholesterol. Where you might find them: olive, canola, sunflower, and grapeseed oil; nuts and nut butters; sunflower and pumpkin seeds; and avocado, among other sources. What you're aiming for each day: about 60 grams total fat (1 tablespoon olive oil or 1 handful of nuts packs in about 14 grams).

◆ **More Good Stuff: Essential Fats**—Omega-3s—More healthy fats! Omega-3s and other types of essential fatty acids have gotten a lot of press, and rightly so. Omega-3s help lower risk or symptoms of heart disease, high cholesterol, cancer, stroke, high blood pressure, depression, digestive disorders, and signs of aging (damn wrinkles), and they boost brain function and reduce inflammation. Here's specifically where to find them: flaxseed and flaxseed oil; walnuts; oily fish, like salmon, mackerel, tuna, sardines, and halibut; tofu and soybeans; canola oil; avocado; milk and cheese from grass-fed cows.

·································

CHEAT SHEET: Fat Portions

- Olive oil and other heart-healthy oils (canola, flaxseed, grapeseed, walnut, avocado, sunflower)—1 tablespoon = 120 calories
- Salad dressing and vinaigrettes—2 tablespoons = 90 to 100 calories
- Butter—1 teaspoon = 36 calories
- Avocado—¼ avocado = 80 calories
- Nuts—small handful, 15 to 20 (50 for pistachios)! = 150 to 200 calories
- Nut butter (peanut, almond, cashew, soy)—2 tablespoons = 190 calories
- Cheese—4 to 5 dice, 1 ounce, 1 deli slice = 80 to 110 calories

·································

Cheater's Secret: Use a full-fat salad dressing and be thrilled about it. I hate to be wasteful, but go ahead and chuck all the fat-free dressings sitting pretty on your fridge door. I know regular fat anything goes against every grain in a perpetual dieter's body. That's precisely the point—we're done with lame, unsuccessful dieting. So say good-bye to fat-free raspberry vinaigrette because: 1) You're not getting any of the benefits of a healthy oil 'cause there isn't any in there! 2) that healthy oil has been replaced by extra sugar and carbohydrates. Ingredients lists should be short, with items you recognize. Reach for plain old olive oil and lemon or a vinegar of your choice, or a full-fat vinaigrette like balsamic or red wine. If you must have your ranch once in a while, reach for a light version or have the real thing in moderation (just a drizzle). Creamier dressings, like blue cheese, Thousand Island, and ranch, have more saturated fat in them and tend to crank up extra calories fast. See page 127 for recipes for super-easy homemade dressings.

Cheater's Secret: Stick to an ounce of cheese at a time. Yes, you can eat cheese without gaining a zillion pounds. There's no way around it—cheese is delicious, and we can easily go a wee bit overboard on it. A serving the size of 4 to 5 dice sounds small, and if you're a glass-half-empty kind of person, it is small. But it's all about the quality and flavor of the cheese and how you arrange it on a plate. Cut a piece of cheese off a block that's about the width of your thumb, and then cut it into a few thinner slices, and magic—you've now got three or four decent-size squares or rectangles of cheese. Lay them on a small plate with some apple slices, grapes, or whole grain crackers, and that's a nice-size snack under 200 calories. Fat-free cheese is typically tasteless and plasticy, so for snacking and sandwiches, work with either a portion of reduced-fat cheese to lighten up on saturated fat and shave off about 30 calories, or use a modest portion of real-deal cheese. For use in cooking, salads, and when you're having people over for wine and cheese, pull out the good stuff . . . Brie, Gouda, Manchego . . . wherever your taste buds take you. Cheeses like Parmesan, Pecorino Romano, Gruyère, blue cheese or Gorgonzola, feta, and goat cheese pack in the flavor, so you can use just 2 to 4 tablespoons to bring life to a meal. Harder cheeses, like Parmesan, Pecorino, and Gruyère are perfect for grating, so again, you're getting a lot of flavor without a lot of calories. Creamy goat cheese is a godsend—it takes like heaven and is naturally lower in fat and calories (about 80 calories and 6 grams of fat per serving; there are 4 servings in one small log). You'll find a hunk of good quality Parmesan, Pecorino Romano, and goat cheese in my fridge at all times. Don't skimp on quality with cheese, or you may sacrifice flavor and hence feel the need to nibble more. (Refer back to the SnackWells theory . . . same thing applies for fat-free feta cheese!) If you're lactose intolerant, you might find you're able to digest harder cheeses more easily, as they contain less lactose than softer cheese. Lactase is the enzyme needed to break down dairy products, and some of us just don't have that much of it.

- **Alcohol**—Lest we forget to discuss alcohol and ideal portions per week. A good glass of wine is one of my favorite indulgences, but one or five too many a week (or a night) will zap your weight loss efforts in a flash. Cut back your total wine, cocktail, or beer intake per week by at least 25 percent to aid the shedding of pounds—this could play a major factor in your feeling that much trimmer by the end of Week 1. In the grand

CHEAT SHEET: Perfect Portions Recap

I'm not going to tell you to ask the waitress to pack up half of your entrée before the meal's even served—that's absolutely ridiculous and a wee bit socially awkward, but here are a few quick tips in general when it comes to portioning:

• Leave a few bites behind on your plate—aim for five, or if portions are large, leave a quarter to half of your meal behind or have it wrapped up to go.
• Be like my dad—swap a regular plate for salad-size in the comfort of your own home
• If you're feeling particularly anal, occasionally measure out or weigh portions on a basic kitchen scale (they're cheap). Sometimes it's helpful to have a solid visual picture in mind. Don't worry too much about fruits and veggies.
• Decrease alcoholic drinks per week by 25 percent. You've got to admit, it's really a pretty reasonable adjustment.

scheme of things, decreasing your libations per week by 25 percent isn't that much—it comes out to between one and four drinks for most of us. Cheaters always get their way, but the key is to step up your game and play more intelligently. You can have your alcohol and drink it, too, but drink a bit less. You'll quickly see the results without impinging on your social life all that much. More details on alcohol and how best to cheat while getting your drink on to come in Chapter 5, but here's a quick synopsis and serving sizes of the least caloric drinks, all between 100 and 120 calories: 5 ounces of red or white wine or champagne, 12 ounces of light beer, 1 ½ ounces (1 shot) of hard liquor, like vodka, gin, whiskey, or rum. A few go-to drink picks that are slightly more scale-friendly include wine, champagne, light beer, vodka with club soda and lime, or liquor on the rocks.

Cheater's Secret: If you like the bubbly, you're in luck. Sparkling wines like champagne, Prosecco, and Lambrusco are some of the lowest-calorie drinks around, averaging about 96 calories per 5-ounce champagne glass, which leaves you a little more room for another glass.

The Cheater's Triangle

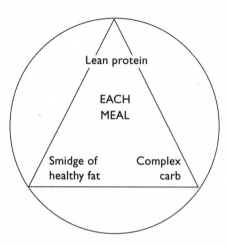

*Fruits and veggies are a constant.

The Cheater's Triangle is the basic building block of the Cheater's Diet. The triangle's an idea that helps put something as ambiguous as satiety into a visual picture, and if you keep a balanced triangle as you eat throughout the day, it'll help ensure that your blood sugar is rock-steady, that your portions are perfect, that you don't leave the table hungry, and that your scale is headed in the right direction meal after meal. When your blood sugar level is sailing smoothly, it works like a charm on your metabolism. You'll really feel a difference in your energy and hunger levels. By following the triangle, you'll uncross wires that have been tangled up for years by one failed diet, wacko eating craze, and starvation/deprivation attempt after another. So without further ado, here's how the triangle works:

The idea is to hit each point on the triangle at every meal and most snacks. Teamed together, fruits and/or veggies act as the base of the meal, filling you up without a ton of calories, while the addition of a little healthy fat, a bit of complex carbs, and some lean protein clinches your sense of satiety and kicks up your energy for the next few hours. It sounds utterly complicated and clinical, but it will start becoming instinctive once we get rolling. For example, a simple snack of an apple and a good hearty tablespoon of peanut butter hits it dead-on. Don't overthink it; this isn't a *MacGyver* episode. The weekly meal calendar in each chapter lays out sample meals and snacks so you can crack the code on your own. *Disclaimer:* Every one of us is different, and our bodies work to their own tune (mine happens to be playing Michael Jackson's "Billie Jean" fairly frequently, but that's just me). Listen to your body's signals as your own wires start uncrossing themselves and trust yourself. You might find that the Cheater's Triangle theory works best for you at certain times during the day—that you're fine with just a piece of fruit or a handful of nuts for an afternoon snack or that your body feels best with some protein and a double dose of vegetables in the evening. Give yourself the freedom to test things out and investigate. Our bodies understand real, fresh food. Let your body guide you and it'll inevitably tell you what it needs.

Plate Your Food

Another shockingly simple rule of thumb that you might just find ingenious: Put your food on a plate BEFORE you start chowing down! In other words, plate your food. We've all been victims in the kitchen, standing in front of the open fridge munching on cookies-and-cream ice cream straight from the carton, spooning peanut butter straight from the jar, cutting off slivers of cheese until half the block has disappeared, or taking handful after handful of Wheat Thins or Doritos straight from the bag. That's the easiest way for a single portion of anything—healthy or not—to become multiple portions in five minutes flat. Try to add up those calories and you might not be so happy. Your solution—plate it! Putting things on a plate, in a bowl, or in a cup allows you to visually see what's in front of you. It's automatic portion sizing. The key is to stick to that portion and not head back into the kitchen for round two. Know your limits. Open a bag of Chex Mix in front of me and it's all over (even nutritionists have weaknesses).

Waterlogged

Ever gone an entire day running on nothing but coffee and Diet Coke? You're jittery, exhausted but wide awake, and feel sort of like you've been run over. Water to the rescue. Water makes up about 60 to 70 percent of the human body and helps flush out toxins, keeps our organs and digestive system functioning at full speed, and keeps our skin looking dewy and drop-dead gorgeous. You've heard the general guideline of eight 8-ounce glasses a day. You personally might need a little more or a little less. Aim for between 1 and 3 liters a day and you should be golden. If you're an avid exerciser, make sure you hydrate before, during, and after your workout. Water's like the oil that runs a fine-tuned machine (your body!). The research confirming water's impact on weight loss is still unclear. But what water does do is keep your body going as it should—increasing your energy levels (dehydration can make us tired and cranky), unclogging your digestive system (kiss bloating and constipation good-bye), and filling you up on less (it's easy to mistake thirst for hunger). So all of this combined *can* help the whole weight game. A Penn State research study found that consuming water-rich foods like fruits and vegetables promotes more weight loss—21 percent more—than not eating them, even if you eat up to 25 percent more food. (Water-rich foods are typically low-calorie.)

Visualization and volume are still key when you're getting your water. Keep in mind that water can be found in fruits and veggies, broth-based soups, seltzer and sparkling water, unsweetened tea, and yes, even coffee (just watch the coffee intake—caffeine can be a slight diuretic for some, so stick to 1 to 2 cups of coffee a day). If you can't stand the sight of plain water, toss in a slice or two of lemon, lime, orange, cucumber, or fresh berries for some flavor action, and drink up.

The Gift of the Written Word

At the risk of sounding like a boring nutritionist, I must take another moment to praise writing. Recording what you eat and when you eat it can open your eyes like nothing else, which is why I strongly encourage it. Keeping a food diary, a journal, or a food log on your computer can help you get portions down pat, reveal particular patterns throughout the day (like if you're dipping into the office candy bowl unconsciously every time you get up from your desk), and ensure that you're reaching the goals you've set for yourself. Use the food journal to your full advantage. Start writing and keep writing each week—at least for the entirety it takes you to finish this book. We'll do a quick check in on how the food journaling is going and what your week is telling you in each and every chapter. As you strive to meet your weight loss goals, you'll love the accountability.

Set to Scale

A very brief mention about the piece of cold metal or plastic lying on your bathroom floor—the scale. You might shudder at the thought of it. Some days you want to kiss it, others you want to throw it out the window. Should you definitely own a scale? Not necessarily. For some, a scale provides that extra push and a sense of accountability—it's a tool that can be motivating and encouraging . . . or not. It's easy to forget that we gain and lose up to three or four pounds in a single given day. The scale simply gives you a number, and if you're the type of person who's going to agonize about it day in and day out, I'd suggest not stepping anywhere near that thing but two or three times a month (not two or three times a day, and definitely not during the three days before your period!). It takes time for your body to shed poundage. Some of us are quick losers initially, and some of us take our sweet time. Either way, you're taking weight off, and it's going to stay off. The most important measurement is really how you feel in your clothes and in your own skin. If you are an avid scale user, aim to weigh yourself max once a week and step on it around the same time of day for consistency. Most of us are at our lightest first thing in the morning in the buff.

Okay, we've got the fundamentals down—meal timing, portions, and water. Now glance one last time at your week. Focus on those dinners, brunches, and nights out and count them up. If it's too many to count, not all is lost; you'll be able to make any situation work for you with strategic cheating. Again, you're choosing two meals out during the week as your *cheat and eat* special occasion meals. Order what looks incredible on the menu, try to keep portions in mind, and share dessert if you're in the mood. I won't use the word "blowout," but if it had to happen, this would be where to do it. When you're eating out at other times during the week, stay on top of your game when it comes to your order and your portions. By eating out five or six times a week, the whole special occasion idea goes out the window. We'll work through restaurant eating further down the road, but let's get you set with solid basics first. A quick note on the booze, also to be discussed in detail in Chapter 5: Apply the same strategy to alcohol that you use with dinners. You're curbing your drinking by at least 25 percent, but figure out what method works for you to achieve that—whether it's setting a target number of drinks to work with in a given week, or choosing specific nights to have a few. If you're a nightly boozer—and I personally like my wine—aim for three nights drip-dry, or between about six to eight drinks maximum over the course of the week.

Calories Shmalories

How many are you supposed to be consuming on a given day? Honestly, there's no one straight answer. We're all different, have faster or slower metabolisms, and have varying calorie needs depending on how much or how little physical activity we're getting. And at the end of the day, what does a blanket number like 1500 or 1800 really mean to you? My guess is not too much. It can, however, be unbelievably helpful to be cognizant of how many calories are in particular ingredients or meals and to have a general idea of what you're looking at over the course of a day. Overall, don't drive yourself nuts with the numbers. Plant your focus on what's on your plate and how much of it you're eating. This makes eating much less scientific and calculated and a lot more enjoyable. If you're a diehard numbers girl, though, here's an easy breakdown.

- If you're petite, shoot for an average of 1200 to 1500 calories per day.

- If you fall in the middle ground, like me, at five foot three to five foot seven, work with about 1300 to 1600 calories per day.
- If you're five foot eight and up, aim for an average of 1500 to 1800 calories per day.
- If you exercise sixty or more minutes four to six times a week, work with the upper range of calories noted, and if you need to tack on another 100 to 200 calories per day, do so. For visual guidance, you'll notice set target calorie ranges at each meal and snack in the sample calendar at the start of each chapter.

Cheater's Secret: Calories in, equal calories out. One single pound is equivalent to 3500 calories. So if your goal is to lose one pound per week, you'll want to shave off 500 calories per day. Sounds like a lot, but 500 calories adds up fast. Get a sandwich for lunch and take off one extra slice of cheese, swap the mayo for mustard, and lose the extra bag of pretzels, and bingo, you're down almost 500 already. A huge shocker—consuming just 100 extra calories per day pans out to ten extra pounds gained per year! What's 100 calories? One extra piece of cheese, one extra handful of cocktail nuts, three Twizzlers, that little mini bagel left over from a morning business meeting, that extra late-night beer on the weekend. Damn those sneaky calories. Thankfully, they're just as easy to swap up and shave off as they are to sneak on. Knowledge is everything, so keep reading.

Skinny Genes

Some people are just born naturally slender—regardless of how many calorie-laden cheeseburgers, frozen margaritas, and pieces of chocolate cake they consume. By comparison, you may feel like you wound up in the deep end of the gene pool. But this is life, and we're all pretty amazing in our own right. I'm a big fan of giving thanks for what your mama gave you—acknowledging it and owning it. I inherited some nice curves on my hips and my backside, and it took me a while, but I love it. The point of this chapter and the chapters ahead is to help you improve the health and natural beauty of *your* body—to give you the tools and tricks of the trade to boost your well-being, maximize your love of delicious *and* nutritious food, have you rocking out in the kitchen, and losing a few in the process. Now let's get cooking.

Back to Basics: Getting to Know Your Kitchen / Simple Meals in Twenty Minutes or Less

"Use my oven—to cook? My apartment's so small, I've converted my oven to storage space for shoes."

—Eileen

Now for the good stuff—a girl's got to eat, after all. It's time to get acquainted with your stovetop and oven. If you're a virgin in the kitchen, don't worry—there's a first time for everything. And if you're already a seasoned gastronome but have trouble streamlining healthful, quick meals, the remainder of this chapter has you covered and will help you pull together the dinner recipes laid out in Week 1's sample week of meals.

But before we get cooking, it's worth mentioning that recipes are adaptable. Yes, there are lots of recipes throughout this book, but if you don't have every single ingredient on hand or forget to add something, don't stress and take liberty in experimenting (and cheating!). Cooking isn't about following a recipe to the tee, it's about mastering techniques and methods and really allowing yourself to test out flavors, cooking times, and ingredients. It's about swapping garlic for a shallot and eventually getting comfortable enough to eyeball a tablespoon of olive oil or a dash of salt or a sprinkle of sugar (yes, real sugar!). Remember that every stove is calibrated a bit differently, so if you need to turn the temperature up or down depending on the status of your dish (under- or overcooking), definitely do so. And if you botch one of the recipes in this book, or any recipe for that matter, who cares? You're learning, creating, and connecting that much more with your food, and that's absolutely invaluable. So, with that introduction, let's start with a refresher course of the basics and build from the ground up. The uncomplicated recipes that follow will take you through the bare-bone basics of simple weeknight cooking—for those nights when you get home from work late, are exhausted, ravenous, and just want to sit down to a quick, tasty meal. Instead of calling the Chinese takeout place, preparing a speedy meal in under twenty minutes will save you money (more for your next shoe purchase), save you time (banging it out yourself is quicker than the delivery dude), and save you a good number of calories (research shows that women who eat out or order out five or more times a week typically consume 290 calories more per day than women who eat out less frequently). If you do the math, that could potentially turn into twenty-nine extra pounds per year.

> *Cheater's Secret:* Keep things balanced when it's a basic weeknight and you're at home. Work in your two fun *cheat and eat* meals for the week on other nights out where you can ease up on the calorie consciousness and enjoy the ride.

First things first—one of the best things you can possibly do for yourself and your kitchen is to invest in a single good chef's knife. Yes, they can get a little pricey, around $100 to $120, but a solid 8-inch knife makes a world of difference and makes cutting, chopping, and cooking your own meals so much easier. Head to your local kitchenware store and test-drive a few different brands to see what feels most comfortable when you grasp the knife handle and how heavy or light you like it. Henckels, Wusthof, Shun, and Global are higher-end cutlery brands; Chicago Cutlery is a more economical option but also a solid brand. Apron on, knife in hand—you're on your way to becoming master of your domain in the kitchen . . . baby step by baby step. The recipes and ideas that follow will help you get through a hectic week when cooking a full meal seems virtually impossible. Nothing is impossible, though, when you're cheating—planning ahead and playing smarter.

Boiling

No, I'm not kidding. We're starting with the real basics. The recipe below allows you to start with something as simple as boiling water and work your way upward. From eggs to pasta, vegetables to potatoes, soups to rice, chicken to lobster, boiling is a plain and simple cooking method—water and ingredients, and that's about it.

CHEAT SHEET: Measuring Up

- Tsp = teaspoon
- Tbsp = tablespoon
- lb = pound
- 4 ounces = ½ cup
- 8 ounces = 1 cup
- 16 ounces = 1 pound
- 32 ounces = 1 liter (liquid)

Hard-Boiled Eggs

Hard-boiled eggs take literally 10 minutes, will stay fresh in the fridge for up to a week, and they're great as a filling snack or part of a light meal at 70 calories and 6 grams of protein a pop. Wondering what the down-low on eggs is? Poor eggs have gotten a bad rap for years. Despite what you've heard, they don't affect our cholesterol, and the yolks actually pack in tons of nutrients you don't want to pass up, like vitamins B$_{12}$ and D and disease-fighting antioxidants.

THE GOODS
    1 or more large or extra-large eggs (brown or white, both are great—the color just depends on the breed of the hen)
    Salt (optional)

THE BREAKDOWN
    1. Place the egg(s) in a medium saucepan and cover with cold water, about 1 inch above the eggs.
    2. Turn the heat to high and bring to a boil. You can add a dash of salt to the water to make the eggs easier to peel.

3. When the water begins to boil (that stage of heavy bubbling), immediately remove the pan from the heat, place on a cool burner, cover, and allow to sit for 10 to 12 minutes.
4. Drain and run the eggs under cold water to stop the cooking process, otherwise you'll get those nasty green, smelly yolks. You can store the eggs in the fridge for up to a week.

The Facts: (per XL egg) 90 calories; 6g fat; 2g saturated fat; 7g protein; 0g fiber

Cheater's Secret—Unscrambled Eggs: Go ahead and eat the *entire* egg, yolk and all. You'll be way more satisfied and happier with what you're eating, which assists the weight loss and weight maintenance process in the long run. Researchers found that individuals who ate two eggs at breakfast lost twice as much weight and had greater levels of satiety and sustained energy. The full egg tends to be much more satisfying that just the white alone, which might explain why you can take down five egg whites and still feel hungry or like you're missing something.

Again, the egg yolk got slammed for supposedly raising cholesterol. In actuality, a real-deal, whole egg won't raise your cholesterol. (It's foods high in unhealthy saturated fats, like heavily marbled red meat, butter, processed foods, super-creamy dairy products, and fried foods, that can cause your cholesterol to shoot through the roof if you eat too much of them.) Egg yolks boast serious nutrients that promote eye health, brain development, and even weight loss. In addition, eggs are an excellent, inexpensive source of lean protein to fill you up fast when you're looking to watch your wallet a little.

Steaming

Next up is steaming, otherwise known as the "clean as a whistle," low-calorie cooking method for just about anything, particularly veggies. Don't cringe. Among all methods of cooking, steaming is the one most often associated with bland, boring, barfy "diet" food. Yeah, if I ate plain steamed vegetables and flavorless chicken night after night, I'd be pretty miserable and unsatisfied, too. But

CHEAT SHEET: Quick Kitchen Crib Sheet

Al dente—Cooking pasta "to the tooth" so that it's tender but slightly firm to the bite

Chop—To cut food into bite-size pieces

Dice—To cut food into teensy ¼ inch cubes

Mince—To cut food into even teensier pieces

Julienne—To cut food into thin, matchstick-like strips

Mirepoix—The traditional combo of diced carrots, onions, and celery to flavor a dish (check out the roast chicken recipe on page 216)

Mise en place—From the French "everything in place," mise en place basically means to have all of your ingredients and cooking utensils prepped, set out on the counter, and ready to roll to make the cooking process that much simpler and streamlined.

Sear—To brown the outside of meat or fish quickly using high heat

Simmer—To cook liquid just below the boiling point so that tiny bubbles continuously form

Zest—To remove the outer skin of citrus fruit in fine strips or shavings (a zester or grater is perfect for this)

steaming does have a lot of redeeming qualities, and you can dress up whatever you're cooking with a basic dressing or marinade, some grated lemon zest, a tablespoon of shaved Parmesan cheese, or simply olive oil and garlic, to name a few. Steamed veggies serve as a quick and healthy accompaniment to a speedy weeknight meal when paired with the whole roasted chicken or grilled salmon fillet you picked up from the grocery store on your way home from work or the veggie burger or turkey meatballs that are stashed in your freezer. So let's steam up some asparagus, green beans, or broccoli, basic enough to start and have you get the hang of it.

Simple Steamed Vegetables and Potatoes

If you don't own a steamer basket or rack, think about making a valuable investment. They typically cost no more than $10 or so. If you don't *have one on hand, you can still make the best of it. Fill a medium pot with about an inch of water, bring to a boil or a simmer (a low boil, mini bubbles), add veggies in the basket or straight in the pot, cover, and cook for 3 to 15 minutes, depending on the vegetable. Veggies like carrots, asparagus, broccoli, and cauliflower will take about 6 to 8 minutes. More delicate veggies like zucchini, green beans, mushrooms, and snap peas require a shorter time to steam, usually about 4 to 5 minutes. Even more delicate greens like spinach, kale, and Swiss chard take just 2 to 3 minutes. And sweet potatoes and regular potatoes go for the long haul, taking about 10 to 15 minutes, cut into ½ inch slices or small chunks. Without a basket, you're technically not really "steaming," but your vegetables will still cook up nicely in the end without allowing too many nutrients to be leached out into the cooking water, thanks to quick cooking times.*

Makes 1 (or potentially more) serving

THE GOODS

Fresh vegetables of your choice, such as carrots, snap peas, broccoli florets, cauliflower, green beans, asparagus, potatoes, zucchini, mushrooms, and more

Make as small or large a quantity as you wish, depending on the amount of servings you're aiming for. If you're going solo on an average weeknight, 1 ½ to 2 cups of veggies tossed into a steamer basket is a solid portion to work with per meal. Or plan ahead and steam an extra serving or two for lunch or dinner the next day.

THE BREAKDOWN

Place your vegetables of choice in a steamer basket over boiling water. Cover the pot and steam for 3 to 15 minutes, depending on the type and quantity of vegetable.

VARIATION: *If you're really in a hurry and don't own a steamer basket, you can dump the vegetables right into a pot of boiling water, fully submerged this time so they'll cook even more quickly. This technique is called blanching and takes about half the time as steaming. Just be watchful not to overcook your veggies and leach the good nutrients and color out . . . nobody likes limp, mushy asparagus or gray green beans. Just like steaming, you can blanch virtually any vegetable of your choice. If you're looking to make a lot of veggies ahead of time to keep them around for a few days (preparation and planning is key to cheating!), plunge the vegetables into a bowl of ice and cold water for 20 to 30 seconds right after blanching them. This stops the cooking process and helps veggies keep their bright color. Ever wonder how they keep crudité platters looking so vibrant and crisp? Ice baths are the big secret!

Steamed Artichokes with Garlic and Lemon

If you're looking to score a few easy compliments, this is a great recipe. It's unbelievably effortless, fun to eat, and it looks quite sophisticated on a plate. Not to mention that artichokes are loaded with antioxidants, folate, magnesium, and vitamin C. Artichokes are known to help cleanse, or detox, the liver (point of interest for all of you who like to drink and party), and they pack in a quarter of our daily recommendation for fiber, 6 grams apiece. A single artichoke bears a mere 60 calories, which leaves you some room for a little garlic butter to dip the leaves in—yum.

THE GOODS

3 or 4 whole fresh artichokes (cut off about an inch at the top and trim the sharp tips of outer leaves; cut off the base and remove the small outer leaves if you like)
1 ½ lemons, halved
2 whole garlic cloves
1 garlic clove, minced and pressed with knife into a paste
2 to 3 tablespoons unsalted butter, melted

THE BREAKDOWN

1. Fill a large pot or a steamer with an inch of water and bring to a boil over medium-high heat.

2. Toss in 2 lemon halves and the 2 whole garlic cloves. Arrange the artichokes in the pot, tips facing up. Cover and steam for 25 to 35 minutes, until the bases are soft and the leaves can be pulled off easily.

3. To make the dipping sauce, melt the butter in the microwave or on the stove in a small pot. Add the garlic paste and juice from ½ lemon. Pour the butter into a small serving bowl or individual mini ramekins and serve with the artichokes.

The Facts: 140 calories; 8g fat; 5g saturated fat; 4g protein; 8g fiber

Sautéing

To sauté simply means to quickly and lightly pan-fry food over high heat, using just a bit of oil or, on occasion, butter. Sautéing is ideal for speedy cooking, so small, thin pieces and strips of protein and vegetables work best to allow everything to cook through evenly. No one likes undercooked chicken. You'll typically want to coat your pan with a bit of oil, or you can try low-sodium broth, water, or wine to keep your dish from sticking.

Cheating Green: Wondering whether you should use a nonstick pan? You might have heard rumors about the small but potential risk of Teflon and nonstick pans emitting chemicals that when heated increase the risk of flulike symptoms, birth defects, and cancer. The good news is that technology has come along and companies like Calphalon and All-Clad are making perfectly safe nonstick products. To be cautious, don't use nonstick pans for anything that requires more than medium heat and don't preheat the pans. Personally, I use a mix of both—some nonstick and some more traditional pots and pans like stainless steel, copper core, or cast-iron pots and pans. Cooking might take more of a watchful eye with them, but I think they brown food much better so you get a great golden color. That said, nonstick pans can make life incredibly easier in the kitchen.

Balsamic-Glazed Steak and Steamed
Asparagus with Lemon Zest

Remember the revised portions we're now working with. Each piece of steak should be about ¼ pound, or 4 ounces. If you're cooking for you and your man, he'll likely need a serving of 5 to 8 ounces—if the dude's bigger than you, it's totally logical that he needs a little more. If you're not into red meat, swap steak for chicken breasts, which are generally sold in packages that total about a pound, so split each ½ portion in two and you've got leftovers or lunch. Use the extra for a sandwich, wrap, or salad. The balsamic vinegar will give the steak or chicken a nice golden-brown coloring and a slightly sweet-tangy flavor.

Makes 4 servings

THE GOODS

1 pound or 4 4-ounce lean steaks (like filet mignon, top sirloin, or tenderloin) or 1 pound boneless, skinless chicken breasts
¼ teaspoon salt
¼ teaspoon freshly ground black pepper
2 teaspoons extra-virgin olive oil
1 small onion, peeled, halved, and sliced into half-moons
3 to 4 tablespoons balsamic vinegar
2 teaspoons sugar
6 spears of asparagus per person or per serving (so if you're cooking just for yourself, go with 6 spears; for 2 people, 12 spears, and so on)
Zest of ½ lemon

THE BREAKDOWN

1. Season the steak with salt and pepper. Heat oil in a large sauté pan. Add steak and cook meat to desired doneness, about 4 or 5 minutes on each side for medium to medium-rare. Place steak on a plate and set aside. *If you're going the chicken route, you can cut the breasts into strips or leave them whole before

cooking. Cutting them in pieces or pounding the whole breast flat with a mallet will allow for a quicker cooking time. Sauté chicken on medium-high heat for 5 to 7 minutes on each side.

2. Add onions to the sauté pan and cook on medium-high heat for about 10 minutes. Add in balsamic vinegar and sugar and boil until the vinegar reduces slightly and becomes a glaze, about 2 to 4 minutes.

3. For the asparagus, rinse and trim the ends (but not the pointy tips) off 6 spears of asparagus per person. Fill a medium pot with 1 to 2 inches of water and bring to a boil or simmer. Place a steamer basket in the pot if you have one (if you're without a basket, you can steam the asparagus standing upright in simmering or boiling water).

4. Once the water comes to a boil, place the asparagus in the steamer basket or stand it upright in the pot, cover, and cook for 4 to 5 minutes.

5. Drain the asparagus and transfer it to your plate. If you've got a lemon lying around, grate a teaspoon or so of lemon zest over the asparagus. Add a drizzle of olive oil if you like, and maybe a sprinkle of sea salt and freshly ground pepper.

6. Plate steak and asparagus, spoon onions and balsamic glaze over steak, and serve.

The Facts: 240 calories; 9g fat; 3g saturated fat; 28g protein; 3g fiber

Store-Bought Rotisserie Chicken with Sautéed Spinach and Baked Sweet Potato

Though it might seem a little plain and straightforward, this is a great meal for the average weeknight when you don't have time to think about dinner and your fridge is feeling a little neglected.

On your way home, hit up your local grocery store and grab a preroasted chicken (most grocery stores will have them in the prepared foods section). Rotisserie chickens can save you a ton of time in a pinch and will last you at least two or three meals—dinner for the night and then lunch

for the following day (use the extra white meat to toss into a salad for a simple lunch you can bring to work). You'll learn how to effortlessly make your own roasted chicken in Chapter 4.

Makes 1 serving

THE BREAKDOWN

1. Grab your chicken from the grocery along with a head of spinach and a sweet potato if you don't already have them at home. Once home, unwrap the chicken and cut the white meat off of the breast and skip the skin. Remember we're aiming for about 3 to 4 ounces (think of your handy-dandy fist). If you're a fan of the dark meat, just keep in mind that it's slightly higher in fat and calories.

2. Rinse off the sweet potato, and if it's enormous, cut it in half. There are two ways you can go about cooking it. Long version: Wrap it up in aluminum foil and toss into an oven preheated to 400°F for 40 to 60 minutes, until soft to the touch. Clearly, this can take a while. Short version when you're starving: Prick the potato with a fork a few times, wrap it in a paper towel, and pop it in the microwave to cook for 4 to 5 minutes, until soft. This isn't the greenest option, and you'll likely get better flavor and texture in the oven, but the microwave's a speedy solution.

Cheating Green: Play it safe and try to skip plastic wrap in the microwave to avoid the release of chemicals or carcinogens. Use a paper towel to cover food instead.

3. While your sweet potato is cooking away, rip up some fresh spinach leaves (3 to 4 cups or one third of a large bunch. Sounds like a lot, but the spinach will shrivel up and cook down to a smaller amount than you might think), place in a bowl, and fill gently with water. Swish the leaves around to rinse any dirt off and pat dry. In a medium sauté pan or skillet, heat a tiny bit of olive oil, 2 teaspoons, just enough to coat the pan very lightly for a small amount of food. If you're

making more spinach, you'll need a little more oil; you can also add a tablespoon of water to the pan to keep calories on the lighter side. Turn the heat to medium, and, if you wish, throw in a minced garlic clove, or invest in a garlic press and save your fingers from the knife. Cook the garlic for about 30 seconds, being careful not to let it brown or burn, and then toss in your spinach and sauté for about 2 minutes, until the spinach wilts.

4. Place the sweet potato and spinach on your plate with the chicken and you're done in under 15 minutes. If you're feeling frisky, add a tiny dab of butter to the sweet potato or a little drizzle of honey and cinnamon, or my personal favorite, a tablespoon or two of shaved Pecorino Romano cheese for a sweet-savory bite.

The Facts: 400 calories; 14g fat; 2.5g saturated fat; 39 protein; 8g fiber

VARIATION: *If you're a vegetarian or not a fan of chicken, swap the chicken out for a grilled portobello mushroom or a simple veggie burger. Brush the mushroom with a little olive oil, throw it on an outdoor grill, a grill pan, or simply in a skillet, and cook that sucker up. Same for the veggie burger, but skip the oil brushing.

VARIATION: *Tired of boring old steamed or sautéed spinach? Try other types of dark leafy greens, like kale, Swiss or rainbow chard, and collard greens. A few possible flavor add-ins include: 1 tablespoon chopped sun-dried tomatoes and ½ teaspoon garlic, ½ teaspoon lemon zest, 1 tablespoon Pecorino Romano or Parmesan cheese, or even 1 tablespoon diced pancetta (yes, bacon!). Amounts are per serving per person.

Sautéed Kale with Raisins and Pine Nuts

Don't have kale lying around in the fridge? Swap it for spinach or another dark leafy green, like Swiss chard.

Makes 1 serving

THE GOODS
  2 teaspoons extra-virgin olive oil
  ½ bunch or 4 cups kale, stems cut and discarded,
     leaves torn
  ½ garlic clove
  2 teaspoons raisins or currants
  1 to 2 teaspoons pine nuts

THE BREAKDOWN
  1. Heat the olive oil in a large sauté pan over medium heat. Add
     the kale and garlic, and sauté until the kale begins to wilt, 2 to
     3 minutes.
  3. Add the raisins and pine nuts and sauté for 2 to 3 minutes
     more.

The Facts: 200 calories; 10g fat; 1g saturated fat; 8g protein; 5g fiber

From Sauté to Stir-Fry

Chinese takeout gets a healthy makeover. Stir-frying is one of the
fastest cooking methods around—it's essentially sautéing. If you
don't have a wok, don't stress. A large skillet will do the trick just
fine. Choose your protein of choice—tofu, sliced chicken breast,
peeled shrimp, or pieces of lean flank steak or sirloin beef tips. Cook
just to brown the outside of the tofu, steak, chicken, or shrimp for
1 to 2 minutes. Place your protein of choice to the side in a bowl
and toss in whatever vegetables sound appealing to you. Add your
protein back to the pan with the veggies and cook another 4 to 8
minutes, more for steak and chicken, less for shrimp and tofu, until
done.

It's helpful to keep frozen vegetables around for emergencies—
look for Asian stir-fry vegetable mixes if you like, but just make
sure they're plain rather than sauced up with extra sugar and
sodium.

Ginger-Soy Stir-fry with Tofu and Vegetables

Makes 2 to 3 servings

THE GOODS

8 ounces extra-firm tofu packed in water
1 tablespoon low-sodium soy sauce
2 teaspoons honey
2 tablespoons water
1 ½ teaspoons cornstarch
1 tablespoon cold water
3 teaspoons peanut or canola oil
1 to 2 small cloves garlic, minced
2 teaspoons minced fresh ginger (if you've got it around, great; if not, keep cooking—it's not a deal breaker)
1 red bell pepper, seeded, cored, and cut into thin matchstick-like strips (julienned)
1 cup snow peas
1 carrot, peeled and julienned
⅛ teaspoon red pepper flakes (optional)

THE BREAKDOWN

1. Drain the tofu and press between two paper towels to remove excess moisture. Cut into cubes and place in a small bowl.
2. In another small bowl, whisk the soy sauce, honey, and water together and pour over the tofu. Marinate for 10 to 15 minutes. Mix the cornstarch and cold water together to form a paste.
3. Heat 1 teaspoon of the canola oil in a large sauté pan over medium-high heat. Add the tofu to the pan and sauté for 1 to 2 minutes, until lightly browned. Set aside.
4. Add the remaining 2 teaspoons of oil to the pan along with garlic and ginger and sauté for 30 seconds. Add the vegetables and sauté for 2 to 3 minutes, until tender.
5. Add the tofu back to the pan, along with any remaining marinade and the red pepper flakes, if using, for a little spice. Cook for about 2 additional minutes. Stir in the cornstarch mixture

and cook for a couple of minutes to thicken the sauce. Serve as is or with ½ to 1 cup of cooked brown rice or 1 cup soba noodles per person.

The Facts: 400 calories; 7g fat; 0.5g saturated fat; 18g protein; 9g fiber

VARIATION: *Rice, cooked and conquered . . . Brown rice can be a bitch to cook, so you may need to do it a few times to get the hang of it. Add 1 cup of dry rice to a medium saucepan and toast the rice on medium-low heat for about 2 minutes to bring out flavor. Add 2 ¼ cups of water or low-sodium chicken or vegetable broth and bring to a boil, uncovered, over medium-high heat, stirring once. Reduce the heat to medium, cover, and cook for 40 to 45 minutes. Yes, it takes a while. One cup of dry rice should make 2 cups cooked (4 servings). To save a little on time, pick up some precooked brown rice from your grocery's salad bar/prepared food section if they've got it.

Chicken (or Beef) and Broccoli Stir-fry with Black Bean Sauce

Makes 4 servings

THE GOODS
   1 tablespoon Asian fermented black beans (you can find them at Asian markets or Whole Foods, or for a fast substitute, use 3 tablespoons jarred black bean sauce)
   1 garlic clove, minced
   1 tablespoon low-sodium soy sauce
   2 teaspoons cornstarch
   2 tablespoons cold water
   1 tablespoon plus 2 teaspoons peanut or canola oil
   1 pound skinless, boneless chicken breast or 1 pound flank or sirloin steak, sliced into 1- to 2-inch-thick strips
   1 small head broccoli, cut into small florets
   ½ cup low-sodium chicken, beef, or vegetable stock
   ½ teaspoon sugar

THE BREAKDOWN

1. Soak the fermented black beans for 10 minutes in a bowl of cold water, then rinse to remove excess salt.
2. Mash the garlic with the soaked black beans and stir in the soy sauce.
4. Blend cornstarch and cold water to form a paste and set aside.
5. In a large sauté pan or a wok, heat 1 tablespoon of the oil over medium-high heat and add the chicken. Stir-fry for about 3 minutes, until it loses its pinkness on the outside. Remove from the pan.
6. Heat the remaining 2 teaspoons of oil over medium-high heat and add the black bean mixture. Add the broccoli and stir-fry for 1 to 2 minutes.
7. Stir in the stock and sugar and return the chicken to the pan. Reduce the heat to medium and cook, covered, for 3 to 5 minutes.
8. Stir in the cornstarch paste to thicken the sauce. Serve with brown or jasmine rice, ½ to 1 cup cooked.

The Facts: 400 calories; 10 fat; 2g saturated fat; 33g protein; 6 fiber

---

FROM SAUTÉ TO STIR-FRY: STIR-FRY SWAPS

(Makes 4 servings)

1. Choose your protein—16 ounces (1 pound) of:
- Tofu
- Chicken breast or tenders cut into 2-inch pieces or strips
- Flank steak or lean pork cut into 2-inch pieces or strips
- Shrimp

2. Choose your veggies:
- 2 carrots, cut into matchsticks
- ⅓ pound sugar snap peas, snow peas, or green beans, trimmed
- 5 to 6 stalks asparagus, ends cut off and cut into 1- to 2-inch pieces
- Red or green bell pepper, cored, seeded, and cut into 2-inch pieces
- Button, shiitake, or canned straw mushrooms (brush any dirt off, cut bottoms off, and slice)
- Yellow onion, diced (peel skin off and chop)
- 2 to 3 scallions, chopped
- ½ cup water chestnuts, baby corn, or bamboo shoots

- 2 to 4 cups bok choy, kale, spinach, or Asian greens, washed and torn
- 2 to 4 cups broccoli florets

3. Spice it up with a stir-fry sauce or flavorings:
- Black Bean Sauce—(see recipe on page 53)
- Ginger-Soy Sauce—(see recipe on page 52)
- 2 teaspoons sesame oil, 1 tablespoon low-sodium soy sauce, 1 minced garlic clove, and 2 teaspoons cornstarch/2 tablespoons water mixture added at the end
- 2 tablespoons low-sodium teriyaki sauce or hoisin sauce, 1 minced garlic clove, and 2 teaspoons cornstarch/2 tablespoons water mixture added at the end
- Thai lemongrass sauce—2 tablespoons dark brown sugar mixed with 2 tablespoons Asian fish sauce and 2 tablespoons minced fresh lemongrass, 2 minced garlic cloves, and 2 teaspoons minced fresh ginger. Add 1 to 2 tablespoons chopped Thai basil and 2 tablespoons chopped cilantro in the last 2 minutes of cooking (you can find Asian fish sauce, fresh lemongrass stalks, and Thai basil in some grocery stores or at your local Asian market).

4. Use flavor add-ins:
- 1 to 2 minced garlic cloves
- 1 to 2 teaspoons minced fresh ginger
- ⅛ teaspoon red pepper flakes, 1 seeded and diced Thai chile, or Asian chili sauce (such as Sriracha)
- 2 to 3 tablespoons chopped cashews or peanuts (toss in at the last minute of cooking or use as garnish)

Baking

We're moving on from the stovetop to turning the oven on in this first chapter. If you've been using your oven as a storage space, now would be a good time to clear it out. Baking is a simple and healthy cooking method. If you've got visions of banana bread, brownies, and biscuits running through your head, know that baking can be much more versatile. It's a perfect cooking method for fish, poultry, lean meats, and veggies. No need for much added fat with this technique—just put everything into a pan, put it in the oven, and you don't have to do much more than let the oven's dry heat do its magic. Not having to slave over a hot stove for hours gives you that much more time to read your mail, do laundry, catch up on your must-see TV shows, or finish up work you brought home.

Baked Shrimp with Feta and Tomatoes and Whole Wheat Penne

This is one tasty recipe, and you'll be pleasantly surprised by your chef skills upon first bite. To make this weeknight meal snappy, the sneaky trick here is to purchase some prepeeled and deveined shrimp, so all you have to do is snap the tails off and toss them. For quality of taste, I usually go with fresh shrimp, but when time is a factor, the precooked frozen ones will do just fine. You'll want to adjust cooking times, though—cook frozen, thawed shrimp for 2 to 3 minutes instead of 5 in the pan before transferring everything to the oven.

Shrimp are also great grilled or sautéed in a pan that's lightly coated with olive oil—they cook up easily and quite quickly. To prevent them from turning rubbery, cook for about 3 minutes on each side, until the shells or flesh turn completely pink.

Makes 6 servings (cut the recipe in half if you're cooking for yourself and have some left over for the following night)

THE GOODS

  1 tablespoon extra-virgin olive oil
  4 garlic cloves, minced
  2 28-ounce cans whole tomatoes, drained and coarsely chopped
      (or the equivalent of fresh plum tomatoes if they're in
      season)
  ¼ teaspoon freshly ground pepper
  Salt
  ⅓ cup chopped fresh parsley (optional)
  2 pounds large shrimp, peeled and deveined
  1 ¼ cups crumbled feta cheese (use the GOOD stuff! I prefer
      Greek or Bulgarian feta—try it if you can get it)
  1 to 2 tablespoons fresh lemon juice
  1 16-ounce box or bag whole wheat penne pasta

THE BREAKDOWN

1. Preheat the oven to 400°F and fill a large pot for the pasta about halfway with water and bring to a boil.

2. Heat a large sauté pan over medium-high heat, add the oil and garlic, and sauté for 30 seconds or so.

3. Add the tomatoes, pepper, a dash of salt, and ¼ cup of the parsley, if using. Reduce the heat to medium-low and simmer for 10 minutes.

4. Add the shrimp and cook for 5 minutes (2 to 3 minutes if the shrimp is frozen and precooked).

5. Pour the mixture into a 9 x 13-inch glass baking dish and sprinkle with the feta. Bake for 10 minutes, or until the cheese browns just slightly and is fully melted. Sprinkle with the remaining parsley and drizzle with the lemon juice.

6. When water comes to a boil, add the penne and cook for 12 to 15 minutes, until al dente (*al dente* means "to the tooth," so the pasta is firm when you bite it).

7. Try portioning out ¾ to 1 cup of pasta, so you know what the serving visually looks like. Top it off with 4 to 5 shrimp and some sauce.

The Facts: 310 calories; 11g fat; 5g saturated fat; 32g protein; 4g fiber

> *Cheater's Secret:* Get your veggies. Start your meal with a simple salad of mixed greens or arugula, about 2 cups worth, dressed with 2 teaspoons (a quick drizzle) of olive oil and a squeeze of fresh lemon juice or balsamic vinegar.

Baked Lemon-Garlic Cod with Pea Puree and Baby Potatoes

This recipe appears gourmet and fancy, but it's surprisingly uncomplicated. If you don't have time or the ingredients to make the pea puree, skip it. The basic baked fish recipe alone can serve as an easy entrée for you to pair with a side salad or vegetables and a healthy carb like the baby red potatoes. Just a few fresh ingredients will always make things taste beyond better and will look gorgeous on your plate.

Makes 2 servings

THE GOODS

Fish
¾ pound fresh tilapia or cod (2 small fillets)
1 lemon
¼ cup minced fresh chives
2 tablespoons minced garlic scapes (scapes look like curly scallions; you'll find them in the late spring and early summer at your local farmers' market or Whole Foods)
⅛ teaspoon cayenne pepper (optional)
2 teaspoons extra-virgin olive oil

Pea puree
1 pound fresh shell peas, shelled (about 1 ¼ cups shelled peas)
1 ½ tablespoons unsalted butter
½ cup minced fresh chives
¼ to ⅓ cup minced garlic scapes
Juice of ½ lemon
¼ teaspoon sea salt, or to taste
1 to 2 tablespoons cooking water from the peas

Potatoes
8 small baby red potatoes
1 teaspoon olive oil
2 tablespoons minced chives
Salt and freshly ground black pepper

THE BREAKDOWN
1. Preheat the oven to 400°F.
2. Place the tilapia or cod in a 9 x 9-inch baking dish. Cut the lemon in half, squeeze the juice over the fish, and drop the rinds into the baking dish for additional flavor. Sprinkle the chives, garlic scapes, and cayenne pepper over the top of the fish.

3. Drizzle with the olive oil and bake for 15 to 20 minutes. Turn on the broiler and broil for 2 to 3 minutes, until the fish is cooked through and lightly browned on top, checking frequently so the fish doesn't burn.

4. While the fish is cooking, make the pea puree: Cook the peas in a medium saucepan of boiling water, then drain, reserving the cooking water.

5. Melt the butter in a medium sauté pan over medium heat. Add the chives and garlic scapes and sauté for 2 to 3 minutes, until softened.

6. In a food processor or blender, combine the peas, chive-scape mixture, lemon juice, salt, and cooking water. Puree until well blended. Taste-test and add additional salt if needed.

7. To make the potatoes, bring a large saucepan of water to a boil. Add the potatoes, reduce the heat a little, and boil until they can easily be pierced with a knife, 15 to 20 minutes. Toss the potatoes with the olive oil, chives, and salt and pepper to taste.

The Facts: 440 calories; 16g fat; 6g saturated fat; 38g protein; 8g fiber

Baked Cauliflower Gratin with Thyme

This recipe is extremely easy to make and fits right into the whole cheating mentality. Gratin? Isn't that usually super-heavy, creamy and cheesy? Sometimes yes, but this recipe's so light because it's packed with veggies. Cauliflower's a cancer-fighting cruciferous vegetable and is loaded with vitamin C. Use the general outline of this recipe and if you like, swap in your favorite seasonal vegetables like tomatoes and zucchini in the summer or potatoes in the fall. Make the cauliflower more colorful by using a mix of white, yellow, or purple cauliflower (yes, purple!) if you can find it. This dish does take a bit longer than twenty minutes, so make it earlier in the week or on a Sunday when you have time and you'll have it as a simple side dish to serve up on a couple of harried weeknights.

Makes 8 servings

THE GOODS

2 teaspoons extra-virgin olive oil, plus more for drizzling
1 yellow onion, thinly sliced
1 to 2 garlic cloves, minced
1 large head cauliflower, trimmed and thinly sliced or cut into
small florets
¼ cup low-sodium chicken or vegetable broth
1 tablespoon fresh thyme leaves
½ teaspoon salt
Freshly ground black pepper
⅔ cup Gruyère cheese (or substitute freshly grated Parmesan
cheese)
½ cup whole wheat bread crumbs

THE BREAKDOWN

1. Preheat the oven to 375°F.
2. In a medium sauté pan, heat the olive oil over medium heat,
add the onions, and sauté until translucent, 5 to 7 minutes,
adding the garlic during the last minute.
3. Spread the onions and garlic evenly over a 9 x 13-inch baking
dish. Arrange the cauliflower and pour in the broth. Sprinkle
the thyme, salt, and pepper to taste over the cauliflower and
drizzle with a bit more olive oil, about 2 teaspoons.
4. Cover the dish with aluminum foil and bake for 25 to 30
minutes. Remove the foil, sprinkle with the cheese and bread
crumbs, and bake uncovered for another 30 minutes, or until
the cheese is bubbly and browned.

The Facts: 110 calories; 4.5g fat; 2g saturated fat; 6g protein; 3g fiber

More Quick and Dirty Weeknights: Eggs Done Easy

Sometimes work, personal commitments, or happy hours get the
best of us. When I come home on the later side and am dying for
dinner but don't want to have something too heavy late at night, I

often opt for eggs—scrambled, omelets, whatever's easy and light-speed fast, because I'm hungry. Breakfast for dinner is always great. Start with the basic equation of 1 to 2 eggs or 1 egg plus 1 to 2 whites. Either option is fine. You might find that 2 whole eggs is a little too filling. It's just fine to leave some behind on your plate. No one's forcing the clean-plate-club rule on you. If you prefer a mix of a whole egg and egg whites, that's fine, too. Never separated an egg before? Crack it in half and jiggle the yolk and white between each half of the shell until the white falls out into your bowl and you're just left with the yolk. Toss the yolk and keep going. If you're cooking up an omelet, add about 1 teaspoon of water for every 3 eggs/whites to keep the omelet light and fluffy. If you're scrambling eggs and like them a little creamier, you can add a teaspoon or two of milk, though you'll want to add 2% or whole milk to get that richer texture (a teensy bit of fat does the job sometimes, and in this case, it's such a small amount you still come away with an incredibly light, healthy meal). Then add in whatever you've got lying around the fridge (a few chopped cherry tomatoes, 1 to 2 sliced mushrooms, a sprinkle of chopped onion, 1 tablespoon salsa, 2 to 3 tablespoons cheese, 1 to 2 teaspoons fresh herbs, etc.). And if you're totally out of veggies, go for scrambled eggs straight up. You can make any situation work to your advantage. There are more omelet and egg ideas on page 247 to 249.

Eggs with Fresh Chives and Mozzarella

Makes 1 serving

THE GOODS
    1 whole egg
    2 egg whites
    Salt and freshly ground black pepper
    1 teaspoon unsalted butter or olive oil
    2 tablespoons grated part-skim mozzarella cheese (or substitute
        goat cheese)
    1 teaspoon minced fresh chives

THE BREAKDOWN

1. In a small bowl, whisk together the eggs and whites with a wire whisk or fork until blended and frothy. Season with salt and pepper.
2. In a small (8-inch) sauté pan or skillet, heat the butter or oil over medium-high heat. Add the eggs and cook for 30 to 45 seconds, until they start to set on the bottom. Use a good spatula to scramble lightly, moving the eggs around the pan to cook evenly.
3. Add the cheese and chives and cook for another 30 to 60 seconds, until fully cooked, then turn the heat off before the eggs start to brown. Serve with a slice of whole grain toast and/or a basic green salad.

The Facts: 170 calories; 11 fat; 5g saturated fat; 17g protein; 0g fiber

Scrambled Eggs or Omelet with Sautéed Mushrooms and Herbs

Makes 1 serving

THE GOODS

1 teaspoon unsalted butter
1 tablespoon chopped onion
2 tablespoons chopped mushrooms
½ teaspoon minced fresh thyme or basil
1 whole egg
2 egg whites
Salt and freshly ground black pepper
1 teaspoon olive oil (if making an omelet)

THE BREAKDOWN

1. Melt the butter in a medium nonstick skillet over medium heat. Add the onion, mushrooms, and thyme and sauté for 3 to 4 minutes, until the onions are translucent.

2. Beat the eggs and whites until frothy and season with salt and pepper. Add them to the mixture and scramble them.
3. For an omelet, do the reverse: Set the onion-mushroom filling aside. Whisk the eggs and whites until frothy and season with salt and pepper. Heat 1 teaspoon of olive oil in a small non-stick pan and add the eggs. Stir the eggs slightly until the edges set. Cook until the omelet is almost cooked through, using a spatula to lift the sides and let the runny egg flow under, about 2 minutes. Once the omelet is almost completely set, spoon the filling down the middle in a thin line. Fold both sides of the omelet toward the middle over the filling and serve.

VARIATION: *Change things up and add ¼ cup chopped zucchini to the mushroom mixture, or add 2 tablespoons of cheese atop the filling just before folding and serving.

The Facts: 180 calories; 13 fat; 4.5g saturated fat; 14g protein; 0g fiber

Week 1 Refresher Course—Key Goals

❑ Resize portions—3 to 5 ounces protein, ½ to 1 cup rice/pasta/ grain, 1 cup/piece fruit, 1 to 3 cups veggies/salad (aim to cut total portions by 15 to 25 percent and set your plate up as: ½ fruits/vegetables, ¼ lean protein, ¼ healthy, complex carbs).
❑ 2 servings of fruit per day; aim to have vegetables with lunch AND dinner.
❑ Drink 1 ½ to 2 liters of water per day.
❑ Don't skip meals—you'll lower your calorie-burn capability!
❑ Cheat it up each week with one or two indulgent meals (order what you wish, but still consider portions) and one or two treats (between 200 and 300 calories each).
❑ Exercise one or two days more than what you do currently and/or increase intensity.
❑ Cut your alcohol intake per week by at least 25 percent.
❑ Food journaling . . . DO IT!

CHAPTER 2—WEEK 2

Eating at Work and Working Out at the Gym

"My gym has a sauna and I use it. Does that count for exercise?"

—Lisa

WEEK 2 GOALS

- Make a staple grocery list (ten to fifteen items long) for easy meals and snacks, shop for it, and stick to it.
- Curb Splenda and artificial sweeteners—your body doesn't like fake stuff. Aim to cut your daily intake by at least half. Reach for I to 2 packets per day (or less) and continue weaning yourself off. Or you could always go cold turkey!
- Bring three to five basics (such as fruit, yogurt, nuts, and all-natural granola bars with 3 or more grams of fiber) to work and keep them there for snacks and emergencies. Replenish when your stash gets low.
- Build in time for the gym or physical activity at least three or four times a week and write it out on your trusty food and exercise calendar.
- Pack snacks when you're traveling and have a small energizing snack before a workout.
- Cook at home at least once this week and test-drive a new recipe that gets your taste buds excited.

Staying on top of your game and eating smartly and healthfully during a hectic workweek isn't easy. Your boss is a classic micromanager and is constantly breathing down your neck, you're balancing three huge deadlines due before the end of the week, two

8 a.m. conference calls, and an unexpected business trip smack in the middle of the week. Or, like some of us, you're your own boss and are constantly stressed for any number of reasons, number one being that you're always on the clock. There's not enough time in the day to go to the bathroom, let alone eat . . . and if you drink all the water you've been meaning to, you'll just have to go to the bathroom even more. But you're already reaping the benefits from the first chapter and are starting to feel and/or see the difference. Whether you're twenty-five or forty-five, your energy should be up and you should feel a little lighter overall. We're all different, and the scale may take more or less time to get moving. Some things, weight loss being high on the list, are harder to crack over the age of thirty, but don't worry, the scale will most definitely move in the right direction if you keep "cheating" and stick with each week's plan of action. You might already notice that your work pants are a tad bit looser this week, and you'd like to keep it that way. Actually, you'd like to chuck the damn pants and buy some a size or two smaller—but one day at a time. Just as you're striving to create a more manageable health- and food-friendly environment at home, let's translate this goal to the job site as well, because if you think about it, you probably spend more waking hours behind your computer, buried in a stack of reports, or in a conference room than anywhere else. Good food can enhance your work life in more ways than you'd think. From increasing productivity to boosting energy and focus, you'll be the sharpest, slickest shooter in the boardroom in no time. Donald Trump would be proud.

The Plan

By week's end, you'll have effectively tackled the workweek and sorted out your schedule to allow for easier, healthier eating habits. You'll also continue to implement Week 1's goals while building upon them—it may seem like a lot, but use Week 1 as your foundation and keep going week by week. The prior week's goals will eventually become engrained and you won't think twice about them. So go to page 70 for a quick little recap of Weeks 1 and 2, short and sweet.

Week 2: Sample—Work/Life/Gym Balance

based on 1400-1600 calories

Week 2:	Monday	Tuesday	Wednesday
BREAKFAST 300-400 calories 7-9:30 a.m.	Start the week off on a good note, as work deadlines could get crazy—HIT THE GYM in the a.m. Have a banana pre-workout, then I cup whole grain, high-fiber cereal with skim low-fat milk and fruit	You're scrambling to get to work—grab a piece of fruit and the low-fat yogurt you stashed in the office fridge. Toss in I tablespoon of the sliced almonds that are in your desk drawer.	9 a.m. meeting and you forgot to bring breakfast. Pop into Starbucks for the Egg White, Spinach and Feta Wrap (280 calories, 9 grams fat) or hit your local deli or the office cafeteria for I egg, scrambled or hard-boiled, I slice whole grain toast, and fruit
SNACK About 100 calories 10-11 a.m. (If you're not hungry, skip it!)	10 cashews, almonds, or walnuts—keep a stash in your desk drawer	I ounce cheese, such as a string cheese, Bonne Bell/Laughing Cow, or the real stuff	Meeting ran long, but the egg at breakfast did the trick and held you until lunchtime
LUNCH 400-550 calories 12-2 p.m.	Your favorite salad joint— 1) greens of your choice, 2) protein such as grilled chicken, salmon, plain tuna, lean steak, hard-boiled egg, beans, or tofu, 3) your pick of fresh veggies and/or fruits, 4) a sprinkle (1 to 2 table-spoons) of 1 or 2 of the following: cheese, dried fruit, nuts, olives, and avocado 5) 1-2 tablespoons vinaigrette or olive oil and vinegar	Leftovers—not super-exciting, but certainly economical! Remainder of chicken, broc-coli, and brown rice. Fiber-rich, filling, and energizing for the rest of the afternoon	Local lunch spot—I scoop tuna salad (even if it's not low-fat) with lettuce, tomato, and sprouts on I slice whole grain bread, I cup roasted tomato or minestrone soup or a broth-based soup of the day
SNACK 100-200 calories 3-5 p.m.	All-natural granola or fruit-nut bar like Kashi TLC or Larabar (also conveniently stashed in your desk)	Semi-stressful day at work and a sweet tooth hits: 2 squares dark chocolate and a small skim or soy latte (the milk in the latte will fill you up, while the chocolate satisfies your craving!)	Pre-gym snack: Plan ahead and keep a jar of natural peanut butter at work. 2 whole grain crackers with I tablespoon peanut butter and I cup grapes or fruit. *HIT THE GYM after work

Thursday	Friday	Saturday	Sunday
Beware: travel day from hell. You prepped ahead and packed snacks for the trip but ran out without breakfast and are stuck at the airport. Grab a small skim or low-fat latte, a granola bar (you can find Nature Valley in most airports), and a banana and you're in the clear.	Quick and simple break-fast at home: 1 cup whole grain cereal, banana and/or berries, and milk	Sleep late and go for an EXTRA-LONG WORKOUT AT THE GYM. Light meal pre-gym—½ whole wheat English muffin with 2 teaspoons natural peanut butter and straw-berry slices	45 minute RUN 1 cup melon chunks pre-run and 2 glasses of water (drinks from the night before leave you a tad foggy)
The bag of unsalted almonds you packed (aim for 8 to 12 total)	½ cup (4 ounces) low-fat cottage cheese		
Catered business lunch (you can make the best of any situation): ½ tomato, basil, and mozzarella sandwich on a baguette, ½ plate full of mixed green salad with whatever vegetables are tossed in. Drizzle (1 to 2 tablespoons) of balsamic vinaigrette or the dressing on hand. If it's creamy, use it sparingly.	You know you've got an indulgent dinner with friends, so keep lunch on the lighter side. Salad with your pick of protein, veggies/fruit, 1 to 2 tablespoons of 1 or 2 of your tasty "extras," and a small whole grain roll. Remember to get the dressing on the side so you can portion it.	At home, turkey wrap: 1 whole grain wrap (with 3 or more grams of fiber), 3 or 4 slices of all-natural or fresh roasted turkey breast (like Applegate Farms), Dijon honey mustard, 1 ounce cheddar cheese, apple slices	Brunch out: ½ whole wheat or everything bagel with 2 tablespoons cream cheese and 2 ounces smoked salmon, 1 to 2 cups fruit salad, and coffee
CHEAT TREAT #1 You're surrounded by a wasteland of office cookies and brownies: ½ brownie and the apple you stashed in your carry-on. Phew.	½ bag of trail mix from the office vending machine	1 cup baby carrots or fresh cut vegetables with ¼ cup roasted red pepper hummus	Go GROCERY SHOPPING and set up your ongoing Staple List. 5 ounces low-fat Greek yogurt with 1 to 2 teaspoons honey or strawberry preserves

Continued

Week 2:	Monday	Tuesday	Wednesday
DINNER 400-600 calories 7-8:30 p.m.	Worked a little late and ordered in at work. Chinese: egg drop or wonton soup (½ container) plus 2 cups or ½ order of steamed chicken with broccoli with ¾ cup brown rice and 2 to 3 table-spoons garlic sauce on the side (not the most exciting, but you've got other indul-gent meals later in the week)	Business dinner out: Roasted chicken with sautéed vegetables and baby roasted potatoes (the potatoes and chicken covered most of the plate and are larger portions than needed, so leave ¼ of each behind)	Pack for work trip and make a quick dinner at home. Mediterranean Chopped Salad (page 121) with toma-toes, avocado, chickpeas, and feta, ½ whole wheat pita cut into triangles, brushed with olive oil, sprinkled with dried oregano and garlic powder and toasted
SNACK 100-150 calories 8:30-9:30 p.m. (If you're not hungry, skip it. Work in desserts and treats when you really want them and they're damn worth it!)	Piece of fruit	Filling dinner out; skip the snack.	2 squares dark chocolate
WATER	1 ½ liters	½ liter (crazy day—note to self: keep a water bottle at desk!)	2 liters
ALCOHOL/ OOPS!		Business dinner means high potential for being over-poured on wine: 2 glasses red wine	
EXERCISE	60 minutes at the gym		Some sort of group class: body conditioning, yoga, spinning, etc.

Thursday	Friday	Saturday	Sunday
Delayed at the airport and you're not a happy camper. Meal options are limited, but you're bound to find a relatively harmless grilled chicken sandwich or salad. Scout out your options with confidence and a fresh set of eyes.	Exhausted from a long week: Order in a light sushi dinner with miso soup and seaweed salad (or mixed green salad with ginger dressing), 1 salmon avocado roll and 2 pieces yellowtail sashimi if you think you'll still be hungry	CHEAT MEAL #1 Pot luck dinner party at friend's house (you're on salad duty; if all other food is heavy, fill up on salad and watch portions elsewhere): 2 wheat crackers with Brie, 4 olives, Salad with Strawberries, Goat cheese, and Pine Nuts (page 123), 1 small piece lasagna	Recipe test-drive: 4 ounces Asian Grilled Steak or Lamb Chops (page 112) with 1 ½ cups steamed snap peas and asparagus drizzled with 1 teaspoon low-sodium soy sauce, 1 teaspoon toasted sesame oil, 1 teaspoon rice vinegar, and ¼ teaspoon sesame seeds
Got home late; skip the snack and opt for sleep!	Piece of fruit	CHEAT TREAT #2 1 cup/small scoop of coffee gelato	You loved dinner, are super-satisfied, and don't need dessert. Skip it!
2 liters plus a large seltzer at the airport. Staying hydrated when flying keeps the bloat down!	2 liters	1 ½ liters	1 ½ liters plus iced tea, unsweetened
½ brownie from office catering, and it wasn't even good.		2 to 3 glasses wine or 1 martini or vodka-soda	
		60 minutes of exercise, your choice—whether at the gym, tennis, a sports league, etc.	45 to 60 minute jog/run

A Look at the Week Ahead:

Create a Ten- to Fifteen-Item Staple Grocery List and Stick to It
Building out your weekly staples allows you, without fail, to be prepared with good stuff in your fridge and pantry. Low-fat yogurt, natural peanut butter, whole grain toast, three vegetables, three fruits, skim milk, chicken breast, eggs, Parmesan cheese, chickpeas, and dark chocolate for dire situations. Right there I've just given you fifteen to work with. That much less room for potential pitfalls, like going without a simple breakfast or coming home at 8 p.m. to an empty fridge and feeling compelled to call the pizza delivery guy.

Slash Your Splenda and Artificial Sweetener Intake
Cut it in half or work down to one to two packets per day. Sweeteners are, first off, fake, and they mess up your digestion, can increase cravings for sweet things and carbohydrates, and may actually contribute to weight gain over the long term. Drop them as best as you can and you'll notice a difference, I swear.

Bring Three to Five Basic Snacks to the Office
Keep them stashed at your desk or in the office fridge. Keeping a healthy snack, like nuts or all-natural granola bars, at your desk prevents that 3 p.m. sugar crash when you'd typically run to the vending machine for a candy bar or empty-calorie pretzels.

Hit the Gym Three or Four Times This Week
Maintaining consistency with exercise and planning it into your week ahead of time provides you with a set schedule. It's an addictive cycle—you'll feel better and will in turn want to continue eating better.

Be Prepared When You Travel
Pack a well-balanced snack (like those laid out in the upcoming pages). And be sure to have an energizing snack before the gym that includes healthy, complex carbs so you don't tire out after fifteen minutes. A solid snack will help boost your intensity level during workouts and your calorie-burn ability.

Get to Know Your Kitchen Better and Cook at Home at Least Once This Week

Delivery and takeout can often become too "convenient," with larger portions than you really need. Making more meals at home gets you excited about your food and keeps things tasty and more healthful at the same time.

Week 2—Cheater's Shopping List:

- ❑ Vegetables: 3 to 5 (or more) vegetables for the week: tomatoes, lettuce, asparagus, sugar snap peas, baby carrots, red onion, avocado (technically a fruit!)
- ❑ Fruit: 2 to 4 types (or more), your pick (enough to get you through 5 to 7 days, 2 servings a day): apples, bananas, berries, melon
- ❑ Protein: 4 ounces of flank steak or lamb chops (or 16 ounces for full recipe), ¼ pound Applegate Farms or fresh roasted turkey for wraps and sandwiches
- ❑ Healthy carbs: whole grain cereal (more than 5 grams fiber, less than 7 grams sugar), whole grain bread, whole wheat pita, all-natural granola (less than 10 grams sugar)
- ❑ Diary/calcium: feta cheese, block of cheddar cheese, 3 to 4 low-fat plain yogurts or cottage cheese, skim or soy milk
- ❑ Other: 1 can chick peas
- ❑ Fresh herbs and spices: garlic, dried oregano, sesame seeds
- ❑ Seasonings and oils: sesame oil, Dijon mustard, 1 lemon
- ❑ Snack stuff and staples (for work/home): all-natural peanut butter, container of unsalted nuts, Laughing Cow/Baby Belle cheese, all-natural granola bars/fruit-nut bars (like Kashi TLC, Larabar, Kind bars), hummus (if you don't already have it)
- ❑ Ingredients for spinach salad for your friend's dinner party: baby spinach, strawberries, pine nuts, goat cheese
- ❑ Dessert/treat: dark chocolate

Week 2: Your Weekly Food Journal

Week 2:	Monday	Tuesday	Wednesday
BREAKFAST 300-400 calories *(Note your hunger level on a scale of 1 to 10 after each meal!)*			
SNACK less than 100 calories *(If you're not hungry, skip it!)*			
LUNCH 400-550 calories			
SNACK 100-200 calories			
DINNER 400-600 calories			
SNACK 100-150 calories *(Work in desserts and treats when you really want them and they're damn worth it!)*			
WATER			
ALCOHOL/ OOPS!			
EXERCISE			

Thursday	Friday	Saturday	Sunday

So let's get down to business. Here's your rollout for Week 2, which should be much easier to decipher than your last expense report.

First Things First, Know Your Surroundings

Before we start discussing any sort of meal or snack options for a typical workweek, do me (and more important, yourself) a favor and take a walk outside of your office building. In a three- to five-block radius, or within a five- to ten-minute car ride, what potential breakfast, lunch, snack, and coffee options are at your disposal? And I don't mean the crappy oversize sub place around the corner. Places that provide good quality, decently healthful, nongigantic portions of fresh food, sundry staples for snacks, or amazing coffee. Knowing what's available around you might lead to the discovery of some better lunch alternatives, a little market where you can pick up fruit, nuts, or some yogurt in emergencies, or a coffee place that serves up a nice mental break and breather at 3 p.m. in addition to great coffee, tea, and your favorite all-natural granola bar. Do a lap and take a new look at what's around you.

Breakfast: Early Morning Energy

You know you're no longer hightailing it to work without a decent breakfast—getting your metabolism running in the morning is imperative. So does this mean you just got the green light to down your beloved mammoth-size blueberry muffin or egg, cheese, and bacon on a buttered roll each morning? Not so much. You're trying to shed pounds, not give yourself a sugar high or a heart attack. And to your benefit, and the benefit of your job security, a well-balanced breakfast really does generate long-lasting energy to start your day and boosts your sharpness and productivity. (Sorry, the caffeine in your morning Venti coffee isn't the most viable solution. Too much caffeine with no food in your stomach means serious jitters and no ability to concentrate.)

**CHEAT SHEET: Weekday Breakfasts
That Actually Work**

- I to 2 slices whole grain toast or I whole wheat English muffin with I tablespoon all-natural or organic peanut butter with banana or strawberry slices
- I cup, or I packet, plain cooked oatmeal with fresh berries and I to 2 teaspoons brown sugar (or diced apple and cinnamon), sprinkled with I tablespoon sliced almonds (if desired)
- I to I ½ cups whole grain cereal (remember to look for brands with more than 5 grams fiber and less than 7 grams sugar) with fresh fruit and skim or soy milk
- 6 ounces low-fat plain or vanilla yogurt with fresh fruit and 2 table-spoons to ¼ cup all-natural granola (look for the brand with the lowest sugar content, ideally 10 grams or less)
- I egg, I to 2 whites (hard-boiled or scrambled, with minimal butter or olive oil) with I slice whole grain toast and a small fruit salad (I to I ½) cups; feel free to throw some veggies into scrambled eggs if you have the option
- 4 ounces low-fat cottage cheese with fresh fruit or diced tomato (I'm a fruit girl myself, but go savory if you like it) with I slice whole grain toast plain or with I to 2 teaspoons all-natural jam

Flashback to the Cheater's Triangle. When trying to pull together your first meal (and every meal to follow) of the day, a "healthful" breakfast is one that combines a little protein (like skim or soy milk, eggs, or yogurt), a healthy complex carb (like oatmeal, whole grain toast, or fruit), and a wee bit of healthy fat (like peanut butter or the fat in low-fat yogurt or eggs). Don't let this be more complicated than it needs to be. See the handy sidebar above for some basic rock-star breakfast examples that hit each point on the Cheater's Triangle and can all be easily obtained in your kitchen, the office cafeteria, or your neighborhood deli or breakfast spot.

Spill the Beans: Coffee, Caffeine, and Weight Loss

You've heard the claims: Drink green tea and you'll magically shed three dress sizes. Caffeine boosts your metabolism through the roof. Or, on the flip side, your friend who's always on top of the latest dieting trends proclaims, "I'm totally cutting off coffee, it's sooo not healthy."

Bottom line, coffee and caffeine do have a lot of good to give, but they're not a magic pill. You need to drink about 4 to 5 cups of caffeinated green tea per day to reap the metabolic benefits. Preliminary research *does* show that sipping on 2 cups of black coffee a day may stimulate the nervous system to give metabolism a nudge, burning about 50 to 75 extra calories per day, but I wouldn't solely rely on that to keep you trim and healthy. The good news is that a few cups a day may help lower cholesterol and can decrease heart disease and diabetes risk over the long term. Expectant mothers should take precaution with caffeine intake—aiming for under 300 milligrams of caffeine a day (that's about one tall Starbucks coffee, which tends to be higher in caffeine content than other coffee brands by nearly 20 percent). And if you've got a sensitive stomach, I'd be wary with the caffeine as well. Caffeine can stimulate digestion and aid your bathroom routine (to put it discreetly). This is incredibly helpful if you're challenged in that area, but if you're a delicate flower, that coffee will run right through you, literally, sometimes causing pain, unnecessary bloating, and/or heartburn. Needless to say, sprinting to the nearest bathroom can be an embarrassing experience.

Coffee Buzz Basics
There is a reason Starbucks and Dunkin' Donuts have now posted the calorie information on their coffees and coffee drinks—many of them are loaded with sugar and empty calories. A Grande White Chocolate Mocha Latte with whipped cream has 500 calories and 22 grams of fat? Yes, it's a small meal and will tack on the pounds, but most people continue to down them without a second thought. You tend to steer clear of them anyway, and thankfully, you can still weave your way through any coffee house and leave with a content, caffeinated, low-calorie smile on your face. If you're a diehard

half-and-half fan, okay, no need to begrudgingly bump down to skim milk. For half-and-half and whole milk, drizzle it in, a tablespoon or two, so you can easily moderate calories and saturated fat. Otherwise, skim or plain soy milk's your answer. Me personally, I go for whole milk, ideally organic when it's available. I prefer to forgo any potential added hormones in the milk. It's likely your Starbucks carries organic milk; just be sure to request it.

For all you Vanilla Skim Latte lovers, nice work getting in a boost of calcium, but you've also got some hefty sugar going on there—35 grams of sugar for a Grande to be exact. After canceling out the sugar that's naturally found in milk, you're left with about 4 extra teaspoons of sugar from the vanilla syrup. That's a lot when we're ideally keeping added sugar to about 12 extra teaspoons, 48 grams or under, per day. No need to rack your brain doing the math each time you order; just try to keep flavored syrups to a minimum, maybe a weekend thing, and ask the barista for 1 to 2 small pumps so you get the flavor without blowing it. And speaking of lattes, thanks to the milk, they can actually serve as a filling, calcium-rich snack or as part of a light breakfast if you're running on the go. Remember to order them with 2%, soy, or skim if you're a frequent buyer.

As for artificial sweeteners and sugar-free syrups, more on both topics down the road, but bottom line, if you're a yellow, pink, or blue packet addict, start weaning yourself off now, PLEASE! Though the pink, blue, and yellow stuff is approved by the FDA, one little packet of raw natural sugar (the brown stuff) or even refined white sugar is just 16 calories . . . it's refined, but at least it's real if you're going to have it. You can spare the 16 calories. Notice, however, that one packet of regular sugar is far *less* sweet than one packet of artificial sweetener; one Splenda packet is about 600 times sweeter than regular sugar—600! Even the newer no-calorie sweeteners on the market that are more natural, like Stevia, PureVia, and Truvia, which are derived from a plant native to South and Central America, are still 300 times sweeter than regular sugar. I find them a bit more manhandled in their white powdery form. You'd think they'd be a great option with zero calories, so what's the real downside?

Having a lot of artificial or manhandled natural sweeteners in your diet (from your coffee or tea, to your yogurt, to your afternoon diet soda, to your gum-chewing habit) can often heighten your flavor palate for sweet things and carbohydrates . . . whether calorie-free or not, which may impact the overall calories you consume in a given day and potentially can impact weight gain. You may not realize it, but that intense sugar-sweet or carb craving you constantly have is likely influenced by all the sugar-free sweeteners you're taking in. The minute I raise this point with clients, I can immediately see the lightbulb going off in their heads. If you want to kick sugar altogether but still want a bit of sweetness in your coffee, you might try agave nectar, a natural sweetener from the agave cactus that looks like honey and doesn't cause blood sugar to spike as much as white sugar (it's a great alternative for diabetics or those who are blood sugar–sensitive). Agave nectar's still pretty darn sweet—1 teaspoon has about 20 calories—so just a tiny drizzle should do the job.

Cheating Green: Get a little greener when pouring your morning cup of joe. You can save some trees by using a recycled coffee cup and cardboard cozy—many shops, Starbucks included, now use cups that are made in part with recycled paper. Even better, save a few more trees and save yourself a few bucks by brewing your own coffee at home and transporting it in a reusable thermal mug. Go a shade of green darker by buying fair-trade coffee, which ensures that family farmers in underdeveloped countries receive a fair price for the coffee beans they harvest. Fair-trade products, coffee and chocolate being two of the most prominent, support environmentally sustainable farming practices, fair labor conditions, and community development. Look for the fair-trade seal on coffees at your grocery store, neighborhood coffee shop, or online at Web sites such as groundsforchange.com and equalexchange.coop. A new, even greener, term has hit the streets—"direct-trade," which is even more socially conscious than fair-trade, as it creates a direct link between coffee roasters and growers and often sets higher-than-market pay minimums. Get direct-trade coffee delivered to your doorstep from companies like terroircoffee.com, counterculturecoffee.com, and intelligentsiacoffee.com. And of course, you can always go with a locally produced brand and support your own community.

Power Lunch: What to Eat During the Week

The Down-Low on Sandwiches (Don't Be a Hater)
Now that you've downed your morning coffee and sailed through a client meeting, we can move on to lunch (it's been about four hours, so you should be starving . . . that means your metabolism's burning like we want it to!). I can't quite pinpoint when or why sandwiches got such a bad rap, but countless women I talk to fear for their lives just looking at one or think they're pure evil, put on this earth as a lame, weight-inducing lunch option. Rest assured, the sandwich is not out to cause you harm. In fact, it's often fewer calories than any number of gut-busting "healthy" salads out there. A few pieces of lettuce drowning in ranch dressing and strewn with fried chicken strips, a hunk of cheese, and croutons don't exactly do much, unless you're aiming for a "light" thousand-calorie lunch. And if you're a "sandwich girl," someone who never is satisfied with a salad, no matter how gorgeous and fresh its ingredients are, then really what's the point? Sandwiches have grown to be the epitome of classic workweek lunch fare, and that's okay. They're a quick way to meet all of your nutrient and energy needs midday so you can refuel and plow through an afternoon of work. Some whole grain bread, a little protein (turkey, chicken breast, light tuna salad or hummus, tofu, cheese, veggie burgers, or portobellos for my vegetarians out there), and whatever fresh or grilled vegetables you're in the mood for. That's a well-balanced meal in my book. Sometimes you crave a sandwich, sometimes you crave soup or a salad. Deal with it—a slice or two of bread won't kill you and may actually cause you to eat less over the remainder of the afternoon. The Cheater's tricks to make sandwiches more manageable are the following, plain and simple:

The Bread: Go for whole wheat, seven grain, whole wheat sourdough, rye, pumpernickel, or a hearty, artisan-baked bread. Try to get more whole grain breads in when possible to boost up fiber

CHEAT SHEET: Power Lunches

- **Talking Turkey:** 2 thin slices whole wheat or walnut-raisin bread with 3 slices all-natural or fresh roasted turkey, Dijon mustard, I slice Swiss or Provolone cheese, lettuce, and tomato.
- **Veggie Tartine:** I slice nine grain or sunflower seed bread topped with I ounce feta cheese and toasted, then topped with 2 tomato slices, 3 thin avocado slices, and 2 fresh basil leaves (if you have them). Sprinkle with salt and pepper. Tack on a piece fruit.
- **Sushi Standby:** I cup miso soup and side salad (or I cup edamame) with I sushi roll of your choice—even the spicy tuna, as the amount of mayo used is minimal. (Choose brown rice if you can get it.)
- **Salad Love:** Your pick of greens plus 3 to 4 ounces lean protein such as grilled chicken, beans, or a hard-boiled egg plus ¼ to ½ cup each of at least 2 fresh veggies and/or fruits, I to 2 tablespoons of avocado, cheese, nuts, sunflower seeds, dried fruit, and I to 2 tablespoons vinaigrette or olive oil/vinegar/lemon.
- **Tuna Salad Revisited:** ½ to ¾ cup tuna salad (a tennis ball–size scoop) in a whole wheat or sprouted grain wrap (look for 3 grams fiber or more) or a 6-inch whole wheat pita with lettuce, tomato, and sliced red onion. Or go the sammie route, with an open-faced version on rye and toss the top slice of bread.
- **Panini-esque:** ½ grilled chicken breast sandwich on whole wheat sourdough or Italian country bread with roasted tomato and I to 2 teaspoons pesto. Add a cup of veggie or split pea soup.
- **Souped Up:** I cup hearty lentil or chicken soup or veggie/turkey chili with a side salad or a small whole grain roll.
- **Clean and Simple** (the "I have a date tonight" lunch): 3 ounces grilled salmon or tofu with I ½ cups steamed (or lightly sautéed or roasted) veggies and ½ cup couscous or quinoa salad.

content and vitamins and minerals. Whole grain breads are slow burners when it comes to carbohydrates, meaning they'll keep your blood sugar, energy, and satiety rock-steady for longer. The darker the bread, likely the more fiber and nutrients it's got. That said, a great piece or two of sourdough, ciabatta, French baguette, or challah is too good to pass up on occasion. Keep bread slices on the thinner side for the perfect portion. Some delis and sandwich shops can serve great whole wheat, but if it's monster-size, it's usually more than we need—like four pieces of bread packed into two. Speaking of four pieces of bread, that's typically the number of pieces of bread crammed into your average bagel. Bagels have 400 to 500 calories rather than the 100 to 150 in a single slice of seven grain bread. If you're doing a bagel, make it good, make it rare, shoot for half, and if you're really determined, scoop out the inside. You'll save maybe 50 calories at most, but it's something, and it leaves you that much more room for a light schmear (about 2 tablespoons) of cream cheese and lox.

When in doubt eating lunch out, chuck the top piece of bread and opt for an open-faced sandwich (a chic "tartine"), or just do a half sandwich. This is a brilliant move if you're dying for your favorite sandwich or panini that's a little more indulgent—like a tuna melt, chicken salad, turkey Reuben, or a tomato, basil, and mozzarella press. Halve that sucker, serve it up with a nice side of greens or a cup of soup, and you've got a great meal that's within a much saner calorie range. If dolled-up sandwiches like these are your weak spot, order them once a week or every other week to keep the scale moving downward or comfortably stable as it should be.

> **Cheater's Secret:** Choose a hearty, denser bread and you'll be much more satisfied off of a single slice. In working with countless clients, I've found that your typical sandwich loaf bread from the supermarket isn't too filling—my theory is that if you can squish a piece of bread in your hand quickly, that's what's going on in your stomach. Your digestive system is plowing through that slice at light speed and oftentimes is still leaving you hungry. Grainier, seedier, heftier breads tend to be more filling. Also, watch your croissant and brioche intake. They're buttery and delish but heavy on the calories. Save them for when they're irresistible (like when you're in France!).

The Inside Goods: Fill 'er up. Pack your sandwich with a lean animal protein of your choice or go straight veggie with hummus, tofu, or a filling combo like avocado and a single slice of cheese. Next, stack on whatever vegetables or fresh fruit you want. Top things off with a slice of cheese (rather than the three or four they give you at the local deli) or some sliced avocado for a heart-healthy boost. A few things to watch—you know the drill:

- Mayo heaven. Egg, chicken, and tuna salads can pack in a lot of extra calories if they're loaded down with mayo. Lighten up a sandwich by making it at home and using a small amount of real-deal mayo, about 2 teaspoons per serving (canola and olive oil–based mayos are a tad healthier) or some light mayo. Or if you're out, go for the half sandwich option and boom, you're enjoying your favorite chicken salad without feeling heinously guilty about it.
- Grilled vegetables. They can double as sponges and suck up a little too much olive oil. Just beware—if they're sopping, step aside.
- Cold cuts. There is a wide array of cold cut options out there, many of which are packed with excess sodium, nitrates, and other preservatives. I don't know about you, but I've never been a fan of slimy, spongy meat—just too darn scary. Obviously, you don't always have an option when ordering a sandwich out, but when you're able to, order fresh roasted turkey, chicken, or ham sliced super-thin. A number of grocery stores roast turkeys in-house and you can get fresh cut slices by the pound right at the deli counter. Otherwise, Applegate Farms is a well-known brand to look for, as it's nitrate-, hormone-, and preservative-free and lower in sodium than most others.

Sauced and Spread: Your sandwich is almost complete. For the finishing touch, spread on a touch of mustard (get adventurous with Dijon, spicy, raspberry-flecked, etc.), a *tiny* touch of mayo or a flavorful aioli (French mayo made with garlic and olive oil), as it's calorie-dense, a thin layer of hummus (in flavors like roasted red pepper and garlic), or get fancy with a small smear of fresh pesto or olive tapenade, about 2 teaspoons or so. Or drizzle some balsamic vinaigrette over your sandwich for a light twist. Notice how we're blowing up your flavor options here, incorporating both calorie-free (mustard) and calorie-dense (mayo, pesto) condiments into the picture, but we're doing it stealthily while still building a nutritious sandwich. Nothing's off-limits, so you walk away happy, satisfied, and still chipping away at those extra pounds.

All Wrapped Up: Think wraps are by far more healthy and lower in calories than sandwiches? Not always the case. Wraps can be deceiving, ranging from 100 calories to 300. And oftentimes, the whole wheat or spinach wrap you just ordered has very little wheat, spinach, or fiber—totally washed up. If you're keeping them at home, look for those that contain 3 grams of fiber or more, and if you're lucky, 4 to 5 grams of protein as well. I like sprouted grain and multigrain wraps that have some substance to them. Ezekiel, Aladdin, and Damascus Flax and Wheat Roll-ups are a few good brands, or check out a local brand at your grocery or health food store.

Salads Don't Have to Be Boring: How to Set Up a Tasty One

On the flip side of the sandwich scenario described above, let's quickly chat salads as another smart lunch option. Just like with so many foods, depending on ingredients, size, and preparation, salads can serve as a nutrient-rich light meal or a caloric catastrophe. If you're eating out and you've got nutrition information handy on a menu, we're aiming for around 400 to 600 calories tops. Otherwise, here's a basic setup step by step that will have you happily crunching and munching away for an average 500 calories.

1. The greens—Mixed greens, romaine, arugula, spinach... whatever your heart desires. The darker the leaf, the more nutrients and fiber. Great for stimulating healthy digestion and packed with filling fiber, a cup of greens tallies a whopping 7 calories—thought you might like that. As deliciously crunchy as iceberg lettuce is, it's got close to zero in terms of vitamins and minerals, just a whole lot of water.

2. The goods—Add in some protein to keep you full and rev up your metabolism. Again, we're talking a fist-size portion or so. Grilled chicken, beans, salmon, plain tuna, lean steak, beans, hard-boiled eggs, edamame, and grilled or steamed tofu, among others.

3. Veggies and fruit—Toss in whatever fruits and vegetables you like. Aim to come up with at least three to four different salad combos so you're consistently changing things up over the course of the week. I find it easiest and most inspiring to think about the different fruits and vegetables that are in season and build various creative salad combos around them. Why seasonal produce? It's typically cheaper, often travels a much shorter distance, so it saves on gas miles, making your salad's carbon footprint that much smaller, and seasonal produce has much more flavor and more nutrients. Find information on when your favorite fruits and veggies are in season on page 330.

Here's a mini sampler of seasonal salad combos:

Winter: Spinach salad with grilled salmon, orange or grapefruit segments, and avocado with an Asian or citrus vinaigrette

Spring: Mixed greens with hard-boiled eggs, asparagus, shaved Parmesan, and walnuts with a simple olive oil and lemon dressing

Summer: Arugula with watermelon, feta, chickpeas, and olives tossed with balsamic vinaigrette

Fall: Mixed greens with grilled chicken, beets, Granny Smith apple, goat cheese (or Gorgonzola), and walnuts (or pecans) with champagne vinaigrette

4. The fun stuff—Top off your salad with a few flavorful extras—they're a little higher in calories, but sometimes they can make or break an incredible salad, so don't be scared of them! Think of these as your flavor poppers. If you're getting a salad at a choose-your-own place, ask the salad guy for a small sprinkling of one or some of the following (if you

like): nuts, sunflower or pumpkin seeds, dried fruit, avocado, and cheese. By requesting a smaller amount, you'll end up with 1 serving of goat cheese instead of 4. Aim for about 1 to 2 tablespoons each of the sprinklers, or ¼ of the avocado. If you're served up a salad with a hunk of blue cheese or avocado, leave some behind. No one's forcing you to eat it.

5. The dressing—Go for a real-deal vinaigrette or good old olive oil and vinegar. Or get fancy and test-drive other heart-healthy, aromatic, and flavored oils such as walnut and avocado. Most non-fat dressings boot out all the healthy olive oil and replace it with filler carbohydrates and sugar. Again, that little drizzle of good fat will keep you satisfied and you will be less likely to finish your meal and wonder what's next. If you're already getting some fat from nuts, avocado, or cheese and want to be a bit thoughtful about extra calories, a squeeze of fresh lemon juice or some vinegar will work just fine. Kick the creamy stuff, as it packs in a lot of calories and saturated fat. If you're a die-hard ranch or blue cheese girl, have it on the side on occasion, or try some lighter creamy dressings made with plain yogurt or make-your-own Caesar (see page 129) (it's the real deal, and it's damn good and super-easy). When in doubt, ask for the dressing on the side. I tend not to worry too much when I'm eating at a nicer restaurant, but at your typical quick lunch place or chain restaurant, drizzling the dressing yourself can be quite helpful and will likely save you 50 to 250 calories. You should be able to perfectly dress your salad with about half to three quarters of a small dressing container, about 1 to 2 tablespoons' worth, to get precise on you. Don't kill yourself; you'll master the art of eyeballing it in no time.

Check out the end of this chapter for a smattering of killer salad recipes.

Cheater's Secret: Leave some salad on the plate if it could clearly feed three people. Even though it's healthy, anything in excess will keep weight on. Keep in mind that those "small" salads you get from your local lunch place or at many chain restaurants can be GINORMOUS! You can pack a lot into a small salad container—it's like they're cramming the world in there. If you were to dump that salad out onto a plate, you'd likely get two meals. (And if it's helpful particularly for lunch portions, use a salad plate for your guide.) But when you're stuck lunching at your desk, furiously typing bite after bite, it's easy to unconsciously lick the container clean. Aim to leave a quarter of the salad behind and try to ease up and take a break from work for five to ten minutes to actually taste and look at what you're eating and gauge your hunger level. That said, I've found a lot of us have an easier time slowing down and eating less when a salad's not all chopped up in itsy bitsy pieces already—when we actually have to do a little work, cutting and chewing, and we can really visually see the components of the salad on our plate. Sounds weird, but this all slows you down and helps you fill up faster on the right portions. And I truly think that visual presentation is one of the secret keys to success of eating really well and hitting a healthy weight. Try having a salad where you have to cut the chicken breast and can distinguish between the cheese, avocado, and tomatoes rather than having everything jumbled. It makes a difference.

What to Eat to Nail It

This is a PG-rated book—don't get any ideas from that subhead. I'm talking about eating for maximum brain power, focus, clarity, and conviction when you've got a serious presentation, meeting, pitch, conference call, annual review with the board of directors . . . or even when you don't. So what should you eat to make sure you're playing your A-game and boosting up cognitive function? The answer is the "brain trust"—foods high in antioxidants, healthy fats, and complex carbs for sustained energy. Foods rich in compounds called antioxidants not only help fend off cardiovascular disease, cancer, stroke, and signs of aging, but they also keep your memory and mental capabilities sharp and ready to fire—research shows certain antioxidants may decrease the development of Alzheimer's disease.

CHEAT SHEET: A-Game Meals, Breakfast Through Dinner

- 1 slice whole grain bread with 1 tablespoon all-natural or organic peanut or almond butter and banana slices, plus 1 small skim latte
- 6 ounces low-fat plain yogurt or 4 ounces cottage cheese with 1 cup fresh or frozen berries and 2 tablespoons chopped walnuts, flaxseed, or granola
- 1 cup veggie chili and 1 slice whole grain toast with 3 to 4 thin avocado slices
- Tuna Niçoise salad or 3 ounces plain tuna with 3 cups greens, ¼ cup each chopped tomato and olives, ½ cup green beans, ½ cup boiled potatoes, and ½ hard-boiled egg with 2 tablespoons vinaigrette
- 3 to 4 ounces grilled salmon with 1 ½ cups sautéed broccoli or roasted Brussels sprouts and ¾ cup wild rice
- 3 to 4 ounces pork or beef tenderloin with blackberry sauce, 1 ½ cups sautéed spinach, and 1 fist-size baked sweet potato (quick sauce— ½ cup berries simmered with 1 tablespoon red wine, 1 teaspoon lemon juice, and 1 teaspoon berry preserves)
- 3 to 4 ounces baked chicken breast dipped in egg and coated with a mixture of 2 tablespoons finely ground walnuts, 2 tablespoons whole wheat breadcrumbs, ¼ teaspoon minced thyme, ¼ teaspoon minced garlic, and salt and pepper to taste, served with green beans and ¾ cup quinoa or barley pilaf with scallions and diced dried apricots

Foods high in vitamins A, C, and E are antioxidant superstars. Vibrant, colorful fruits and vegetables like berries, dark leafy greens, bell peppers, tomatoes, watermelon, oranges, cherries, artichokes, broccoli, and Brussels sprouts are loaded with antioxidants. Nuts and beans are a great source as well. And to many people's pleasant surprise, your morning cup of coffee gives you a nice jolt of antioxidants. Serving for serving, coffee beats out blueberries and is the top source of antioxidants for most Americans. Green, black, and white tea fall in line as well as antioxidant-rich beverages.

In addition to antioxidants, the caffeine in coffee and tea acts

CHEAT SHEET: Top Antioxidant-Rich Foods

1. Small red beans	11. Strawberries
2. Wild blueberries	12. Red Delicious apples
3. Red kidney beans	13. Granny Smith apples
4. Pinto beans	14. Pecans
5. Blueberries	15. Sweet cherries
6. Cranberries	16. Black plums
7. Artichokes and artichoke hearts	17. Russet potatoes
8. Blackberries	18. Black beans
9. Dried plums (prunes)	19. Plums
10. Raspberries	20. Gala apples

as a natural stimulant that can enhance memory, focus, and alertness. But too much of a good thing can put you over the edge. You know the deal—when you've had nothing but eight cups of coffee all day, have a raging headache, and are nearly jittering right out of your seat, barely able to concentrate on anything. Bottom line—have your Grande Americano or coffee in the a.m. and possibly another small cup or two later on; just don't go crazy and become a caffeine junkie. It's not so fun for your health, your digestion, or your breath. With the possible exception of infamous celebrity stylist Rachel Zoe, who's rarely caught on camera without her Venti Starbucks cup, your body can't function on java alone.

Back to brain food, those good fats, unsaturated and omega-3s, can also enhance cognitive function. Cold-water fatty fish, such as salmon and tuna, as well as nuts, flaxseed, avocado, and healthy oils like canola and olive oil are no-brainers to help you nail that big presentation. In terms of eating during the day, it doesn't have to be complicated. And don't forget that complex carbs and whole grains can provide you with long-lasting energy. Refer to page 90 for a sample day of brainiac meals and snacks (and take notice that Red Bull—or any of its artificial, man-made cousins—is nowhere in sight).

CHEAT SHEET: Home and Office Staples

Snacks and Breakfast

Protein, Dairy, and Carbs:

Nuts—Keep a small tub in a desk drawer. DON'T leave the tub out and open if you're prone to mindless munching while typing away or talking on the phone. Grab a small handful (10 to 20) for a snack.

All-natural granola bars, like Kashi TLC, Nature Valley, 18 Rabbits, Clif Nectar, Larabar, Kind, Think Organic, Gnu Flavor and Fiber

Low-fat yogurt—Keep a few extra in the fridge (ideally they're plain— some good brands include Stonyfield Farms, Horizon, Fage 0% or 2%, or try soy or goat's milk yogurt or a small local brand)

Portable, storable cheeses—String cheese, single-serve cheddar cheese (like Horizon, Cabot, or Cracker Barrel), Babybel, or Laughing Cow

Whole grain crackers or crisps—Wasa, Kashi TLC, and Finn Crisps (they may look strikingly similar to cardboard, but you might be surprised and like them with a little PB, jam, hummus, or cheese spread on. They're higher in fiber than many other crackers and will fill you up fast)

All-natural or organic peanut, almond, or cashew butter

Oatmeal—Single-serve microwavable packs, such as McCann's Irish Steel Cut, Arrowhead Mills, or Quaker, or a multigrain hot cereal (get plain rather than flavored and flavor and sweeten it yourself with cinnamon, fresh fruit, a sprinkle of raisins or dried cranberries, a drizzle of honey, and/or a spoonful or two of brown sugar or all-natural jam)

Box of whole grain cereal or granola (toss granola into yogurt for a quick breakfast or snack)

Fruit and precut veggies—Always a clutch option and not to be forgotten. Bring what's in season and it will stay fresh for the workweek, such as apples, oranges, bananas, grapes, peaches, baby carrots, bell pepper strips.

Consider bringing in a smaller-size plate and/or bowl to keep at work if it's helpful with portioning. It might sound slightly neurotic, but if it works for you, who cares!

Breakfast—Low-fat plain yogurt with berries or banana and 2 tablespoons chopped walnuts or ground flaxseed meal (it's like wheat germ . . . nice and nutty and crunchy—don't be scared!) OR 1 to 2 pieces of whole grain toast with all-natural or organic peanut butter and sliced banana (I swear, this is a breakfast of champions—energy-packed and so tasty).

Lunch—Spinach salad with grilled salmon or tuna and orange segments. Pile on veggies of your choice, such as red bell peppers, tomatoes, and artichoke hearts. Drizzle a heart-healthy boost of balsamic vinaigrette, about 2 tablespoons.

Snack—An apple or cupful of cherries and 10 pecans, or ⅓ cup trail mix, or 1 slice whole grain bread with sliced avocado and 1 teaspoon each olive oil and lemon juice for a super-energizing snack.

Dinner—Grilled or roasted chicken with veggies and a cup of roasted butternut squash or ½ cup whole wheat couscous or wild rice pilaf with dried cranberries and walnuts.

Office Supplies

Take a moment to take stock of your working environment. Certain things are essential at your desk—pens, a stapler, your computer, your phone with ten-way conferencing, a bottle of Advil for those really heinous days, and a pair of ass-kicking high heels that scream "I mean business" for emergency meetings. Now add food to that list. Stashing your desk and the office fridge with a few staples can save you from being ambushed by afternoon candy bar raids and bagel breakfast meetings, and from going cross-eyed staring at your computer for too long on an empty stomach. Throw a few extra items into your basket at the grocery store, pack them up, and bring them in to your workplace. You've just made your staples accessible and have eliminated the chance of forgetting your brown bag each morning when you're running out the door. At the end of the day, it's just an efficient way of doing business.

Risky Business: Recognize Your Workday Weaknesses

Most of us have had to complete a self-evaluation at some point or other in our careers. Painful and tedious as they are, they allow you to think about your performance on the job, your strengths and weaknesses, and day-to-day functions, responsibilities, and routines. Cut to lunchtime and beyond. Stop for a moment and assess daily patterns or trouble spots that you might experience at work. Any of these situations sound familiar?

a) There's at least one office birthday a week, which means you're headed straight for the cupcake, frosting-smothered piece of cake, or double fudge brownie . . . and then headed back again to nibble on the leftovers. Though the baked goods aren't typically over the top and are distinctly stale, for some reason, you just can't resist. Half hour later you're racked with a sugar crash and are nodding off at your desk.

b) The office receptionist always keeps a bowl of mini chocolates and peanut M&M'S filled to the brim. You unconsciously take a quick detour for a candy or two each time you hit the restroom. Keep in mind one or two can quickly multiply to five or six over the course of the day. An extra 50 or 100 calories turns into 250 or 300 calories easy, which can jump to 25 to 30 pounds gained per year if eaten daily (or lost if not eaten). Damn those bite-size Snickers and Milky Ways!

c) You entertain quite a bit for work and have at least two to four business lunches, dinners, or drinks each week. You're hitting up nice restaurants and your meal's expensed. Of course you're having an appetizer, entrée, dessert, cappuccino, or cocktail *and* wine. You're playing with bigwigs, so it's near social and business suicide to simply order just a salad, but you often come away from the table totally stuffed and totally tipsy and know you've likely overdone it.

d) The office kitchen is constantly filled with "healthy" junk—snacks that essentially don't provide any added value in terms of nutrients and energy. Pretzels, baby oatmeal cookies, chocolate-coated protein bars, gummy fruit snacks, snack mix, 100-calorie packs of Oreos and chocolate chip cookies, sugar-free hot cocoa, every diet drink you could imagine . . . nothing that truly appeals to you or that actually satisfies you when you're dying a slow death at 4 p.m., but you'll stock up anyway and go back for round two to barely get through the rest of the afternoon.

e) You're often stuck at the office working late and order dinner at your desk, lovely as that sounds. You're so miserable and annoyed that food becomes the reward and distraction for the evening and you're prone to ordering something heavier and eating just about all of it. Too bad you're left feeling lethargic and incredibly unproductive and have to attempt to bang out a deadline before midnight.

If any of those situations strike a chord, there are always sneaky ways to get around them. Simply recognizing your usual patterns is an easy first step. Staying mindful and conscious throughout the day and tackling lunch and dinner situations smartly takes some time to master, but it can make a world of difference. Keep a written list in your food journal of what your Achilles' heels are at work— there are bound to be one or two. Set some basic ground rules for yourself and stick to them—remember it takes up to three weeks for a habit to become engrained, so keep trucking. If the office birthday treats aren't the best cupcakes you've ever laid eyes on and they're bound to send you on a "sugar crash and burn," skip them. This by no means precludes you from singing happy birthday to your coworker and socializing with colleagues. If the cupcakes do look utterly phenomenal, please have one! Or have part of one and balance it out with the healthy snack waiting at your desk (like a piece of fruit or a yogurt, or even a small skim latte) so that you prevent the sugar crash syndrome and can finish your work for the day without a massive headache.

The receptionist's candy dish . . . out of the picture. Just like the cupcakes, make candy nibbling really worth it. Fun-size or mini Snickers and Milky Ways on a daily basis do not qualify (sans a few at Halloween—it's just part of the holiday and at least the candy's already portioned). Cheating is most definitely worth it, however, when there's the occasional decadent Belgium double chocolate truffle lying around the office. Or on those random two or three days a month when you simply must have a shot of chocolate to get through the afternoon, run out to the chocolate boutique around the corner and get a phenomenal truffle or single piece of dark chocolate almond bark. If you're going to cheat, do it right.

Back to those business lunches and dinners. Again, look at your week ahead and try to prep for them, particularly if you know you've got a heavy-hitting weekend of dinners out ahead of you. You're on business, not vacation, so give some thought to what you're ordering. Stick to something simple but good—roasted chicken, broiled or grilled fish, pork loin, or filet mignon (it's typically the leanest, smallest cut of steak in most restaurants), maybe start with a salad or light appetizer (something not fried or laden with butter or a creamy dressing). It can be helpful to do some homework and take a sneak peek at the menu ahead of time so you don't overstress while attempting to hold an intelligent conversation. Keep an eye on that bread basket (same theory as the office cupcake—if it's not the best bread ever, why bother?). Moderate the alcohol—if it's lunch and you don't need it, skip it. If it's dinner and professionally obligatory, have a glass of wine or a lighter cocktail like vodka and club soda, a martini, or something on the rocks (it's hard to chug the straight stuff). Just sip slowly and watch how frequently the server is refilling your glass—the last thing you want to do is start slurring your words in front of your boss or a potential new client. Most of all, remember what your portions should look like—it's not as easy after a stiff drink!

As for the office kitchen, to sum up, think about the snacks you've brought in yourself that are satisfying, energizing, and actually quite tasty. No more 4 p.m. sugar slumps that have you running to the kitchen or snack machine for something with empty calories and zero nutrients. The snacks similar to those described in the previous pages, like a handful of nuts, a granola bar, or a skim latte and a piece of fruit, won't leave you hungry for more and will allow you to rip through the rest of your work and jet out the door at a decent hour.

And finally, the late-night office ordering . . . don't take out your frustration on your food. Sabotaging yourself after a solid day of good eats won't make your work happen any faster. Set aside twenty minutes, even ten will do, to think about what you're ordering and how much of it you're eating. Try your best to sit back, slow down, and taste your food, even when you're cramming out a deadline. If it helps, eat somewhere besides your desk if you can, otherwise set your computer to sleep and put your work aside during your meal. I harp on this point for good reason. You'll end up enjoying your food much more and eating less of it because you're focused on it rather than on your keyboard. You'll be ready to refocus so you can go back to your work with a clear head and a well-fueled tank.

> "Those 100-calorie packs of Oreos weren't even REAL Oreos, I felt totally cheated."
>
> —Carla

Suited Up: Afternoon Snacks

You can successfully check breakfast and lunch off the list. We're now approaching the witching hour. The clock strikes 3 or 4 p.m., and if you don't get your hands on some chocolate or a Diet Coke, it's likely you'll turn into your evil twin, and it isn't pretty. This is otherwise known as low blood sugar, the afternoon sugar slump, or carb crash. Whatever you want to call it, it can be avoided, as can your Wicked Witch of the West persona that comes with it. Your body's signaling that it's ready for some refueling . . . with real food. Grab a decent snack (see Box, facing page) and you'll boot that candy bar, chocolate, or coffee fix. And if you've already had a serving or two of fruit earlier in the day, your sugar cravings should noticeably start subsiding. Why? Your body's getting what it really needs from a wholesome source—shocker. Usually this is the time of day when you're scrounging for something a little more fun and "snacky." Definitely doable. Check out the sidebar for a list of snacks to refresh and reboot you. Obviously these are just a handful of options; feel free to get creative once you get the hang of it. Notice again that we're really aiming to provide a simple, tasty snack to balance your blood sugar and keep it steady. An apple alone or with a tablespoon of peanut butter, a piece of dark chocolate and a decaf skim latte, or a few whole grain crackers with cheese will do the trick.

CHEAT SHEET: Talking Snack Smack

(all snacks between 100 and 200 calories)

Solid everyday snacks:
- Fresh fruit
- Apple with 1 to 1 ½ tablespoons natural or organic peanut butter (or try cashew or almond butter for a change)
- Sliced apple or cup of grapes plus 1 ounce cheese, such as cheddar or Gouda, string cheese, Laughing Cow, or Babybel
- Fresh cut veggies plus ¼ cup hummus
- 15 Kashi TLC crackers with 2 tablespoons hummus or spreadable bean dip
- 2 to 3 whole grain crackers plus 1 ounce cheese (goat cheese, light or regular cheddar cheese, etc.) or 1 tablespoon almond butter
- 10 to 20 nuts, such as pecans, cashews, almonds, walnuts, or 30 to 50 pistachios—try to get them unsalted
- 1 slice whole grain toast with ¼ avocado, 1 teaspoon olive oil, and 1 teaspoon lemon juice
- Low-fat plain yogurt or mini cottage cheese with fruit (most delis or convenience stores will carry these)
- All-natural granola bar, such as Kashi, 18 Rabbits, or Nature Valley
- Fruit and nut bar, such as Larabar, Clif Nectar, Gnu Flavor and Fiber, Kind, or Think Organic bars, or make your own at www.youbars.com
- Small bowl of oatmeal with cinnamon and 2 tablespoons raisins or other fruit
- ⅓ cup trail mix (1 solid handful) or 3 dried apricots plus 10 to 12 pecans
- 3 dried or fresh figs and 1 tablespoon goat cheese

Satisfy your sweet tooth:
- 2 squares dark chocolate plus a piece of fruit
- Tall skim or low-fat decaf or regular latte with cocoa powder or cinnamon
- 1 to 2 whole wheat fig bars and a piece of fruit
- 2 graham crackers with Nutella (chocolate-hazelnut spread) and banana slices
- Starbucks iced skim mocha (tall) plus 1 Starbucks chocolate brownie cookie
- Starbucks tall non-fat hot chocolate

Continued

- 2% Greek yogurt with 10 dark chocolate or butterscotch chips
- Small skim cappuccino with 1 almond-vanilla biscotti, dunked

Something salty and savory:
- 4 cups all-natural or light popcorn, such as Newman's Own or Good Health
- 15 whole grain tortilla chips with salsa and/or 2 tablespoons guacamole
- 1 serving whole grain or honey wheat pretzels plus 1 tablespoon nut butter
- Soy crisps, on occasion—IF they fill you up
- 1 cup edamame in pods
- ¾ cup cherry tomatoes plus 3 mini mozzarella balls
- 10 olives (Greek, Spanish, or whatever type you prefer)
- 1 serving whole wheat pita chips with 2 tablespoons hummus

CHEAT SHEET: Snacks on the Run

- Nuts—Those sneaky snack-machine nuts have 2 servings in them. Go for half and stash the rest for later or toss a zip-top snack bag in your purse.
- All-natural granola bars, such as Kashi TLC, Nature Valley, 18 Rabbits, Clif Nectar, Larabar, Kind, or Gnu Flavor and Fiber
- Fresh fruit or precut vegetables (bag them and go)
- Low-fat yogurt (grab one at just about any corner deli)

Exercise: Your Pre-Sweat Fest—If you're gearing up to hit the gym or go for a run after work, you'll absolutely want to fuel up with a smart afternoon snack so you can ensure a more intense workout (read: increase your calorie-burn potential and avoid getting light-headed because your last meal was six hours prior, at noon). If you're sweating it up, make sure you choose a small, power-packed snack that incorporates some easily digested complex carbs. An apple and peanut butter would work, as would a banana and a handful of almonds, or even a quick packet of oatmeal. Your body

CHEAT SHEET: Solid Snacks Before You Sweat

- Apple or banana and 1 tablespoon peanut butter
- 3 whole grain crackers or graham crackers, 1 tablespoon almond or cashew butter, and 1 teaspoon fruit preserves or jam
- Piece of fresh fruit
- ⅓ cup trail mix, such as walnuts, dried cranberries and apricots, and dark chocolate chips
- 1 cup oatmeal with cinnamon and ¼ cup diced apple
- 1 cup fresh veggies with ¼ cup hummus and ½ small whole wheat pita
- Fruit and nut bar (yet again), such as Larabar or Clif Nectar
- 1 small baked sweet potato (sounds odd, but it's great energy food!)
- ½ to ¾ cup mixed bean salad with diced bell pepper and scallion and 2 teaspoons olive oil (beans are a great source of slow-burning carbs; just beware if you have a sensitive stomach)

CHEAT SHEET: Satisfying Staples After You Sweat

- 8-ounce smoothie with low-fat yogurt or milk, frozen berries, or mango and banana
- 1 hard-boiled egg when you're on the go
- 1 cup skim or soy milk and 2 teaspoons chocolate syrup (all-around a great sports recovery drink/snack that fits in protein and a quick shot of carbs)
- A balanced meal, like 3 ounces turkey or lean beef meatballs with ¾ cup whole wheat penne with marinara sauce and 2 cups mixed greens or sautéed broccoli

will convert those slow-burning carbs to sustained energy, so you can have a prolonged, booty-burning workout. If you happen to be an early bird raring to hit a spin class at 6:30 a.m. (myself most definitely excluded), consider popping about 50 to 100 calories of rise-and-shine energy. Many of us have a hard time digesting anything at such an early hour, so keep it simple. A small banana, ½ slice whole wheat toast with 2 teaspoons nut butter, or ½ glass skim or soy milk will do the job just fine. Attempting to work out on an empty stomach means you've got zero fuel in your tank and it might leave you trying to plow through sixty minutes of cardio or toning at a snail's pace.

If you plan to exercise a bit later in the morning and have time to digest a light meal, go ahead and have your standard breakfast or a slightly smaller version of it (about a quarter to a third less cereal or yogurt).

Post-Sweat Fest—You're pumped up and exhausted after tearing it up on the treadmill and hitting a round of weights. It's the perfect time to recharge your body's energy stores and rebuild the muscle fibers you just tore up. Your body's screaming for a serving of healthy carbs to boost the energy you used up (known as glycogen stores). Your body's also craving some lean protein to feed your muscles and fuel your metabolism, which work together to get you that lean, luscious figure you're after. Don't make things difficult for yourself. The answer's surprisingly simple: a normal, well-balanced dinner such as grilled shrimp with spinach salad and roasted baby potatoes or some whole wheat pasta. All your components fit right in the picture. The trick is to eat a balanced meal or, if you're on the go, at least a quick protein-packed snack (like a hard-boiled egg or a yogurt with fruit) within about 1 to 1 ½ hours after your workout. This is your body's sweet spot in terms of utilizing those nutrients and building lean muscle mass with the utmost precision.

Let's back things up for a second. What do you do if you start up a new kick-ass exercise regimen or add in a body conditioning class where you're using heavier weights than usual and your hunger levels are now through the roof? Yes, research does show that weight training increases your body's metabolic rate, meaning it's able to burn slightly more calories throughout the day . . . even when you're just sitting around on your bum. Strength training also helps build lean muscle, and though muscle actually weighs more than fat, it does help to burn up body fat over time and moves you closer to the leaner look you're going for.

With weight training and body toning, your metabolism is revved up and you're naturally going to be hungrier. That or you might feel you're entitled to eat more (or beyond indulgently) because you just worked out. Does this mean you can chow down like a champ? If we're looking at the big picture, not so much. Running or strength training for thirty minutes doesn't erase the oversize blueberry muffin you grabbed afterward, which is likely far more calories than you burned training. Again, the idea of "cheating" revolves around playing smarter and more strategically—empty calorie items generally don't fall into this category. Exercise and eating well go hand in hand, boosting your overall health, energy, and mood.

If you find yourself starving all the time, that's actually a positive signal. It means that you've successfully set your metabolism into high gear and you'll continue shedding the pounds full-steam ahead. The idea is to keep that daily calorie deficit going strong (in a manageable, healthful fashion). I see the plateau occur too often with too many gym-goers. It's either one of two situations:

a) You've been a gym rat for as long as you can remember. You keep the same weekly workout routine, can knock out four or five miles at a clip, and feel like you put in all this effort and nothing budges. What the hell!? Your body's used to what it's doing, so it's just going through the motions. Play smart and change up your workouts consistently, just like you're ideally changing up your meals and snacks to ensure you're getting a variety of nutrients. In the case of your workout, strive to continuously challenge your body in new ways, whether it's trying out a new spin or yoga class at your gym, upping the intensity on the elliptical, doing interval workouts on the treadmill or outside, or training for a 5K, half-marathon, or triathlon. As much as I stay physically active, I'm no fitness expert (the food's my specialty), but keeping your exercise routines fresh and varied will definitely help kick things into high gear.

b) You're just getting into the whole gym thing or have recently added weights/body toning work into the picture and your metabolism and hunger have noticeably heightened. Without realizing it, you compensate by taking on too much extra food—another snack or three, or your portions get a little out of hand at meals, but you're hungry all the time so you don't think twice about it . . . that is, until you step on the scale and you've gained a few. Damn it! By timing your meals and snacks strategically throughout the day and keeping a handy list of foods that really do a great job of filling you fast on small portions, you'll be able to address your hunger pangs, keep your body energized, and keep the scale on a downward trend. I've found that for a lot of people I work with (and for me myself), protein-rich foods really do wonders to curb hunger right after a workout. Even a quick swig of skim or soy milk, a couple of spoonfuls of cottage cheese, an egg, a spoonful or two of peanut butter . . . all small, satiating snacks between 70 and 150 calories that will get you over that hunger hump until your next meal without going overboard on calories or portions.

This notion particularly comes in handy with morning workouts. You kill your 7 a.m. body conditioning class, have your normal breakfast, and are famished by 10. You feel like a bottomless pit. The solution: Shut the door on your hunger fast and furiously with that strategic morning snack. Shut it down, because if you don't, the likelihood of the rest of your day unraveling with a heftier lunch, a sugar and carb attack at 4 p.m., and a massive "bring it on" dinner is high. Just remember to try out a few different snacks so you can determine which is particularly effective for your body and your hunger—the serving of cottage cheese or spoonful of peanut butter might work for me, but maybe a latte or egg is your go-to quick fix.

CHEAT SHEET: "Shut It Down" Snacks
After Exercise

- ½ cup cottage cheese and fresh or frozen fruit
- Hard-boiled egg (it's kind of boring, but it works)
- 1 string cheese or 1 ounce of cheddar and 1 cup of grapes
- Skim or soy latte
- 2 teaspoons to 1 tablespoon nut butter
- 8- to 12-ounce smoothie with low-fat yogurt and fruit
- 1 scrambled or poached egg and ½ whole wheat English muffin
- 1 cup edamame

Cheater's Secret: Just to reemphasize, if you're an early bird and work out in the a.m., have a small, easily digested snack (like a banana) or a light breakfast (like a small bowl of cereal or oatmeal) before your workout. Consuming more fuel enables you to have a more intense workout, which helps you burn more calories to a crisp. If you work out at the crack of dawn and typically can't stomach anything that early, I hear you—I can't either. But even two or three bites of a banana will give your body just enough of a kick-start. Thanks to the caffeine, coffee before a workout can help intensify things, but don't let it take the place of real food and nutrients—your body will get the max benefit and if you've got a sensitive digestive system, coffee probably isn't what you want to be sipping right before a workout.

Sports Drinks—What's the deal with sports drinks and recovery aids like Gatorade and Powerade? Bottom line, if you're exercising sixty minutes or less, water's your pick. If you're running or intensely exercising for more than sixty to ninety minutes, a little Gatorade or Smartwater won't hurt and will help replenish any electrolytes you may have lost. Gatorade is often a pick among athletes and runners because it contains sodium in addition to potassium and helps restock your body's stores that are lost with perspiration. With caloric drinks like Gatorade or Powerade, aim for half of the bottle and see how you feel. Unless you're training for a marathon and it's your twenty-miler day, you're probably fine with about 8 ounces—save some calories for brunch and curb excess sugar. Do keep in mind, however, that Gatorade contains high-fructose corn syrup (a less-than-healthy type of refined sweetener). In small doses it's not a huge deal, but it's definitely something you'll want to watch for on nutrition labels and try to steer clear of when possible. And to finish up, like I mentioned above, for big-time runners and marathoners running more than ten miles at a clip, 8 to 12 ounces of non-fat or low-fat chocolate milk is one of the best recovery drinks out there, giving you a quickly digested shot of lean protein and carbohydrates. More good-quality cheating for you.

Cheating Green: Coconut water's a great alternative for a sports recovery drink. I liken it to nature's version of Gatorade. It's high in potassium and is pretty low on the calories per serving. You can find it at Whole Foods and many health food stores.

Fine-tuning Travel and Checking Traumas at the Gate

Your gym schedule for the week was coming together so nicely, and then you get hit with a midweek business trip out of the blue. (Keep in mind that most hotels have gyms, or if it's a quick trip, pick right back up on the gym schedule when you return home.) Whether you've been shipped off for a quick one- or two-day business trip or you're headed off to a much-needed tropical vacation, the most dreaded part of the trip is often trying to pilot your way through the airport terminal, looking for something relatively healthful and appetizing to eat. Potential disaster zone.

Extra Baggage: How to Compensate for Travel Food, Fast Food, and Eating All Your Meals Out

If you're stranded at the airport with a four-hour flight delay or stuck scouting out food along the interstate while driving, it's time to make the most of a potentially derailing situation. Avoid disaster when you're flying and step away from the Cinnabon stand (just one of those things tallies up at more than 800 calories!) or the greasy Chinese counter. Most airports will have at least one or two options you're able to work with, whether it's a basic deli, sandwich or sub place, Starbucks, or McDonald's. Use your skills to build a decent meal—from a simple turkey sandwich, to a cheese and fruit plate or an egg wrap at Starbucks, to a salad or single burger at McDonald's (you're okay—they're only 250 calories). We'll leave the whole "quality of food and meat" discussion around fast food for another time. I'm a serious supporter of eating the highest quality food with the fewest preservatives or fillers possible—foods and animals that are produced and raised with environmental and ethical consciousness—but sometimes you have to work with what options lie before you and make the very best of it. Which further supports the whole brilliant concept of being prepared and packing your own meal for a long trip.

In comparison to airports, rest stops and fast-food chains along the highway or interstate can be a bit trickier to navigate. It's likely either greasy calorie- and salt-laden fast food, or a middle-of-nowhere gas station with some scary "lunchmeat" sandwiches, an aisle full of every variety of potato chip, pork rind, and candy bar possible, and a bruised, mushy apple or two if you're lucky. Since it's not feasible, healthful, or helpful to your metabolism to starve yourself, look for the path of least resistance and the most nutrients. Pair together what you can find and create a makeshift meal out of, such as a small bag of trail mix or roasted nuts, even if salted, a small bag of white cheddar popcorn, and, if you're lucky, a banana. A combo similar to that will do the job in dire straits, at least until you get to your final destination and can get back to a normal meal schedule. Keep in mind, though, that attempting to fill up on a meal of "snacks" is generally a slippery slope to go down—not exactly satisfying and quite possibly way over your ideal calorie range for a meal. So try to do it as infrequently as possible.

When fast food on a trip is inevitable, try to make smart decisions. This is food that isn't typically worth cheating for (aside maybe from the annual trip to In-N-Out Burger). We all have that random low-budget weakness, whether for McDonalds's french fries or a Krispy Kreme donut, but when you're a frequent traveler, it's important to stay on your standard routine as much as possible, because even with all-out efforts, a few hundred extra calories will surely weasel themselves into the picture each day. You can't control how food is prepared outside of your own kitchen, but you can compensate for it by:

a) making leaner decisions at fast-food chains (like the grilled chicken sandwich or platter, baked potato with a cup of chili, or a single burger sans fries),
b) paying attention to portions like a hawk when eating out and starting your day with a light but filling Cheater's Triangle breakfast (lean protein, bit of healthy fat, healthy carbs) just as you'd do at home, and

c) continuing to get fruits and vegetables in whenever possible and making sure that you're guzzling enough water. This can make or break most travel experiences. The fresh produce keeps you grounded and simulates your routine at home, lightens up the calories at mealtimes, and saves you room for those extras like the mini bag of pretzels on the plane (you were desperate) or the desserts you were "forced" to share with coworkers three nights in a row. Staying well-hydrated wards off any water retention and keeps your digestion running smoothly so you don't get thrown off from the change in time zone or location and end up backed up for four days straight.

Cheater's Secret: Drink your water, at least 1 ½ to 2 liters a day, and eat your fruits and veggies when at home or on the road. Constipation is not fun and can make you feel five pounds heavier in a flash.

Last, when your itinerary has you eating breakfast, lunch, and dinner out in restaurants, yes, you can 100 percent expect meals to be larger in serving size and higher in calories. Your trusty yogurt and handful of granola that you love every morning just went from a reasonable 300 calories at home to 700 calories at the hotel restaurant or a nearby breakfast place. Keep aspects of your daily routine (and your portion sizes) cemented when possible during travel and you'll be able to handle eating out multiple meals in a row without too much baggage on the back end. Again, if you're traveling often for reasons other than a big vacation, remember that it's NOT a vacation. There are definitely times and places, like when you're jetting off to Bali, Tokyo, the Greek Islands, or Brazil for a full-on vacation or even a once-in-a-lifetime work trip, to ease up a little and have a few days straight of more indulgent (though still smartly portioned) meals or exotic delicacies while maintaining your overall healthful foundation. For business and other general travel, obviously if you have a client dinner at the all-out best restaurant in Seattle or Chicago, then by all means make that one of your fun "cheat meals" for the week. The Cheater's mantra is to eat for real life and enjoy it, and then get right back on track afterward.

Escape Routes and Extended Stays—A few other quick tips to ensure smooth travels come to mind. First, pack a snack or a meal. Clearly, you're not going to pack a gourmet meal to stash in your carry-on bag. But a quick and dirty PB&J or turkey sandwich, a small bag of nuts, a piece of fruit or your all-natural granola bar (like Nature Valley or Kashi TLC) or fruit and nut bar (like Larabar, Clif Nectar, or Kind) can be lifesavers in dire travel situations. If you're traveling later in the day and don't have time to make something at home, pick up a healthy sandwich or salad from somewhere you trust near work or home before embarking on your trip, because lord only knows what kind of meal, if any, you might get on the plane. Calorie-wise, airplane meals won't kill you because they're generally small portions—but save yourself from the scary, rubbery chicken breast with faux grill marks and overly salted sauces. If your ankles weren't swelling before from water retention, they sure as hell will be now. Last, the mini plastic-wrapped brownie or cookie that accompanies your meal . . . skip it, no matter how desperate you are for something sweet. We're talking preservative heaven. Save yourself for the pastries in Paris.

Aside from the plane-ride meal or snack, stock your suitcase with a few other food necessities for an extended stay. You're becoming maternal and thinking ahead—embrace it. A box of granola bars, some nuts, a Clif Bar or Larabar for an emergency breakfast—they'll fit snugly into your luggage or carry-on bag. Either way, it spares you from spending way too much money on the mini bar. (Airplane bottles of vodka and M&M'S do not constitute a balanced dinner.)

When you get to your hotel or place of stay, check out your surroundings and the hotel room service and restaurant menu. The one meal you're likely to eat at your hotel is breakfast, and luckily for you, there are always some decent options on the room service menu or at the breakfast buffet. A basic bran or whole grain cereal, like Bran Flakes or Cheerios, oatmeal, yogurt, fresh fruit, whole wheat toast, and poached or hard-boiled eggs are bound to be on every room service menu you pick up or scattered among cold pancakes and soggy bacon at the buffet. Bottom line, you can absolutely make any situation work to your healthier advantage.

CHEAT SHEET: Travel Tactics—Best Bets for Planes, Trains, and Automobiles

- Starbucks—They've literally invaded every airport, train station, and highway rest stop possible. Thankfully they've got some good options, like the protein plate with peanut butter, the Spinach, Roasted Tomato, Feta, and Egg Wrap, Perfect Oatmeal, a fruit and cheese plate, and roasted almonds, to name a few.
- Au Bon Pain—Another airport staple. Make your own sandwich or salad to grab and go, or pick up a yogurt with fruit or some oatmeal for a quick breakfast.
- Newsstands and delis—If you're stuck with a wall lined with candy, chips, and snacks, trail mix and nuts are your new best friends as healthful, satisfying on-flight holdovers. Beware, however—check the number of servings on the bag. Most of them have at least two servings. Go for a solid handful or two and you're golden.
- McDonald's or pizza—Not your finest hour in terms of options, but we'll make it work. Straight shoot it and go for a hamburger or grilled chicken sandwich (they're some of the lesser-calorie options on the menu) and a salad or a slice of veggie pizza and a side salad if you can get it. McDonald's also has yogurt parfaits with fruit, which can serve as an easy and filling breakfast or snack.

If you're traveling for an extended period, more than three or four days, and you have a small fridge or even a small kitchen if you're in a corporate apartment or executive suite, stock it! Make a run to the corner mini-mart or a local grocery store if you can and purchase those few weekly staples that keep you even-keeled and stress-free. For me, it's usually a few low-fat plain yogurts for a morning breakfast or light snack, some fruit, a small bag of granola or nuts, some whole grain crackers, like Wasa or Kashi TLC, and some hummus and cheese—usually cheddar or goat—for a quick satisfying snack. Go a step further and buy a few simple ingredients for a healthy, fast dinner. Five ingredients or less, such as chicken breast, fresh garlic, extra-virgin olive oil, whole wheat penne, and zucchini and you've got a great meal in your hotel without going overboard on groceries.

Cheater's Secret: As a quick point of reinforcement, when you're traveling for business, remain cognizant of portions, particularly at larger meals and buffets. You're there for business, not vacation, which means your meals should strive to look similar to how they would on any other average weekday, particularly if you jet around for business frequently. Navigate as best you can, keep fruit and vegetable intake high, and be on top of your game when you've got multiple business dinners to attend—which means opting for the roasted chicken, the grilled fish, or the filet.

Quick and Dirty: Making a Fast, Healthy Meal After a Hectic Workday

"It's like a full-on salad bar in my fridge. And I kind of love it!"

—Anne

In Week 2 we're building upon the Cooking 101 Basics mastered in Week 1. This week, we're deconstructing dinners, giving you the primary tools to prepare a quick, light evening meal, whether you've just returned from the gym, a late night at work, or happy hour with friends. I've chosen to target the next layer of fundamental (and uncomplicated) cooking techniques—grilling and toasting, beyond just popping a slice of bread in the toaster. Sexier salads are also on deck this week—dress them up in their finest and they make a nutrient-rich, gorgeous entrée or side dish (and it's a guaranteed way to get your veggies in). If you're not big on salads, I'm hoping I can change your mind with the recipes in the pages that follow. Whatever you do, don't put salads in that miserable "diet food" category. They don't have to be designated as "rabbit food," as my dear father sometimes likes to call them. This is the perfect time for cheating—go ahead and deviate from the recipes below, mix and match, and get crazy and creative in the kitchen with the salad ingredients you have on hand. Experiment with flavors, dressings, and seasonal produce to come up with a new combo that's so good you get giddy. You know, that same feeling you get after finding the dress you've been eyeing for months on the sale rack at 40 percent off.

But before we delve into the wondrous world of salads, let's run through a few cooking methods that will help you build and accent a masterpiece of mesclun, mâche, arugula, or endive (a few of your fancy lettuce leaves); of course, spinach and romaine are great, too.

Grilling

It's an average Tuesday night and you're feeling über-productive after a workout and renegade run into the grocery store for dinner makings. Missions 1 and 2 accomplished. In the comfort of your kitchen, unpack your groceries and prepare to cook a simple, fast dinner that will provide that final healthful blow for the day, leaving you proud and satiated. You've lined up all the trusty ingredients for your meal and they're looking really pretty on your crystal-clean countertop. Unfortunately, the ingredients won't cut and cook themselves—so much for wishful thinking. Grab the reins and get cooking. Grilling and broiling are two of the easiest, healthiest cooking methods around. Grilling and broiling both rely on direct, dry heat (coming from below when grilling, broiling from above) in the oven and are super-healthful methods for cooking tender cuts of meat, chicken, and fish, as the fat drips off away from the food.

Take the grill pan out of the box—you know, the one your mom gave you three years ago for your birthday. If you don't have a grill pan, a stainless steel pan or cast-iron griddle pan will do the job just fine, and if you're lucky enough to have an outdoor grill, light it up! Brush the grill or pan with a very light coating of olive or canola oil. Grab your protein of choice, and it's time for physical contact with the grill. Don't move the item until it's seared and grill marks form, at least 2 minutes. The same basic grilling method can generally apply to any type of protein—chicken breast, wings, and thighs, red meat, tofu, seafood, and fish. Grill times will depend on your choice of protein, and in the case of red meat and certain fish, like salmon and tuna, your "rare to well" preference as well as the thickness of the meat (thicker cuts of tougher red meat may take longer). You'll be able to achieve the coveted grill marks by turning over your chicken, beef, salmon, etc., just once. Grilling is also a fantastic, healthful way of preparing vegetables, corn, and even breads, pizza, and fruits for an exotic twist to your meal or dessert.

CHEAT SHEET: Your Grilling Game Plan

1. **Choose 16 ounces (I pound) of your protein of choice (makes 4 servings):**
- Red meat: 97% lean ground beef, lean cut of steak, like sirloin or flank, bison or buffalo burger (which has 75% less saturated fat than beef!), veal, lamb, pork tenderloin
- Poultry: chicken breast or tenderloin strips (choose skinless or take the skin off after grilling if on the bone), chicken wings or thighs, turkey or chicken burger, whole chicken
- Fish and seafood: shrimp, scallops, wild salmon, tuna, swordfish, mahimahi (any thicker, meatier type of fish is great—flaky white fish will fall apart on the grill, as it's too delicate)
- Vegetarian: veggie or soy burger, tofu steak, portobello mushroom

2. **Pick your poison (aka marinade):**
- Plain Jane: 2 teaspoons olive oil, and salt and pepper to taste
- Fast and furious: 2 to 3 tablespoons fresh minced herbs (rosemary, oregano, basil, thyme), the juice of 2 fresh lemons, 2 tablespoons extra-virgin olive oil, and salt and pepper to taste
- Italian stallion—3 tablespoons balsamic vinegar, I tablespoon extra-virgin olive oil, I to 2 smashed garlic cloves, 2 teaspoons honey, ¼ teaspoon red pepper flakes, and salt and pepper to taste
- Major mojo—Juice of 3 limes plus juice of I orange (or ¼ cup orange juice), ¼ cup chopped onion, I to 2 minced garlic cloves, I to 2 teaspoons ground cumin, and salt and pepper to taste
- Asian invasion—2 tablespoons low-sodium teriyaki sauce, 2 tablespoons low-sodium soy sauce, 2 teaspoons honey, I minced garlic clove
- Asian invasion 2.0—2 tablespoons low-sodium teriyaki sauce, 2 tablespoons low-sodium soy sauce, 2 tablespoons Worcestershire sauce, I minced garlic clove
- Greek goddess—I to 2 tablespoons extra-virgin olive oil, juice from 2 fresh lemons, 2 teaspoons chopped fresh oregano, and salt and pepper to taste
- Middle Eastern magic—I cup plain low-fat Greek yogurt, 2 teaspoons olive oil, 2 teaspoons ground cumin and coriander, ½ teaspoon paprika and red pepper flakes, ¾ teaspoon grated ginger, 2 minced garlic cloves, a pinch of cinnamon, and salt and pepper to taste
- Vintage Cuba—½ mango cut and muddled, juice of 2 limes, I minced garlic clove, salt and pepper to taste, and a sprinkle of red pepper flakes if you like

Continued

- Chimichurri sauce for steak and chicken—½ cup packed chopped fresh parsley, ¼ cup packed chopped fresh cilantro, 2 minced garlic cloves, ¼ cup olive oil, 3 tablespoons red wine vinegar, ¼ teaspoon crushed red pepper, ¼ teaspoon ground cumin, and ¼ teaspoon salt. Muddle all items together until semiblended or combine in a food processor and puree until smooth.

3. Rock out with veggies:

- Great vegetables for grilling: asparagus, zucchini, mushrooms, tomatoes, eggplant, corn, onions, bell peppers, squash
- Brush veggies with olive oil and sprinkle with salt and pepper

CHEAT SHEET: Grill Times

- Chicken breasts (skinless and boneless)—4 to 6 minutes on each side (more or less depending on thickness)
- Burgers—3 to 4 minutes each side for medium (turkey, bison, 97% lean beef, lamb, and veggie)
- Lean flank steak (about ½ to ¾ inch thick)—3 to 4 minutes on each side for rare, 4 to 5 minutes on each side for medium, 5 to 6 minutes on each side for well done
- Tenderloin or sirloin (about ½ inch thick)—5 to 6 minutes on each side for rare, 7 to 8 minutes on each side for medium, 9 to 10 minutes on each side for well done
- Shrimp—2 to 3 minutes on each side
- Fish (salmon, tuna, swordfish, monkfish, bass—about 1 to 1 ½ inches thick)—4 to 5 minutes on each side, until the fish gives a little and will flake if you fork it
- Vegetables—5 to 7 minutes on each side (less for thinly sliced vegetables)

To the Touch

For steak and red meat:
Rare—Meat is soft when touched
Medium-rare—Meat is springy to the touch
Well-done—Meat is resilient to the touch

Grilled Chicken Breasts or Shrimp
with Lemon-Herb Gremolata Sauce

Traditional gremolata is a mixture of lemon zest, parsley, and garlic and is often used as a topping for lamb, chicken, and seafood. I've added a slight twist here with the addition of chives and olive oil to create an easy and colorful marinade and drizzling sauce.

Makes 4 servings

THE GOODS

Juice and zest of 1 lemon
½ cup minced fresh parsley
1 garlic clove, minced
3 tablespoons olive oil
2 teaspoons finely chopped chives, plus 1 tablespoon for
    garnish (optional)
Salt and freshly ground black pepper
1 pound chicken breasts (skinless or with skin and bone intact)
    or 1 pound uncooked large shrimp, peeled and deveined
4 to 6 metal or bamboo skewers for shrimp (soak bamboo
    skewers in water for 5 minutes first so they don't burn)

THE BREAKDOWN

1. In a small glass or bowl, combine the lemon juice, parsley, garlic, olive oil, chives, and salt and pepper to taste. Muddle (or smash) the ingredients until semiblended.
2. Place the chicken or shrimp in a large bowl, pour half of the gremolata sauce over, and toss well to coat. Allow to marinate for 30 minutes.
3. Set a gas grill on high for 10 minutes, then lower to medium-high, or preheat a charcoal grill for 10 minutes, or set a grill pan on medium-high heat.
   For bone-in chicken on a gas or charcoal grill: On a lightly oiled rack, grill skin side down for about 5 minutes, turn off burner or move from heated coals, flip and grill for another

15 to 20 minutes, until cooked through and browned. For skinless breasts, cook 8 to 10 minutes total, turning occasionally. For chicken on a grill pan: Grill for about 6 to 8 minutes on each side.

For shrimp (with grill or grill pan): Skewer shrimp in a C shape and grill for 2 to 3 minutes on each side, until the shrimp are pink.

4. Place the chicken breasts or shrimp on a platter, drizzle the remaining gremolata sauce over, garnish with extra chives, and serve.

The Facts: 220 calories; 15g fat; 3.5g saturated fat; 19g protein; 0g fiber

Note: I opted for bone-in chicken breasts with skin on in this recipe because I find that they provide a little more flavor and are a nice change up to your standard skinless, boneless chicken breasts. Sure, the skin's going to have extra fat and calories you don't need, so just peel it right off and go straight for the lean white meat when you sit down to eat. You can always swap boneless, skinless breasts if you prefer them.

Asian Grilled Steak or Lamb Chops

Makes 4 servings

THE GOODS
   3 tablespoons low-sodium soy sauce
   3 tablespoons low-sodium teriyaki sauce
   2 garlic cloves, minced
   16 ounces flank steak or lamb chops (look for meat with the least amount of fat)

THE BREAKDOWN
   1. Combine the soy sauce, teriyaki sauce, and garlic in a heavy-duty zip-top bag. Add the steak or chops, seal the bag, and marinate for at least 1 to 2 hours in the refrigerator. Take the steak out of the fridge about 30 minutes before grilling.

2. Heat a grill pan on medium-high heat. Or preheat an outdoor grill on high for about 10 minutes and then lower to medium-high. Grill the steak for 6 to 8 minutes on each side for medium doneness.

3. Serve it up with a gorgeous green salad or 1 ½ to 2 cups steamed sugar snap peas and asparagus dressed with 1 teaspoon toasted sesame oil, 1 teaspoon low-sodium soy sauce, 1 teaspoon rice vinegar, a pinch of red pepper flakes, and ¼ teaspoon sesame seeds.

The Facts: 180 calories; 6g fat; 2.5g saturated fat; 25g protein; 0g fiber

Basic Burgers (Bison, Beef, Turkey, or Lamb)

Makes 4 burgers

THE GOODS
    1 pound extra-lean ground meat
    2 tablespoons chopped fresh flat-leaf parsley
    2 tablespoons chopped fresh chives
    1 egg
    Salt and freshly ground black pepper

THE BREAKDOWN
    1. Mix together all ingredients in a medium bowl and make 4 patties.
    2. Grill or pan-fry for 3 to 6 minutes on each side, depending on preferred doneness.

The Facts: 150 calories; 6g fat; 2g saturated fat; 24g protein; 0g fiber

VARIATION: *For the lightest burger, try extra-lean ground turkey and save 5.5 grams of fat. Bison is making a huge comeback as an ultra-lean, low-cholesterol red meat—lower in fat, calories, and cholesterol than both beef and skinless chicken! Or get creative and try ground lamb, which makes for a deliciously light Middle Eastern–inspired burger (ditch the egg, parsley, and chives, and instead throw a clove of minced garlic and ¼ cup feta cheese into the lamb burger mixture for a pop of flavor).

VARIATION: *Throwing a cocktail party or having friends over for the Super Bowl? Get chic and smart at the same time with sliders (mini burgers, about 2 ounces each instead of 4 ounces). It's genius because it's automatic portion-sizing!

Fresh, Fast Grilled Vegetables

Use the vegetables of your choice, such as tomatoes, eggplant, zucchini, yellow squash, asparagus, mushrooms, onions, fennel, or red bell peppers. Here's a quick sample.

Makes 6 to 8 servings

THE GOODS
   2 to 3 tablespoons olive oil
   2 tablespoons balsamic vinegar
   2 garlic cloves, smashed
   Salt and freshly ground black pepper
   2 zucchinis, sliced lengthwise in long, thin strips
   1 medium eggplant, sliced lengthwise or in rounds about 1 inch
      thick (lightly sprinkle salt on the eggplant slices to draw out
      any bitterness and acidity)
   1 pint cherry tomatoes
   1 bunch asparagus spears, ends snapped off

THE BREAKDOWN
   1. Whisk together the olive oil, vinegar, garlic, and salt and pepper to taste in a small bowl. Place the veggies in a large bowl or glass dish. Pour the olive oil mixture over the veggies and marinate for at least 15 to 30 minutes or up to 2 hours.
   2. Heat a grill pan or outdoor grill over medium-high heat. Grill the veggies in batches until light grill marks form—about 8 minutes for zucchini and eggplant, 5 minutes for tomatoes and

asparagus. Save about 2 tablespoons of marinade. Arrange the vegetables on a platter, drizzle over the remaining marinade, and serve.

The Facts: 90 calories; 6g fat; 1g saturated fat; 3g protein; 4g fiber

VARIATION: * For super-basic grilled veggies, simply brush them with a bit of olive oil (using a pastry or grilling brush—they're not hard to find), sprinkle with salt and pepper, and throw them on the grill or in the grill pan. Done deal, easy as that.

Toasting

Toasting nuts, seeds, and spices makes for great add-ons to dishes and brings out incredible flavor. If you can get fresh whole spices, they'll typically take you much further than the powdered stuff, which loses its flavor fast. You should really replace ground spices after about a year. Toast whole spices in a dry skillet over medium heat for 3 to 5 minutes, and then grind in a coffee grinder or with a mortar and pestle. As for the nuts, you can leave them whole, chop them, or buy them already slivered or shaved as with almonds. The greatest thing about toasting is that you need just a single piece of equipment—a dry pan or baking sheet.

Toasted Nuts, Plain and Simple

You can toast nuts in the oven on a baking sheet at 350°F for 5 to 10 minutes. Stir the nuts halfway through to prevent burning. If I'm running behind and don't have time to preheat my oven, I'll cheat a little (not surprising) and toast nuts in a skillet. Heat a small or medium skillet over medium heat, scatter your choice of nuts (walnuts, pecans, pine nuts, almonds, etc.) in the pan, and toast for about 5 minutes, until they start turning golden brown. Shake the pan a few times to prevent burning. For seeds like pumpkin or sunflower, either a skillet or baking sheet will do the trick equally well. Same times apply as above.

Toasted Whole Wheat Pita Chips

These are perfect to accompany a light salad or to pair with hummus or an easy dip, like the Roasted Red Pepper and Feta Dip on page 259. Making your own cuts costs and excess calories.

Cut 2 large whole wheat pitas into 8 small triangles. Brush the top of each triangle with olive oil and sprinkle with any of the following spice combos:

- Salt, pepper, and garlic powder
- Salt and fresh thyme or rosemary
- Zaatar (a Middle Eastern spice mixture—check your local international food store or www.kalustyans.com)
- Salt, paprika or chili powder, and garlic powder

Arrange the pita on a large baking sheet and toast in the oven at 400°F for 4 to 5 minutes, until golden brown.

Toasts for Bruschetta or Crostini

Possibly some of the easiest crowd-pleasing appetizers ever, bruschetta and crostini, "little toasts," are great for a large group or just a few close friends. Here's the basic toast recipe. The topping options are endless.

Preheat the oven to 350°F. Slice a regular or whole wheat baguette or ciabatta bread into thin slices and arrange on a baking sheet. Brush the bread lightly with olive oil and toast in the oven until golden, 7 to 8 minutes.

VARIATION: *For garlic toasts, slice a garlic clove in half and rub one side of bread slices with the cut side of the garlic.

TOPPINGS
- Diced fresh tomato and basil—3 medium diced tomatoes, 2 tablespoons chopped fresh basil, 1 tablespoon olive oil, 1

tablespoon balsamic vinegar, and salt to taste. Mix all the ingredients together and spoon atop garlic toasts.

- Goat cheese, fig spread, and caramelized onions—spread a thin layer of goat cheese on plain toasts, followed by a small dollop of fig jam, and top with 1 teaspoon caramelized onions (see Note).
- Brie with cranberry or ginger-pear compote (store-bought) or brandy-soaked raisins
- Butternut Squash Bruschetta with Pine Nuts and Sour Cherries (see page 259)
- Try out other dips and spreads, such as olive tapenade and artichoke and white bean dip (see page 258), grilled or sautéed vegetables, and salmon or tuna tartare. You name it and it can probably top a crostini toast!

Note: Caramelizing is the browning process of natural sugars in foods, or added sugar. Caramelizing creates great flavor and color. To caramelize onions, cut the top off of an onion, remove the peel, and cut the onion in half, keeping the root intact. Take one half of the onion and place it flat side down. Cut the onion into thin half-rings. Repeat with the other half. Heat a large sauté pan over medium heat and melt 1 tablespoon unsalted butter. Add the sliced onion, sprinkle with a pinch of salt, and cook for about 20 minutes, stirring frequently, until the onion is a nice caramel brown color.

The Sexier Side of Salads

I admit it, I love salads. However, I am not a fan of boring, "diety" salads. No "rabbit food," "plain Jane" iceberg and shaved carrot salads allowed in this book. I've pulled together some of my favorite colorful, flavor-packed salads that can serve as a fresh start to a meal, a fast, light entrée for a weeknight dinner, or even a gourmet brown-bag lunch that will be the envy of all your coworkers. I speak from experience here. I've even managed to get my dad to enjoy many of the recipes that follow . . . and that's quite a feat!

Mixed Greens with Pear, Pomegranate, Gorgonzola, and Champagne Vinaigrette

It's become tradition for me to make this salad every year at Thanksgiving; otherwise my family might bar me from sitting down at the table, no joke. The pear, pomegranate, and walnut make a great combo of fall flavors. A few Thanksgivings back, I decided to get a little racy and toss in some whole wheat garlic croutons (see recipe on page 119). I know you're thinking that croutons are nutritional blasphemy. Not in a cheater's kitchen. Anything's possible . . . and healthful. I've swapped regular white bread here for whole wheat, bumping up the whole grain, higher-fiber goodness. Yes, there's a wee bit of olive oil and butter involved, but 2 to 3 mini croutons tossed onto your salad plate won't set you back too much, and these are so tasty.

This salad also gets nutritional bonus points . . . pomegranate seeds are jam-packed with disease-fighting antioxidants, and the walnuts are rich in healthy omega-3 fats.

Makes 8 to 10 servings

THE GOODS
  11 ounces (2 bags) mixed greens or baby spinach
  2 red pears, thinly sliced
  ½ small red onion, thinly sliced
  ⅓ cup chopped toasted walnuts or pecans
  ¼ cup dried cranberries or golden raisins
  ⅓ cup pomegranate seeds
  ½ cup crumbled Gorgonzola cheese (or substitute 4 ounces, or
    1 small log, of fresh goat cheese for a milder flavor)
  About 3 cups whole wheat croutons (recipe follows)

THE DRESSING
  1 ½ tablespoons Dijon mustard
  ¼ cup champagne vinegar
  Salt and freshly ground pepper
  ½ small shallot, minced
  ¼ cup plus 2 tablespoons extra-virgin olive oil

THE BREAKDOWN

1. Toss all the salad ingredients in a large bowl.
2. Place the mustard and vinegar in a small bowl as your base, then season with salt and pepper to taste and add the shallot. Slowly whisk in the olive oil—pour it in a slow, continuous drizzle while continuing to steadily whisk. The mustard helps the oil to emulsify, or blend, with the vinegar (or the lemon juice in other dressings). This way the oil and vinegar won't separate after mixing and you're left with a nice, smooth dressing. The dressing will remain fresh for 3 to 4 days. If you prefer a vinaigrette without garlic or shallots (just oil, vinegar/citrus juice, and/or mustard), the dressing will hold up for a week or more on your countertop.
3. Drizzle the dressing over the salad and toss.

The Facts: 240 calories, 15g fat, 3.5g saturated fat, 5g fiber, 4g protein

Cheater's Secret: For a heartier entrée salad, pop on some protein and top off your greens with a grilled chicken breast (great if you made an extra breast the night before and have leftovers).

VARIATION: *No clue how to remove the seeds from a pomegranate? The easiest way is to cut it in quarters, stick it in a bowl of cold water, and start picking out the seeds with your bare hands. By placing the pomegranate in water, you avoid staining your fingers a lovely shade of fuchsia, as pretty as that sounds.

Herb-Garlic Whole Wheat Croutons

THE GOODS

1 tablespoon unsalted butter
3 to 4 garlic cloves, minced
1 small whole wheat baguette, cut into bite-size cubes
2 teaspoons to 1 tablespoon extra-virgin olive oil
About 2 tablespoons minced fresh rosemary or thyme, or a
mixture

THE BREAKDOWN
1. Preheat the oven to 375°F.
2. Melt the butter in a large skillet over medium heat. Add the garlic and cook for about 30 seconds. Add the bread, drizzle in the olive oil, and sprinkle in the fresh herbs. Stir the bread until well-coated. Turn off the heat and transfer the croutons to a baking sheet.
3. Place the croutons in the oven and bake for about 10 minutes, until golden brown and crisp. Remove from the oven and cool.

The Facts: 60 calories; 2g fat; 1g saturated fat; 2g protein; 1g fiber

Watermelon-Feta Salad with Mint and Arugula

This is one of my go-to summertime salads when watermelon is in season and dripping with sweetness. This salad is perfect for a refreshing starter.

Makes 2 servings

THE GOODS
1 ½ cups seedless watermelon chunks
¼ cup chopped kalamata or Greek black olives
¼ cup crumbled Greek, French, Bulgarian, or locally made feta cheese (Bulgarian and Greek are typically the most salty and sharp among feta varieties, while French is a bit smoother)
1 tablespoon shredded fresh mint
2 cups torn arugula

THE DRESSING
1 tablespoon extra-virgin olive oil
2 teaspoons balsamic vinegar
Salt and freshly ground black pepper

THE BREAKDOWN

1. Toss the salad ingredients except the arugula together in a medium bowl. Arrange the arugula leaves on plates, and top with watermelon-feta mixture.
2. For the dressing, in a small bowl, whisk together the olive oil, vinegar, and salt and pepper to taste. Drizzle the salad with the vinaigrette and toss.

The Facts: 180 calories; 13g fat; 3g saturated fat; 4g protein; 2g fiber

Mediterranean Chopped Salad with Avocado, Tomato, Feta, and Chickpeas with Toasted Whole Wheat Pita Chips

This is an excellent, easy salad for satisfying workweek lunches or a light dinner when you get home on the later side. The avocado packs in healthy fat, the chickpeas give you some protein and fiber to fill you up fast, and the feta gives you some tasty indulgence.

Makes 4 servings

THE GOODS

1 head green leaf or romaine lettuce, chopped
1 ripe avocado, chopped
2 vine-ripened tomatoes, chopped
1 medium-large cucumber, chopped
¾ cup crumbled feta cheese
½ small red onion, diced
1 ½ cups chickpeas

THE DRESSING

3 tablespoons extra-virgin olive oil
Juice of 1 lemon
Salt and freshly ground black pepper

THE BREAKDOWN
1. Toss all the salad ingredients together in a large bowl.
2. For the dressing, in a small bowl, whisk together the olive oil, lemon juice, and salt and pepper to taste.
3. Drizzle the salad with the dressing, toss, and serve.

The Facts: 330 calories; 23g fat; 5g saturated fat; 7g protein; 9g fiber

Spinach Salad with Grilled Salmon, Citrus, and Avocado

This salad gets in a major dose of healthy fats, vitamins, and antioxidants. It's great for cleaning things up and taking a breather after a heavy week of dinners out and/or travel. Call it the Cheater's way of detoxing.

Makes 2 servings

THE GOODS
2 4-ounce salmon fillets (ideally wild salmon rather than farmed)
4 cups baby spinach
1 cup orange or grapefruit segments or slices
½ avocado, sliced
1 tablespoon shredded fresh mint

THE DRESSING
1 tablespoon extra-virgin olive oil
1 tablespoon fresh orange or lemon juice
½ teaspoon minced garlic
Salt and freshly ground black pepper

THE BREAKDOWN
1. Heat a grill pan or skillet over medium-high heat and place the salmon skin side down. Cook for 3 to 5 minutes on each side, until the skin is crisp and the salmon is cooked through.
2. Toss the spinach, citrus, avocado, and mint together in a large bowl.

3. For the dressing, in a small bowl, whisk together the olive oil, lemon juice, garlic, and salt and pepper to taste. Drizzle the salad with the dressing, toss, and serve with the grilled salmon.

The Facts: 360 calories; 22g fat; 3g saturated fat; 25g protein; 7g fiber

Spinach or Mâche Salad with Strawberries, Goat Cheese, and Toasted Pine Nuts

Who would have thought to put strawberries into salad? It works, though, and is absolutely delicious. This salad is fancy enough for a chic dinner party but simple enough for a nice side salad on an average evening. Keep in mind that spinach is a great source of folic acid and vitamins A and K. When you're talking about lettuce and leafy greens, generally the darker the leaf, the more nutrients it has.

Makes 4 servings

THE GOODS
    1 bag baby spinach or 2 bunches mâche (fancy lettuce)
    2 cups sliced strawberries
    4 ounces goat cheese, crumbled or sliced into 8 thin rounds
    2 tablespoons toasted pine nuts

THE DRESSING
    1 teaspoon Dijon mustard
    2 tablespoons balsamic vinegar
    1 teaspoon minced fresh shallot or 1 small garlic clove, minced
    Salt and freshly ground pepper
    3 tablespoons extra-virgin olive oil

THE BREAKDOWN
    1. Arrange the spinach, strawberries, goat cheese, and pine nuts on serving plates.
    2. To make the dressing, in a small bowl, whisk the mustard with vinegar, shallots, and salt and pepper to taste. Slowly pour in

the olive oil while continuing to whisk until blended. Drizzle about 1 tablespoon dressing over each salad, toss, and serve.

The Facts: 160 calories; 14g fat; 1.5g saturated fat; 2g protein; 4g fiber

White Bean and Tuna Salad

This is a fantastic salad for an energizing, protein-packed lunch or a light dinner. I'll often finish it off with a sprinkling of Pecorino cheese, about one tablespoon per serving.

Makes 3 to 4 servings

THE GOODS
   1 15-ounce can cannellini beans, drained and rinsed
   1 can no-salt-added water-packed chunk light tuna (or 1 can
      Italian tuna in olive oil, drained)
   ¼ cup diced red onion
   4 plum tomatoes, diced, or 1 ¼ cups halved cherry tomatoes

THE DRESSING
   2 tablespoons extra-virgin olive oil
   1 tablespoon red wine vinegar
   Salt and freshly ground black pepper

THE BREAKDOWN
   1. Toss the salad ingredients together in a large bowl.
   2. For the dressing, in a small bowl, whisk together the olive
      oil, vinegar, and salt and pepper to taste. Drizzle the salad
      with the dressing, toss, and serve.

The Facts: 210 calories; 8g fat; 1g saturated fat; 17g protein; 5g fiber

VARIATION: *I prefer the taste of tuna packed in olive oil. You can skip the olive oil in the dressing and just drizzle balsamic vinegar for a deliciously light salad.

Black Bean Salad with Fresh Corn, Tomato, and Roasted Poblano-Jalapeño Vinaigrette

This salad brings together Southwestern flavors and is a filling side dish or entrée salad for all you spice and heat lovers. Remember, the black beans are slow-burning carbs and are excellent for extended energy.

Makes 2 servings

THE GOODS
  1 ½ cups cooked black beans
  ½ avocado, diced
  Kernels from 1 ear cooked corn
  2 vine-ripened or heirloom tomatoes, diced
  1 yellow or orange bell pepper, cored, seeded, and diced
  ½ roasted poblano pepper, cored, seeded, and diced
  2 tablespoons dried cherries
  ¼ cup finely crumbled cotija cheese (a Mexican cheese found
    in some grocery stores; you can substitute Monterey Jack
    cheese if it's not available)

THE DRESSING
  2 teaspoons white or red wine vinegar
  ½ roasted poblano pepper (see Note)
  ¼ roasted jalapeño pepper (see Note)
  1 teaspoon garlic clove, minced
  2 tablespoons cilantro, chopped
  Juice from ¼ lime
  ¼ teaspoon salt
  1 ½ tablespoons extra- virgin olive oil

THE BREAKDOWN
  1. Mix all the salad ingredients in a large bowl.
  2. Place all the dressing ingredients except the olive oil in a
     blender. Blend while slowly pouring in the oil through the
     hole in the top.
  3. Lightly spoon the vinaigrette over the salad, toss, and serve.

Note: Roast both peppers over an open flame—use one of your stove's burners and just place directly on burner until the skin blackens and bubbles all over, turning the pepper with tongs to blacken all sides. Place them in a brown paper bag or a covered bowl and allow to steam for 3 to 4 minutes. Rub the skin off each pepper with a paper towel, slice lengthwise, and discard the seeds.

The Facts: 400 calories; 23g fat; 6g saturated fat; 13g protein; 16g fiber

Shaved Brussels Sprout Salad with Pecorino, Walnuts, and Lemon Vinaigrette

Pure deliciousness. And as a nutritional bonus, Brussels sprouts are loaded with disease-fighting antioxidants and a ton of fiber. They are a cruciferous veggie, though, and can be gas-inducing, so don't overdose.

Makes 4 to 6 servings

THE GOODS
> 12 to 16 Brussels sprouts, outer leaves removed if necessary
> ¼ cup chopped toasted walnuts
> ¼ cup shaved Pecorino Romano cheese

THE DRESSING
> Juice of 1 lemon
> 2 tablespoons extra-virgin olive oil
> ½ to 1 teaspoon minced garlic
> Salt and freshly ground pepper

THE BREAKDOWN
1. Using a mandolin slicer on the thinnest setting, shave the Brussels sprouts over a medium bowl—shave down to the stem and then discard the stems. Watch your fingers on the slicer! Place them in a large bowl and toss in the walnuts and Pecorino.
2. Whisk together the lemon juice, olive oil, garlic, and salt and pepper to taste in a small bowl. Drizzle over the salad, toss well, and serve.

The Facts: 120 calories; 9g fat; 2g saturated fat; 4g protein; 2g fiber

All Dressed Up . . .

I can't say enough about homemade salad dressings. Your outlook on salads will change forever if you trade in bottled, bland, gooey, gloppy dressings for those you can make in your own kitchen in just five minutes or less. Ever take a look at the ingredient list on most store-bought salad dressings? It can be pretty frightening . . . and far too complicated. The most straightforward salad dressing really only has two, three, four, maybe five ingredients—not twenty. Bottled brands are often loaded with hidden sugar and preservatives, particularly your "diet-friendly" non-fat dressings (insert sarcasm). If it must be bottled, look for those with good-quality ingredients, the fewer the better (like Newman's Own and Annie's Naturals). When you do have the time, try making your own—it's incredible what fresh ingredients can do. Make a dressing and you'll have it around for at least a week to drizzle over salads or use as a quick marinade for grilled or baked chicken, fish, or vegetables. Aim for 1 to 2 tablespoons of dressing per salad or per meal.

> *Cheater's Secret:* Try out a different heart-healthy oil if you wish to get creative with dressings or marinades. Oils like walnut or avocado can add a whole new flavor component and also help reduce cholesterol levels.

Balsamic Vinaigrette

Makes 4 servings

THE GOODS
1 teaspoon Dijon mustard
2 tablespoons balsamic vinegar
4 tablespoons extra-virgin olive oil
1 to 2 teaspoons minced fresh shallot or garlic
Salt and freshly ground pepper

THE BREAKDOWN

In a small bowl, whisk the mustard with the vinegar, shallot, if using, and salt and pepper to taste. Slowly pour in the olive oil while continuing to whisk until blended.

VARIATION: *Swap the balsamic for red wine or sherry vinegar for a basic red wine vinaigrette.

The Facts: 130 calories; 14g fat; 2g saturated fat; 0g protein; 0g fiber

Simple Lemon–Olive Oil Vinaigrette

Makes 4 servings

THE GOODS

2 tablespoons fresh lemon juice (for a less lemony flavor, drop down to 1 tablespoon)
1 teaspoon fresh herbs, such as mint, chives, or basil (optional)
Salt and freshly ground pepper
3 tablespoons extra-virgin olive oil

THE BREAKDOWN

In a small bowl, whisk together the lemon juice, herbs (if using), and salt and pepper to taste until well blended. Slowly pour in the olive oil while continuing to whisk until blended.

The Facts: 120 calories; 14g fat; 2g saturated fat; 0g protein; 0g fiber

Champagne-Dijon Vinaigrette

Makes 4 servings

THE GOODS

1 teaspoon Dijon mustard
1 ½ tablespoons champagne vinegar
1 teaspoon minced shallot

Salt and freshly ground pepper
4 tablespoons extra-virgin olive oil

THE BREAKDOWN

In a small bowl, whisk together the mustard, vinegar, shallot, and salt and pepper to taste until well blended. Slowly pour in the olive oil while continuing to whisk until blended.

The Facts: 130 calories; 14g fat; 2g saturated fat; 0g protein; 0g fiber

Cheater's Caesar Dressing

Makes 4 to 6 servings

THE GOODS

¼ cup plus 2 tablespoons extra-virgin olive oil
¼ cup freshly grated Parmesan or Pecorino Romano cheese
2 tablespoons fresh lemon juice (the juice of about 1 lemon)
1 garlic clove
½ teaspoon Worcestershire sauce
Salt and freshly ground pepper to taste

THE BREAKDOWN

Combine all the ingredients in a blender or food processor and blend until smooth.

The Facts: 180 calories; 19g fat; 3.5g saturated fat; 2g protein; 0g fiber

VARIATION: *Toss crisp romaine or green leaf lettuce with this dressing and top with sliced grilled chicken breast, steak, or shrimp and an extra sprinkling of Pecorino for a quick, easy, healthfully indulgent meal.

Spiced-Up Red Wine Vinaigrette

This dressing was inspired by one of my favorite hole-in-the-wall Brazilian restaurants in New York's West Village. Try tossing together red or

green leaf lettuce or Boston lettuce, fresh tomatoes, red onion, and hearts of palm and drizzle the dressing over. Beware, it's a little addictive.

Makes 4 servings

THE GOODS
  2 tablespoons red wine vinegar
  1 tablespoon fresh lemon juice
  1 tablespoon minced scallion
  1 tablespoon minced red onion
  2 tablespoons diced tomato
  Salt and freshly ground pepper
  ¼ cup extra-virgin olive oil

THE BREAKDOWN
  In a small bowl, whisk together the vinegar, lemon juice, scallion, onion, tomato, and salt and pepper to taste until well blended. Slowly pour in the olive oil while continuing to whisk until blended.

Ts: 120 calories; 14g fat; 2g saturated fat; 0g protein; 0g fiber

Asian Vinaigrette

Makes 4 servings

THE GOODS
  1 ½ tablespoons cider vinegar
  2 teaspoons low-sodium soy sauce
  1 ½ teaspoons organic sugar or agave nectar
  1 scallion, chopped
  3 tablespoons canola oil

THE BREAKDOWN
  In a small bowl, whisk together the vinegar, soy sauce, sugar, and scallion until well blended. Slowly pour in the canola oil while continuing to whisk until blended.

The Facts: 100 calories; 11g fat; 1g saturated fat; 0g protein; 0g fiber

VARIATION: *For a quick entrée salad that's perfect for lunch or dinner, toss 1 cup shredded red, green, and/or Napa cabbage with 3 to 4 ounces grilled chicken, tofu, shrimp, or steak, ½ cup red bell pepper strips, ½ cup shredded carrots, and 1 tablespoon toasted sliced almonds. Toss with the vinaigrette and serve over 2 cups romaine lettuce or mixed greens.

VARIATION: *For a slightly different flavor twist to this dressing, add ¼ teaspoon minced garlic, 1 teaspoon minced ginger, 2 teaspoons toasted sesame oil, and 2 tablespoons all-natural peanut butter.

Refresher Course—Key Goals from Weeks I and 2

- ❏ Resize portions—3 to 5 ounces protein, ½ to 1 cup rice/pasta/ grain, 1 cup/piece fruit, 1 to 3 cups veggies/salad (aim to cut total portions by 15 to 25 percent and set your plate up as: ½ fruits/vegetables, ¼ lean protein, ¼ healthy, complex carbs).
- ❏ Eat 2 servings of fruit per day; aim to have vegetables with lunch AND dinner.
- ❏ Drink 1 ½ to 2 liters of water per day.
- ❏ Don't skip meals—you'll lower your calorie-burn capability!
- ❏ Cheat it up each week with one or two indulgent meals (order what you wish, but still consider portions) and one or two treats (between 200 and 300 calories each).
- ❏ Exercise one or two days more than you currently are or increase intensity.
- ❏ Cut your alcohol intake per week by at least 25 percent.
- ❏ Food journaling . . . DO IT!
- ❏ Cut artificial sweeteners in half—aim for 1 to 2 packets per day (or less!) and keep weaning down.
- ❏ Bring 3 to 5 basic office staples to work for snacks and emergencies.
- ❏ Be prepared when traveling and pack a meal or snack.
- ❏ Be sure to have an energizing snack before a workout and a balanced meal or satisfying snack afterward.
- ❏ Take a chance with a new recipe and experiment in the kitchen. Cook at home at least once.

Restaurant Road Maps and Holding Out for the Best

"When it comes to bagels, muffins, and the bread basket, I'm just a hot mess."

—Danielle

WEEK 3 GOALS

- Re-plate and re-portion takeout food (take it out of the to-go container and aim for half to three quarters off the entrée portion).
- Map out your restaurant meals for the week and note where to plug in your cheat meals.
- At restaurants, try to leave at least 5 bites, or a quarter to half, behind on your plate. Portions still count when you're out!
- Work in a new type of whole grain, such as quinoa or whole wheat couscous, or a new healthy fat, such as walnuts, into the picture this week and each week going forward. Variety is a good thing.
- Keep fluffy, refined breads like focaccia and bagels to a minimum, once or twice a week max (they won't fill you up and only leave you looking for more). If the restaurant bread basket isn't top-top notch, SKIP IT!

The Plan

With the first two weeks out of the way, you should be feeling pretty great. You're *down* four to eight pounds (remember, everyone takes weight off at different rates—give it time and it'll keep coming) and you're comfortable and confident in the goals you've hit and are sticking to thus far. You can feel a difference in how your clothes are fitting, in your energy levels and sleep patterns, and you're loving getting to know your kitchen a little more personally. There's a growing sense of freedom in "cheating" and eating sanely and smartly rather than the desperate dieting many of us are so accustomed to. Now let's translate that freedom to restaurant eating and dining out. Get excited—there's a world of incredible food waiting for you.

A Look at the Week Ahead:

Re-portion Takeout and Delivery Food
Eating off of an actual plate rather than out of the takeout container allows you to better visualize and assess appropriate portions. You should be comfortably satisfied by half to three quarters of your meal. It's quite economical if you think about it—you'll have leftovers for lunch the next day!

Plan Ahead for Restaurants
Think about your week ahead and write restaurant meals into your week's calendar/food journal. By thinking a bit ahead, you're that much better prepared to plan where treat meals come in and which other meals you'll want to keep cleaner and more consistent with the rest of the week.

Mind Your Portions
Consider portion size when you're eating out. Leave at least 5 bites of your meal on the plate. If the portion is beyond gigantic (two or three times what you know it should be), leave a quarter to half behind. Or better yet, think about splitting an entrée.

Incorporate One New Healthy Fat or Whole Grain
Try a new fat or whole grain in your rotation this week and each week going forward. Take note—you might find that it helps complete the meal and satisfy you that much better, and prevents you from nibbling on extraneous items afterward. You'll end up saving on calories in the long run, trust me.

Week 3: Sample—Eating Out with Ease

based on 1400-1600 calories

Week 3:	Monday	Tuesday	Wednesday
BREAKFAST 300-400 calories 7-9:30 a.m.	Start the week off on a good note—you've got a heavy social slate in the days ahead HIT THE GYM in the a.m. Banana pre-workout Protein-packed satisfying breakfast: 1 egg, 1 slice whole grain toast, piece of fresh fruit	Power breakfast for a long day ahead: 1 slice whole grain toast with 1 tablespoon peanut butter and banana slices 8-ounce glass of skim or soy milk (optional)	Girls night out—HIT THE GYM in the a.m. ½ banana pre-workout At work: 1 cup cooked/ 1 packet oatmeal with 1 tablespoon raisins, 1 tablespoon chopped walnuts, cinnamon, and 1 teaspoon brown sugar
SNACK about 100 calories 10-11 a.m.	Skim latte	Cup of grapes or piece of fruit	Skip it—that oatmeal was filling
LUNCH 400-550 calories 12-2 p.m.	Local sandwich spot: ½ grilled chicken sandwich on hearty whole wheat with avocado, sprouts, tomato, and 1 to 2 teaspoons herbed mayo (scrape some off if there's a lot) Cup of fresh fruit salad	Fancy biz lunch out: Baby greens with beets and goat cheese Grilled branzino (a Mediterranean fish) or tuna ½ small whole grain roll Sparkling water with lemon or iced tea	Make-your-own salad You know the drill: 1. mixed greens, spinach, or arugula 2. some type of protein 3. whatever veggies or fruits you wish to add 4. a sprinkle of 1 or 2 of the following: cheese, dried fruit, nuts, olives, and/or avocado 5. 1 to 2 tablespoons vinaigrette or olive oil and lemon
SNACK 100-200 calories 3-5 p.m.	0% or 2% Greek yogurt and a square of dark chocolate	granola bar or fruit-nut bar	Small plum 25 to 30 pistachios in the shell (great for when you're bored at work and are looking for something to pass the time!)
DINNER 400-600 calories 7-8:30 p.m.	Meal out with relatives in town. It's early in the week and you've got three other dinners and a few lunches out—choose 2 appetizers and call it a night. Butternut squash soup Mussels in white wine broth	Prepare for meals out the rest of the week; have a light meal at home. 4 ounces Poached Salmon with Cucumber-Chive Sauce (page 164) 1 ½ cups sautéed spinach with garlic or Sautéed Kale with Raisins and Pine Nuts (page 50)	CHEAT MEAL #1: Great Italian place with to-die-for homemade pasta Olives for the table Tri-colore salad or insalata mista Share tagliatelle pasta with lamb ragù or pumpkin ravioli
SNACK 100-150 calories (If you're not hungry, SKIP IT! Work in desserts and treats when you really want them and they're damn worth it!)	Skip it	1 to 1 ½ cups fresh berries with 2 tablespoons whipped cream	CHEAT TREAT #1: Share tiramisu or vanilla gelato with coffee (affogato) for dessert
WATER	1 ½ liters	2 liters plus sparkling water	2 liters
ALCOHOL/ OOPS!	Skip the wine at dinner; it's Monday and you've got the whole week ahead of you!		2 glasses of wine
EXERCISE	60 minutes		Some sort of group class: body conditioning, yoga, spinning, etc.

Thursday	Friday	Saturday	Sunday
Had a heavier dinner last night; go for a light breakfast to kick-start your day: 6 ounces low-fat plain yogurt with fresh fruit and 2 table-spoons granola (like Bear Naked or Feed; look for 10 grams sugar or less per serving)	Quick and simple breakfast at home: 1 cup whole grain cereal, banana and/or berries and milk	Sleep late and head to brunch!	60 to 90 minutes of tennis, a bike ride, or physical activity of your choice 1 cup whole grain cereal, banana and/or berries, and milk before exercise
10 to 12 nuts (remember the ones stashed in your desk drawer)	1 ounce cheese, like a string cheese, Bonne Bell/Laughing Cow, or the real stuff		Skip it—you're off biking or slamming tennis balls
Out with coworkers for pizza: Arugula salad with shaved Parmesan to start 1 slice thin-crust pizza piled high with veggies of your choice	Two restaurant dinners down for the week and you've got two more ahead—opt for a light lunch to keep things in check! 1 ½ cups White Bean and Tuna Salad (page 124) with 2 cups mixed greens, romaine, or arugula	Brunch out: Eggs Benedict with Hollandaise on the side plus a side of mixed greens Snag 5 bites of home fries from your friend's plate	Lunch out : Cobb salad with ¼ to ½ of the avocado, bacon, and blue cheese scooted to the side of your plate. There's a lot going on in Cobbs, but they're so darn tasty! Ask for a vinaigrette on the side, aim for 2 tablespoons
½ packet of trail mix from the vending machine	2 to 3 whole grain crackers with hummus or peanut butter ½ apple Get in a quick workout after work before you head out for dinner	Small cappuccino (yes, with whole milk once in a while!) topped with cocoa powder Piece of fresh fruit Do a quick GROCERY run while you have time	15 whole grain tortilla chips with 3 tablespoons guacamole at home
Simple meal at home 2 cups Mom's Minestrone Soup (page 168)	Another night out . . . Mexican, brace yourself Skip the chips and salsa if you can't stop, otherwise aim for 10 to 12 and be done 2 grilled chicken or steak soft tacos or fajitas with green peppers and onions, and 1 tablespoon sour cream ½ cup mixture of black beans and rice	CHEAT MEAL #2: Dinner out with friends 1 small piece rosemary bread with 1 teaspoon butter (well worth it because it's really awesome bread!) Baby greens salad to start Scallops for entrée Share incredible truffle mac 'n cheese three ways	Recipe test-drive: 1 ½ cups Thai Shrimp Curry with Pineapple and Red Bell Pepper (page 161) ½ to ¾ cup white or brown jasmine rice
Movie/TV night at home: 4 cups all-natural popcorn			CHEAT TREAT #2: Go out for 1 scoop of ice cream at the best place in town
2 liters	2 liters	1 ½ liters	1 ½ liters
	1 margarita on the rocks, 1 Corona Light at dinner	2 glasses of wine at dinner	
	60 minutes		60-90 minutes tennis, biking, jogging, etc.

With Bread, Hold Out for the Best
Associate the breadbasket at restaurants with the theme of this chapter: "Hold out for the best." If it's not the greatest bread you've ever seen or tasted, drop it. Cheat when it's really worth it, and keep refined breads to a bare minimum, once or twice a week.

Week 3—Cheater's Shopping List:

- ❑ Vegetables: 3 to 5 (or more) for the week: kale, 2 red bell peppers, 3 tomatoes, carrots, celery, 2 onions, 1 zucchini, 1 red onion, 1 cucumber, 1 can bamboo shoots
- ❑ Fruit: 2 to 4 types or more, your pick (enough to get you through 5 to 7 days, 2 servings a day): apples, berries, bananas, plums
- ❑ Protein: eggs, 1 pound shrimp, 4 ounces salmon fillet
- ❑ Healthy carbs: 2 baby red potatoes, jasmine rice, whole wheat macaroni pasta, whole grain cereal (more than 5 grams fiber, less than 7 grams sugar), whole grain bread, plain oatmeal (single-serve packets or Irish steel cut), granola (look for less than 10 grams sugar per serving)
- ❑ Dairy/calcium: Parmesan or Pecorino Romano cheese, Laughing Cow/cheddar/or snacking cheese of your choice, 3 to 4 low-fat plain yogurts or cottage cheese, skim or soy milk
- ❑ Other: 1 28-ounce can of whole plum tomatoes, 1 can kidney beans, 2 cans cannellini beans, 1 can pineapple chunks (or 1 ½ cups fresh chunks)
- ❑ Fresh herbs and spices: chives, garlic, ginger, cilantro, bay leaves
- ❑ Seasonings and oils: peanut oil, Asian fish sauce, low-sodium chicken or veggie broth, light coconut milk, red curry paste, 1 lime
- ❑ Snack stuff and staples: hummus, guacamole, all-natural peanut or almond butter, whole grain crackers (like Wasa or Finn Crisp, more than 3 grams fiber per serving), whole grain tortilla chips, all-natural granola bars (more than 3 grams fiber), all-natural popcorn, roasted nuts/pistachios
- ❑ Dessert/treat: dark chocolate, whipped cream

See page 138 for "Week 3: Your Weekly Food Journal."

Eating Out with Confidence

Trying out new restaurants ranks high on the list of my favorite pastimes. To my bank account's dismay, I dine out with relative frequency, a couple of times a week typically. Living in New York City is like being a kid in a candy store in terms of incredible restaurant options. I admit I'm a self-professed "foodie-nutritionist" who hunts down newly opened restaurants, hidden neighborhood gems, and the best authentic ethnic places around, like it's my job—actually it kind of is my job. So I hope by now it's clear that I'm not one of those nutritionists who only flocks to health-foody restaurants or organic, vegan, raw joints, although there are some really extraordinary, groundbreaking ones all over the country. And you won't find me, save the last-ditch emergency pit stop on a road trip, frequenting most fast-food places or chain restaurants or high-end five-star restaurants (though that's always nice once in a while). I fall somewhere in the middle—finding the thrill, wonder, and pleasure of good-quality, fresh, seasonal, inventive, and classic food and a warm, inviting environment. If I'm so frequently hunting, tasting, and sipping, how do I manage to keep healthful, tasty eating habits on the straight and narrow? Simple. Like with everything else in this book, it's all about cheating the system and making it work for you.

Let's put things in perspective: If you're someone who fears eating out because you're not sure what to order off the menu, or you're someone who subsists on baby carrots and yogurt all week only to then say "screw the diet" and go buck wild at restaurants, no worries. We're on to a completely new mind-set here. Eating out doesn't have to cause anxiety attacks any longer.

Restaurant Road Map—Final Destination: "Delicious Meal and Perfectly, Pleasantly Full"

Point by point, I've mapped out the tricks of the trade when eating out so you don't have to feel automatically relegated to the salad section or the bone-dry chicken entrée.

Week 3:	Monday	Tuesday	Wednesday
BREAKFAST 300-400 calories *(Note your hunger level on a scale of 1 to 10 after each meal)*			
SNACK About 100 calories *(If you're not hungry, skip it!)*			
LUNCH 400-550 calories			
SNACK 100-200 calories			
DINNER 400-600 calories			
SNACK 100-150 calories *(Work in desserts and treats when you really want them and they're damn worth it!)*			
WATER			
ALCOHOL/ OOPS!			
EXERCISE			

Thursday	Friday	Saturday	Sunday

- **Do your homework . . . ahead of time.** Scope out restaurant menus ahead of time, as it can be incredibly helpful and ease the decision-making process. In social situations, you never want to feel ambushed by options, or lack thereof, on the menu. Sites like menupages.com, healthydiningfinder.com, urbanspoon.com, or the restaurant's own Web site provide you with an insider's peek at the menu. That said, sometimes the element of surprise when dining is equally wonderful. Eventually, I want you to be able to walk right off the street into any restaurant and feel completely comfortable and excited to navigate the menu and make smart, mouthwatering choices. You'll be cheating like a pro in no time.

If you do happen to take a gander at the Web sites of some of your favorite dining establishments, you might be in for shear shock—like you've just finished watching a bad eighties horror flick. Many national chains now have the nutrition information listed directly on their Web sites. Who knew there could be so many calories and more than a day's worth of fat in a stinking chicken salad or that a veggie burger could somehow rack up over 1000 calories!? A tomato bruschetta appetizer with 990 calories? It's just tomato and bread!

No joke—welcome to the land of excess and hidden calories and fat. Surely not every restaurant hits quadruple digits in each of its menu offerings, but sometimes it's easy to get tripped up when you think you're making a healthful decision. Like when you think you're being good and ordering "just the salad." Fried chicken tenders, three servings of cheddar cheese and bacon, and a river of ranch dressing later, you've dug yourself in deep, and for half the calories you probably could have had the petite filet you'd been eyeing . . . along with some broccoli, half a baked potato with a smidge of sour cream, and a few of your boyfriend's fries.

Bottom line: Be mindful when you hit up a chain restaurant like Ruby Tuesday, Macaroni Grill, Chili's, Applebee's, Outback Steakhouse, and Cheesecake Factory, just to name a few. Thankfully, many of these restaurants have started offering half-portions, healthier options under 500 or 600 calories, and list calorie and fat information right on the menu. But regular portions tend to be mammoth, loaded with saturated fat and sodium, large enough to feed a small country. A huge plate of food sitting right in front of you doesn't make it any easier, of course, but hopefully it alerts you to what's *not* an appropriate portion size.

You've got the tools now, so use them to your advantage. You know that if a steak is 8 or 12 ounces, you're aiming for about half of it, same thing with an 8-ounce burger; ask for half and add a little cheese. Get some fresh veggies or a side salad in there somehow and we're starting to get somewhere. There are always cheatable options on the menu—you're not stranded at sea with a measly "diet-friendly" cottage cheese and fruit plate. See, not all hope is lost.

CHEAT SHEET: Restaurant Redo

Ruby Tuesday—Bacon cheeseburger: 1226 calories, 85 grams fat
Redo: Top sirloin with steamed broccoli and mashed potatoes: 539 calories, 28 grams fat
Romano's Macaroni Grill—Parmesan crusted sole: 2190 calories, 141 grams fat | Fettuccini Alfredo: 1220 calories, 93 grams fat
Redo: Caprese mozzarella, tomato, and basil starter plus "skinny" roasted chicken: 570 calories, 26 grams fat, | ½ piece lasagna with side of steamed broccoli plus Italian sorbet and biscotti: 820 calories, 31 grams fat
Chipotle—Chicken burrito with guacamole, sour cream, cheese, and rice: 980 calories, 50 grams fat
Redo: Chicken salad bowl with guacamole, black beans, and salsa: 490 calories, 21 grams fat
Uno Chicago Grill—Individual Chicago Classic Pizza: 2310 calories, 165 grams fat
Redo: ½ BBQ chicken flatbread pizza: 480 calories, 16.5 grams fat
Denny's—French Toast Slam: 940 calories, 53 grams fat
Redo: 1 egg, 2 strips bacon, and hash browns: 410 calories, 28.5 grams fat (à la carte menu) or veggie-cheese omelet with Egg Beaters: 410 calories, 22 grams fat

- **Breaking Bread**. Ah, the beloved breadbasket. For years you've had the mantra of "don't dare touch that evil bread basket" drilled into your head. That's a bit extreme, in my opinion. Can bread tack on a few extra calories and simple carbs to your meal? Yes. Is it the epitome of evil at the dinner table? No.

The French eat bread, cheese, and wine nearly daily ... yet somehow they've magically managed to stay much slimmer and much healthier than their U.S. counterparts. It isn't magic, it's called quality and quantity of what you're nibbling on. The French have a right to be a bit snooty, as they've mastered the fine art of eating the "best of the best," and so should you. Eating the best means you end up eating less because you're actually satisfied, something I often refer to as the satisfaction factor. So let's deconstruct that concept with bread: If the bread is literally the most incredible, amazing, orgasmic-looking loaf of "baked heaven" you've ever seen in your life, HAVE A SMALL PIECE, and if you're really looking to get naughty, dip that sucker in a touch of heart-healthy olive oil or smear on a tiny dab, 1 to 2 teaspoons, of butter (notice the emphasis on small amounts here). Again, if the bread's a pretty sizable piece, equivalent to the thickness of two or three standard slices, break some off—you've still got your entire meal ahead of you. If, however, the bread looks like any other stale, tasteless loaf you wouldn't even use to make croutons, SKIP IT! If it isn't worth it, why bother? I'd personally much rather have a second glass of vino or a few bites of dessert, wouldn't you? If you cheat and play smart, you'll always come out ahead in the end.

Cheater's Secret: Disclaimer—Know your weaknesses and don't be afraid to address them. If bread is one of them, remove the breadbasket from eye line or get it off the table. If you are a bread-obsessed junkie (you know who you are) and it's virtually impossible for you to take just one piece of bread from the basket without scarfing down three more slices, don't even start with a single bite. I'm not preaching willpower, I'm just saving you from torturing yourself and not having room for your actual meal. Walking away from the table feeling puffed up and bloated off too much bread like the Pillsbury Dough Boy is not fun. Focus on your dining companions, spark conversation, take a sip or two of wine, and order a light appetizer like a noncreamy soup, fresh oysters, olives to share, or a salad ASAP.

- **Pick Two.** Structure can be a godsend sometimes. As I mentioned in Chapter 1, if you're a social butterfly who eats out most days of the week, aim to choose two meals per week (brunch, lunch, or dinner) that are deemed your *cheat and eat* freebie meals. These are meals where you can ease up, have the filet mignon or osso bucco if you've been dying for red meat, share a pasta dish or mac 'n cheese when it's really worth it, indulge in your favorite omelet AND the hash browns or bacon. The trick with *cheat and eat* meals is this: As with any other meal, you're still being cognizant of portion sizes by eating only half or three quarters of what's on your giant-size plate or you're sharing an indulgent dish with a friend or someone dining with you. You're also eating more slowly so that you're aware of your satiety level and can put down the fork when you're full. But, and this is a big but, you're employing the Cheater's mentality at the exact same time by feeling completely confident and excited about ordering something that would have been "off-limits" in diets past. Relish the foods and dishes that catch your eye and sound extraordinarily fabulous on the menu. No regrets and no guilty conscience—you're ordering it without a second thought. Setting your sights on two meals like this per week will allow you to keep shedding those pounds, maintain a healthy balance consistently, and really look forward to dining out and exploring new dishes and cuisines.

On other days of the week that require restaurant eating, keep your head in the game and try ordering something similar to what you might make at home (or would like to make), such as the grilled salmon or baked halibut; the roasted chicken with vegetables; the simple filet, baked potato, and asparagus; a turkey burger (half if it's an 8-ouncer) with a side salad instead of fries; the homemade lentil soup and spinach salad with roasted beets, walnuts, and goat cheese; or splitting mixed greens and the whole wheat penne with grilled shrimp and arrabiata (spicy tomato) sauce just to name a few. This evokes the idea of dishes that are a little lighter, simpler, but certainly equally delectable. If you wouldn't think to make it at home (or attempt to), there's a chance it's too heavy, too fried, too calorie-dense, or too high in fat. Just like you would at home, focus your meal on balance and color (i.e., fruits and vegetables), whether this means swapping fries for a side salad to go with your cheeseburger or tacking on some fruit salad to your brunch order. Lucky you, oftentimes it's the most straightforward salad, roasted fish, or braised chicken dish that is the standout signature item on the menu.

- **Bon Appetizer: Eat Two Instead of Ordering an Entrée.** Whoever invented appetizers and hors d'oeuvres was a culinary mastermind. Talk about cheating at its finest. I find again and again, appetizers make up some of the most innovative, thrilling, mouthwatering tidbits on a restaurant's menu. And unlike most entrées, appetizers nowadays are generally perfectly portioned. Again, pick two and you've got a great, complete meal that's within your calorie target but doesn't skimp on flavor. Two appetizers or soup and a salad is a great call for a light weeknight meal out, particularly if you've got five other meals out lined up throughout the week. A few quick examples of appetizer-cum-dinners straight off the menus of some of my favorite NYC restaurants:

  ◆ Asparagus with Parmesan cheese, truffle salt, and soft-boiled egg with Prince Edward Island mussels or tuna tartare
  ◆ Roasted butternut squash soup and roasted beet salad with feta cheese and poached pear

- ◆ Thai chile–seared shrimp with mini tortillas and mango salsa with mesclun greens tossed in balsamic vinaigrette
- ◆ Prosciutto di Parma with fresh fruit and classic minestrone soup with pesto
- ◆ Red snapper ceviche with avocado, orange, and heart of palm salad
- ◆ Seared lamb skewer with sugar snap peas, apple, bacon, and blue cheese

- **Portion Distortion: Make Portions More Manageable.** The vast majority of restaurant portions are two to four times larger than what a normal serving should be, and they've been steadily increasing since the 1970s. The portions in many large-scale chain restaurants or family-style places are large enough to feed a small country. Just a little scary. Unfortunately, no one's making things easier on you. It takes some serious mindfulness at mealtimes to think about what's on your plate and how much you should aim to consume. But it most definitely can be done. And it can be done without completely embarrassing yourself, requesting that the waitress immediately wrap up half of your plate before she even sets it down on the table—slightly socially awkward.

Let's be honest, you're not going to listen to me tell you to "leave half of your plate behind." Yeah, right. But you might make a habit stick if you aim to leave just five bites behind on your plate, or 15 to 25 percent of your meal. That's pretty darn reasonable. If you're one who likes to pick and will just keep nibbling off your plate, make a signal to yourself that the meal's completed—excuse yourself to use the restroom, finish the last few sips of your wine or beverage, focus on conversation. It sounds a little kooky, or maybe slightly neurotic to some, but it is effective. Figure out what your automatic "stop sign" at meals is and . . . surprise, stop! The only thing I wouldn't suggest is putting your napkin down on your plate. I just find it a bit rude if others are still eating, and I hate to see gleaming white cloth napkins get all dirty and sauced up.

You can manage portions that much better by allowing your food to settle and giving your stomach time to speak to your brain signaling that you're full. This typically takes about fifteen to twenty minutes and hinges around the *muy importante* concept of eating SLOWLY. I've mentioned this before, and nutritionists harp on it all the time, but it's really true and makes an incredible difference in how much you eat and how fast you become satiated. (A quick note for all you science nerds—two little hormones called leptin and ghrelin work in tandem to regulate hunger and satiety cues.) Eating quickly at lightning speed can also impact digestion, bloating, and gas. Don't "dump truck" your food, and you'll feel so much better getting up from the table.

- **Selfishly Chic: Help Steer Group Orders in Your Direction.** Let's talk for a moment about eating out in group settings and sharing. You thought you left peer pressure behind in high school, but clearly you were incorrect. Every time you go out with a particular group of friends or some pushy coworkers, they inevitably want to order a number of "interesting" (aka unappealing) dishes for the table or they scoff at you and obnoxiously comment when you order something that isn't deep-fried or dripping with butter. First off, maybe they have latent food issues they've yet to dig up and they're just pissed off because they know they, too, should be ordering something lighter, who knows. Let it go. Second, who cares what others think? If you want to order a certain way off the menu, it's your prerogative. No one's force-feeding you chili nachos, jalapeño poppers, and fried cheese sticks. Sometimes it's okay to be selfish in social situations. Order what you wish, what you feel comfortable with and excited by. Your friends can still share stuff, you're not preventing that. On the flip side, sharing dishes family-style can be really fun and provide for a diverse tasting of the menu. Keep things balanced with a few light dishes and some that are a bit heavier. Speak up and contribute a suggestion or two to the group order so you feel totally pumped about what's coming out of the kitchen. If it's just two or three of you, share one or two appetizers and one or two entrées. More tasting done on less food means perfect portions.

- **The Order.** We could easily come up with countless combinations of what to order at a given restaurant. Here's the Cliffs-Notes version with a few basic suggestions for each meal.

◆ **Breakfast/Brunch**
  —Eggs Benedict/Florentine—Get the hollandaise sauce on the side, and assess your satiety after 1 to 1 ½ eggs and English muffin halves. Pair it with fruit salad and/or mixed greens.
  —Homemade granola, yogurt, and fruit—Get the granola on the side so you can portion it yourself, about ¼ cup or a handful. Or for a heartier brunch meal, go with ½ cup.
  —Omelet—Go ahead and order a regular, whole-egg omelet—you'll fill up much faster and likely eat less (those yolks are really satisfying!). Egg whites are okay, too, if you prefer them. Pile on the veggies and ask for them to go light on the cheese if you get it. If you receive an omelet that's oozing with cheese, push some aside—no one's forcing you to eat all of it! Aim for half or three quarters of the omelet if it's enormous, and pair it with one slice of whole wheat, multigrain, rye, or sourdough toast, mixed greens and/or fruit salad. Add one to two pieces of turkey bacon on occasion if you're a fan. Dying for hash browns or fries? Ask nicely and snag a few bites off a dining companion's plate.
  —Pancakes, French toast, waffles—If you're going to indulge, do it smartly. Go for one well-size pancake, a piece of French toast, OR a waffle instead of two or three, and a drizzle of maple syrup, about 1 to 2 tablespoons.

Cheater's Secret: Ask for a side of yogurt and fruit with pancakes or waffles so you actually have something that will fill you up (the protein in the yogurt and the fiber in the fruit). If you can get whole wheat, multigrain, or buckwheat pancakes or waffles, go for it!

◆ **Lunch**
   —½ sandwich on multigrain or whole wheat bread (at least 75 percent of the time) and soup or a side salad
   —A full sandwich or open-faced (ditch the top piece of bread) and add a side of fresh fruit or mixed greens
   —Soup and salad combo—Choose a broth- or bean-based soup, like lentil, minestrone, chicken and vegetable, black bean, roasted tomato, carrot-ginger . . . the list could go on. Watch out for bisques and creamy soups.
   —Entrée salad—Just make sure you've got some sort of protein going on to help fill you up and beware of behemoth-size entrée salads that could feed two or three people or more. Many restaurants will serve half sizes, which is a great call. If there are multiple calorie-heavy toppings (more than three), such as nuts, cheese, avocado, croutons, dried fruit, tortilla strips, remember that your goal is about 1 to 2 tablespoons of each, but usually there's double that amount. Some sample orders: Greek salad with grilled shrimp or chicken; steak salad; grilled salmon, chicken, or tofu salad; seared tuna or tuna Niçoise salad, Cobb salad (there's a lot going on here—watch the amounts of avocado, blue cheese, croutons, and bacon and aim for half of each or less. This salad is an easy 800 to 1000 calories—think halvesies and you'll still be perfectly full).

Cheater's Secret: At nicer restaurants, I wouldn't worry too much about heavy-handed salad dressings, as usually salads are lightly dressed. Don't overstress about asking for the dressing on the side 100 percent of the time.

◆ **Dinner**
   —Appetizer/Starter: Salad, soup, or a light appetizer such as beef carpaccio, shrimp cocktail, tuna tartare, grilled

calamari, oysters, steamed dumplings to share, hummus or baba ghanoush to share, with ⅓ or ½ piece of pita bread

—Entrée: A world of options awaits you. When possible, strive to have your plate look similar to your setup at home: ½ of mostly vegetables, ¼ protein, ¼ healthy carb. Most restaurants flip that equation and bump up protein and carb quantities and skimp on the veggies. Remember that vegetables fill you up on fewer calories (unless they're drowning in butter or oil). Order a salad to start or a side of sautéed spinach or steamed broccoli with garlic if you're concerned there's not enough in your entrée choice. Recall to memory the portion size of protein and carb servings that you're working with (3 to 5 ounces protein; ½ to 1 cup or a small fist size for carbs). Look at your entrée, assess the actual portion, revise in your head, pick up the fork, and execute your foolproof plan of action.

- **Red Flag Roadblocks.** Here are some key words to look for and steer clear of on menus—the vast majority of the time. Obviously, if you've encountered the best place in the country known for fried chicken, have a piece of fried chicken—one or two, not five. This list of hidden calorie pitfalls will make deciphering a menu a little easier and a lot more healthful.

  - ◆ **Naughty Words.** Fried, pan-fried, breaded, battered, buttered, buerre sauce (butter), Alfredo, carbonara, cream sauces, creamy dressings like ranch, blue cheese, and Thousand Island, super-oily sauces, au gratin (typically a heavy cheese-butter sauce), bottomless (duh), smothered, loaded, casserole (often involves heavy cream sauce), bisque (creamy soups), tempura (fried Japanese food)
  - ◆ **Sideline It.** Right in tune with the idea that cheating makes everything possible, below are some high-calorie items, sauces, toppings, etc., to sideline (read: request on the side, rather than in or on your entrée). This way you don't have to give up the stuff you enjoy, but you're able to moderate

things and better control how much goes into your meal. Just be nice and put on your biggest smile when asking the server. If we're talking some serious sidelining—I'm thinking back to the apple pie scene in *When Harry Met Sally*—consider ordering something a little less complicated or chill out and enjoy the heavier meal as one of your two *cheat and eats* for the week. Being known among friends as the neurotic, high-maintenance orderer or pissing off your server is not in our game plan. Here are a few items to sideline, when possible, and use sparingly if at all: Hollandaise/Béarnaise sauce, Caesar dressing (making it at home or having a noncreamy version is definitely doable, though), sour cream, mayo, aioli, guacamole, a heavy dipping sauce, "special sauce," blue cheese, ranch and honey mustard dressing, whipped cream

Cheater's Secret: Be careful with ketchup if you're an addict. Two or three packets is fine, but above and beyond that, you're taking in a whole lot of added salt and high-fructose corn syrup (unless the ketchup's organic or homemade). One teensy packet of fast-food ketchup contains 5 percent of your daily sodium recommendation (2300 milligrams for a 2000 calorie per day diet)!

- **Green Light, Go.** We're thankfully turning the tables on naughtiness. No one likes a "Debbie Downer" laundry list of things you should have in moderation. Here are some key words to make a beeline for when perusing the menu.

  ◆ Steamed, poached, grilled, braised, baked, broiled, lightly sautéed, seared, roasted, marinated, stir-fried, wine sauce, vinaigrette, ceviche, carpaccio (thinly sliced raw beef or fish), tartare (raw meat or fish), salsa, reduction, relish, compote

- **When in Doubt, Ask.** Plain and simple. If you're wondering about how a certain dish is prepared or what's in the sauce that accompanies it, just ask. No harm done.

- **Keep Unexpected Treats to Three to Five Bites.** This is a downright sneaky cheater's tip, if I do say so myself. The three to five bite rule is for those sticky situations like when deliciously scrumptious (and creamy) mashed potatoes land up right below your perfectly roasted chicken breast or when your best friend orders your favorite chocolate mousse for dessert. First, damn her for being such a good friend. Second, take three to five bites of your mashed potatoes, or the mousse, or whatever's out to taunt you. Knowing that you *can* actually taste something indulgent without the world ending makes everything that much more pleasurable and lifts that gray cloud of "dieting hell" that's been overshadowing you for far too long. Go ahead, take a bite.

- **The Dish on Dessert.** Give me chocolate or give me death. Dessert, like death, is inevitable . . . and irresistible. Just as with your two *cheat and eat* meals of the week, you've got two tasty treats to work with per week. If dessert looks delectably dangerous (in a good way), order it and share it with the table. Make it memorable and so good that it really is to die for. Don't order the mixed berries or sorbet if you're not so into them. You'll end up fooling yourself and eating most if not all of it because you're not satisfied, then 250 calories later, you're cursing the raspberry and lemon sorbet you finished off when you could have saved 100 calories and been much happier with four bites of impeccable sticky banana-toffee bread pudding, apple-almond crisp, or chocolate molten cake.

- **Walking Away Perfectly Full.** It's a bit of an odd concept, but leaving the table just "perfectly full" is really what we're striving for here. A former client of mine who had recently moved to the United States from Italy mentioned that the Italian style of eating always stresses leaving a meal just perfectly sated, almost slightly hungry (remember your brain will get the satiety message shortly after the meal's complete). Her message stuck with me, so I repeat it here. Many other cultures adhere to this message as well—eat until you're 85 to 90 percent full. It really encourages you to listen and connect to your hunger and satiety cues—not an easy task to retrain your brain but certainly a valuable one.

Dating and Eating: Holding Out for the Best

We all know how dinner-date situations can play out. Your nerves are racked up against the wall and you're doing your best not to say something stupid or spill red wine all over yourself or your date. If your date's a catch, you may not have any appetite whatsoever. If your date is more miserable than waiting in line at the DMV, anything on the menu is fair game, regardless of who's paying. Either way, you're trying to act calm, cool, and confident as you scan the menu, though somehow nothing's really registering while you attempt to keep up conversation. What do you do in situations, date or no date, where the pressure's on and you've got to pull off an ironclad order? This is when perusing the menu ahead of time definitely comes in handy. Otherwise, when in doubt, keep it basic and look to what the restaurant's known for—whether it's the roasted chicken, steak (you know to look for the filet), fish, or something vegetarian. If the entrée salads actually look amazing, go ahead and order one. If your date is up for splitting entrées or sharing a few different small plates, go with the flow and try to keep things balanced, depending on your preferences, making at least one dish light and ideally vegetable-heavy. Sharing makes the dining experience that much more intimate, and it will sneakily keep portions in line at the same time. Even if a dinner situation goes totally awry (the grilled salmon comes swimming in a sea of butter), you're prepared, you know your portions, and you know you'll be right back on the wagon with breakfast the next morning. Confidence in ordering and in eating, as in life, speaks volumes, and that's what's important.

So cheat it up (not literally—this guy might be a keeper) when you're out with a new dating prospect. If your relationship journey takes you to the world of ethnic eating, where menu items you've never heard of before are plentiful, don't freak out. Sure, unfamiliar cuisines and dishes can be daunting sometimes, but they can also be incredibly exciting and delicious. It's one meal, so have fun with it and expand your taste buds—just keep portions in mind and take note of what other meals you're eating out for the remainder of the week. Check out the Cheat Sheet below for some go-to healthy options at ethnic restaurants.

CHEAT SHEET: Ethnic Eating

Thai/Vietnamese

Yum: Summer rolls, steamed dumplings (split an order and have two or three), Thai papaya salad/green salad, marinated beef or chicken salad, chicken or beef satay skewers, lemongrass tom yum soup, lettuce wraps, Thai barbecue chicken, grilled lemongrass chicken/salmon/shrimp, steamed or grilled fish, red or green curry. (Classic Thai curry is a great *cheat and eat* order. Yes, I realize that Thai curries are made with coconut milk, which is high in fat and calories. But there's typically little oil involved in these dishes, so you can strain the veggies and chicken/shrimp/tofu out and spoon some of the sauce over. The sauce is usually so spicy that you'll just need 2 to 3 tablespoons to seal the deal on flavor.)

Yikes: Spring rolls (fried), sautéed dishes (too much oil and heavy sauces often overwhelm the veggies and protein in the dish. If it's a higher-end restaurant, you can more easily test the waters, as cooking methods are usually more refined and a little lighter), fried rice (enough said), pad Thai (I know, it's so delish, but it's usually the biggest offender on the menu, at 1000 calories or more per dish. Aim to have it once in a while and balance it out by sharing a lighter dish).

Cheater's Secret: Your goal is to get 2 to 3 servings out of the side of rice that comes with your meal. Consider requesting brown rice when you're able to for a boost of fiber. I find regular jasmine rice so aromatic and flavorful that it's my preference. Although it's white, I just keep tabs on my portions and have a third to half of the little takeout container, about ½ cup. Take on a new skill and learn to use chopsticks. Not only is it fun, but using them helps slow down how quickly you eat, speed racer!

Japanese/Sushi

Standby order #1: Miso soup or salad and/or shared edamame and 1 roll of your choice (try to keep those tempura rolls in check, and if brown rice is an option, request it!). If you're still hungry, order 2 to 4 pieces of sashimi.

Standby order #2: Soup or salad and 2 appetizers, such as beef negimaki and shumai (mini dumplings) (you might be full after 4 out of the 6 shumai—just a disclaimer to put the chopsticks down).

Standby order #3: Soup, salad, or shared edamame and 1 entrée, such as chicken teriyaki or miso glazed cod

Standby order #4 (for when you really need another roll): Soup or salad, plus 1 roll of your choice and 1 naruto roll (wrapped in cucumber rather than rice)

Yum: Miso soup, greens, edamame, shumai (share them), oshitashi (spinach with sesame seeds), tuna tataki, salmon/tuna tartare, naruto sashimi rolls (rolls wrapped in cucumber rather than rice), seaweed salad (a little on the salty side, but once in a while won't hurt ya), yakitori skewers, beef negimaki, salmon/chicken teriyaki, miso cod, maki rolls, chirashi (watch the amount of rice), sashimi, teppanyaki

Yikes: Tempura, heavy sesame and mayo sauces, excess soy sauce (use the low-sodium stuff)

Cheater's Secret: Don't be deceived by sushi. A single 6- or 8-piece roll can easily add up to 300 calories, and that can do you in if you're eating three rolls at a time, 900 calories later. The amount of protein that adds up in one little roll is pretty minimal and may leave you looking for more. If you're hungry, tag on 2 to 4 pieces of sashimi to your standard order—one roll of your choice (even the spicy and crunchy ones a few times a month) and start with miso soup and a salad or a cup of edamame.

Mexican

Yum: Tortilla soup, tamales, fajitas (aim for 1 or 2 tortillas and have some of the additional chicken/shrimp/steak and veggies on the side), enchiladas (just watch the sauciness and cheesiness—enchiladas suiza generally has cream), pulled pork carnitas (typically pretty lean), shrimp/salmon veracruz, soft tacos (aim for two, they're usually pretty simple as far as the toppings), grilled, roasted, or mole chicken, guacamole (it's healthy fat—aim for about ¼ cup maximum), black beans and pinto beans, quesadillas (these are a little iffy, as they can often come oozing with heavy cheese, not to mention two tortillas instead of one)

Cheater's Secret: If you adore quesadillas, add in whatever veggies you can, split the order between two to three people, and get a lighter dish, salad, or appetizer along with it. Balance really is everything in this game.

Yikes: Flautas, taquitos, tostadas, and chimichangas (all are fried). If you're getting a salad and it comes in a tostada "bowl," skip it and just go for the greens and crumble one handful of tortilla chips into the salad—you'll easily save 300 to 500 calories. Suiza (cream sauce), refried beans, skip the sour cream or get it on the side and use sparingly, the never-ending basket of chips and salsa (set a goal of 10 chips and you're done).

Cheater's Secret: I could eat chips, salsa, and guacamole till the cows come home, I love them so much. Obviously, I set some ground rules. Set a number of chips (say 7 to 12) and make that your max point. Better yet, skip the saturated fat in the fried

tortilla chips—a lot of restaurants now offer fresh cut vegetables
to go with guacamole and salsa.

Italian

Yum: Minestrone, pasta e fagioli, antipasto, olives, caprese salad
(fresh mozzarella, tomato, and basil—share it and go for 1 to 2
slices of mozzarella), tricolore or arugula salad, fresh tomato and
basil bruschetta (share it), tuna, salmon, or beef carpaccio, grilled
calamari and octopus, mussels, lighter pastas with tomato or wine
sauce (try to choose those with veggies and shrimp/seafood, beans,
or chicken to actually fill you up!), grilled/roasted chicken, steak,
seafood and fish dishes, 2 pieces of thin crust pizza (tack on some
vegetable toppings!)

Yikes: Fettuccine alfredo, fritti (fried), penne alla vodka (cream sauce),
carbonara (cream-bacon sauce), chicken Milanese (breaded), eggplant and chicken parmesan (breaded and fried), the plentiful basket of focaccia or ciabatta bread with olive oil (you know the deal,
1 small piece if it's the best of the best!)

The Perfect Pizza Order: Most definitely start your meal with
a nice-size salad or bowl of minestrone soup to fill up before the
pizza comes out (because pizza alone generally takes a whole lot to
wipe out hunger). If you can easily go through 3 or 4 slices of pizza
at a clip, bring the portion down to a more reasonable 1 to 2 slices.
Order thin crust or even whole wheat crust when possible. As for
toppings, you know vegetables are always fair game, as is fresh basil
and creamy buffalo mozzarella. Choose higher-calorie, higher-fat
items like sausage and pepperoni less frequently . . . let's say 50 or
25 percent of the time instead of 100 percent.

Indian

Yum: Mulligatawny soup, roti (whole wheat bread), tandoori chicken
(or anything from the tandoor—it's spiced and grilled), chana
masala (chickpeas), dal (lentils), chicken or vegetable biryani, raita
(yogurt sauce), roasted fish, lamb, chicken, or meat dishes

Yikes: Chicken tikka masala (cream tomato sauce), malai (cream
sauce), samosas (fried), aloo gobi, too much naan bread (the fluffy,

spongy bread you can't get enough of—again, reach for 1 small piece or don't start. Remember you've also got basmati rice that comes with your dish. Choose one and be done.)

Middle Eastern/Mediterranean

Yum: Israeli salad (tomatoes and cucumbers), Greek salad with feta, olives, pickled vegetables, fattoush salad, hummus, baba ghanoush, grape leaves, kofta (spicy meatballs), lamb or chicken kebabs, tabbouleh salad, foul (fava beans), lamb or chicken tangine, whole wheat pita (have half of one), Merguez sausage (share it two or three ways—it's delicious but fatty), grilled chicken, meat, and fish entrées

Yikes: Falafel (fried), the basket full of pita to go with your hummus (it's easy to keep dipping and munching straight from the hummus plate until both have magically vanished—take a third or half of the pita and 3 to 4 spoonfuls of hummus, put it on your plate, and then dig in), baklava (it's one of my favorite desserts ever but can be loaded with butter—perfect time to employ the three to five bite rule!)

Spanish Tapas

I love the small plates and small portions, but watch the fried stuff and dishes dripping with oil. Pick 2 or 3 fun things you love (like chorizo or tortilla Española) and then try to keep the rest of the order on the lighter side and get a few vegetables in the mix.

Yum: Spanish olives, tortilla Española (egg and potato omelet), gambas al ajillo (shrimp sautéed with garlic), mussels in red wine vinaigrette, paella, marinated mushrooms, and white asparagus

Yellow-Light Moderation: Chorizo, Serrano ham, albondigas (meatballs in tomato sauce), Mahon and Manchego cheese, patatas bravas (spicy potatoes—steer clear if they're fried), dátiles rellenos (dates stuffed with cheese and wrapped in bacon)

Yikes: Croquetas (fried), calamari fritos (fried calamari)

Weeknight Lifesavers: More Meals to Cheat By

We're finishing off Week 3 with a few more speedy dishes and some one-pot meals, getting all the nutritious goodies in one fell swoop without slaving in the kitchen. You've got a hectic social schedule, and after eating out multiple times a week, it's nice to come home and prepare a quick, comforting, healthy meal. Use this week to experiment with braising and poaching, two super-healthy cooking methods that involve liquid (rather than a ton of fat or oil). Braising is an unbelievably easy method for slow-cooked dishes like soups, stews, and hearty meat and poultry dishes, perfect for cold-weather fare. Braising's technical definition is to brown or sear the meat or vegetables in a small amount of fat (like olive oil) to lock in flavor, and then to simmer/cook slowly in liquid. Cooking for a longer period of time at a lower heat helps tenderize the meat or vegetable and bring out its flavor. Meat should be so darn tender that it falls right of the bone. This makes braising an ideal cooking technique for tougher, usually less expensive and fairly lean cuts of meat, like pot roast/brisket, lamb and veal shanks, short ribs, chicken on the bone, or chicken thighs (keep the skin on during cooking for more flavor—you can ditch it when the dish is done to save on fat and calories). You can also braise heartier veggies like leeks, onions, beets, carrots, parsnips, sweet or regular potatoes, cabbage, fennel, and beans like lentils and cannellini beans.

Along with a few braised dishes, we're going to poach up some fish as well as eggs before the chapter's through. Poaching is one of the simplest, most straightforward cooking methods, and it's incredibly light and healthful. Poaching is defined as submerging and gently simmering delicate foods like eggs, poultry, fish, fruit, and vegetables in broth, water, or wine—clean and simple. We'll also throw together a few one-pot meals like soups and stews that you can make ahead of time to have around during the week so that there's actually something in the fridge ready to roll when you come home exhausted after a hellish day.

Braised Short Ribs with Dried Cherries and Red Wine

This is a perfect dish for a wintry evening when you're looking for something warm, hearty, and comforting. And if you're cooking for a guy or a meat lover, this is bound to be a big pleaser.

Makes 4 to 6 servings

THE GOODS
- 1 ½ tablespoons olive oil
- 2 pounds boneless short ribs, extra fat trimmed off
- Salt and freshly ground black pepper
- ¼ cup all-purpose flour for dredging
- 1 to 2 carrots, roughly chopped
- 5 cremini or button mushrooms, roughly chopped
- 1 tablespoon fresh thyme leaves
- 1 bay leaf
- 1 to 2 cippolini onions (or 1 small yellow onion), roughly chopped
- ½ shallot, diced
- 3 garlic cloves, peeled and smashed gently with a knife
- 1 tablespoon tomato paste
- ⅓ cup dried cherries
- ½ bottle dry red wine (I use a wine with dark cherry overtones)
- 2 cups beef stock

THE BREAKDOWN
1. Preheat the oven to 350°F.
2. Heat the olive oil in a heavy ovenproof saucepan or enameled cast-iron Dutch oven (like those from Le Creuset—a Dutch oven is just a heavy-duty pot, usually made of cast iron) over medium-high heat. Season the short ribs with salt and pepper. Dip in flour to cover each side. Brown the short ribs, about 4 minutes on each side. Transfer the ribs to a plate.

3. Place all the vegetables and herbs in the saucepan and sauté for 5 to 7 minutes. Stir in the tomato paste and dried cherries and cook for another minute. Place the short ribs back into the pan, add the wine and beef stock, and bring to a boil.

4. Transfer the pan to the oven and cook for 2 ½ hours, or until the meat is tender, stirring occasionally. Remove from the oven, place the meat on a platter, and boil down the liquid for about 20 minutes on the stovetop.

The Facts: 360 calories; 16g fat; 6g saturated fat; 25g protein; 4g fiber

Chicken with Mushrooms and Red Wine Sauce

Makes 4 servings

THE GOODS

    2 teaspoons extra-virgin olive oil
    1 pound skinless, boneless chicken breast, cut into thinner cutlets and then into pieces
    Salt and freshly ground black pepper
    2 to 3 tablespoons minced shallot
    2 tablespoons unsalted butter
    1 heaping teaspoon all-purpose flour
    ½ cup dry red wine
    ¼ cup low-sodium chicken broth or water
    6 to 8 mushrooms, mix of button and cremini, or whatever suits your fancy, thinly sliced
    2 teaspoons fresh thyme leaves

THE BREAKDOWN

1. In a medium to large skillet, heat the olive oil over medium-high heat. Add the chicken breasts and season with salt and pepper. Brown the chicken on both sides, 4 to 5 minutes, adding the shallot during the final minute. Remove the pan from the heat and set aside.

2. In a large saucepan, melt the butter over medium heat and add the flour to make a roux. Add the wine, chicken broth, and chicken and bring to a simmer.

3. In the pan used to cook the chicken, add the mushrooms and cook with the oil remaining in the pan over medium heat until softened, 2 to 3 minutes. Add the mushrooms to the saucepan along with the thyme. Season with additional salt and pepper if needed. Reduce the heat to medium-low and simmer to thicken the sauce for 10 to 15 minutes.

4. Serve with ¾ cup quinoa, brown rice, or fettuccine, and vegetables.

The Facts (including carb): 240 calories; 11g fat; 4.5g saturated fat; 24g protein; 0g fiber

Thai Shrimp Curry with Pineapple and Red Bell Pepper

I concocted this recipe on a random weeknight and I must admit, I may never order Thai curry takeout again. This dish is incredibly flavorful and spicy enough to clear up any stuffy nose. If you want to tone down the spice, just add less curry paste. (Red curry paste is less hot than green.) I curbed excess calories and saturated fat by using light coconut milk—great flavor, and you can't tell the difference. You can find fish sauce, curry paste, and straw mushrooms in the Asian section of your grocery store or at your local Asian market.

Makes 4 servings

THE GOODS

　　2 teaspoons peanut oil
　　1 small onion, chopped
　　1 tablespoon minced fresh ginger
　　2 tablespoons red curry paste
　　1 15-ounce can light coconut milk

2 tablespoons Asian fish sauce

Juice and zest of 1 lime (or substitute fresh Kaffir lime leaves if you can find them at the supermarket)

1 cup diced fresh or canned (in water) pineapple

2 medium tomatoes, chopped

1 red bell pepper, chopped

½ cup bamboo shoots

1 cup straw mushrooms

¾ to 1 pound fresh shrimp, peeled with the tail left on

1 to 2 tablespoons minced fresh cilantro

1 to 2 tablespoons fresh Thai basil leaves cut into chiffonade (see Note)

1 or 2 cilantro sprigs for garnish

THE BREAKDOWN

1. Heat the peanut oil in a large, heavy saucepan over medium-high heat. Add the onion and ginger and cook for 2 to 3 minutes, until the onion is translucent. Add the curry paste, stir, and cook for another 2 minutes.

2. Add the coconut milk, fish sauce, and lime juice and zest. Stir until well blended.

3. Add the pineapple, tomatoes, bell pepper, bamboo shoots, and straw mushrooms. Stir, lower the heat to medium, cover, and simmer for 20 to 25 minutes.

4. Add the shrimp to the pan, mix well, increase the heat to medium-high, and cook for another 5 to 6 minutes, until the shrimp is cooked through, adding the cilantro and basil during the last 1 to 2 minutes of cooking.

5. Serve with jasmine rice and garnish with cilantro sprigs.

Note: Chiffonade is a cutting technique used for herbs or leafy greens in which they're rolled tightly (stack a few on top of each other) and then cut horizontally into very fine, thin ribbons. It's a great technique for fresh basil leaves.

The Facts: 240 calories; 10g fat; 6g saturated fat; 22g protein; 4g fiber

Chicken Cacciatore

Makes 4 to 6 servings

THE GOODS
  2 to 3 tablespoons olive oil
  3 pounds broiler chicken, precut into pieces (or breast and
    thighs on the bone with skin)
  2 to 3 garlic cloves, minced
  1 onion, minced
  2 carrots, chopped
  1 15-ounce can whole or diced plum tomatoes
  1 8-ounce can tomato sauce
  Salt and freshly ground black pepper
  2 bay leaves
  ½ cup dry red or white wine

THE BREAKDOWN
  1. Heat the olive oil in a heavy pot or cast-iron Dutch oven over
     medium-high heat. Add the chicken pieces and brown on all
     sides, 4 to 5 minutes.
  2. Add the garlic, onion, and carrots and cook for another 2 to
     3 minutes.
  3. Stir in the tomatoes and tomato sauce, season with salt and
     pepper, and add the bay leaves and wine.
  4. Bring to a simmer, cover, and simmer over medium heat for 50
     to 60 minutes, stirring occasionally to keep the bottom from
     burning or sticking.

The Facts: 240 calories; 8g fat; 1.5g saturated fat; 23g protein; 3g fiber

VARIATION: *Serve with the pasta of your choice (I tend to go
for a thicker, wider noodle like whole wheat or regular fettuccine or
pappardelle). Or go even lighter and swap the pasta for whole wheat
couscous and a side salad or veggies.

Poached Halibut with White Wine, Lemon, and Thyme

Super-easy, incredibly light, and classically simple, this recipe is a cinch when you're time-crunched. Serve with steamed or sautéed vegetables and roasted potatoes, quinoa, or brown basmati rice.

Makes 2 servings

THE GOODS
    1 ½ cups water
    ½ cup dry white wine, plus more if needed
    2 4-ounce halibut, salmon, cod, or trout fillets
    1 teaspoon fresh thyme leaves
    4 peppercorns (if you have them)
    ½ lemon, sliced into rounds, or to taste
    Salt and freshly ground black pepper

THE BREAKDOWN
    1. Fill a large skillet with the water and wine and arrange the fillets so that they're completely covered by liquid; add more wine if needed.
    2. Add the thyme, peppercorns, if using, and lemon slices to the pan. Bring the liquid to a boil over medium-high heat.
    3. Reduce the heat, cover the pan, and simmer for 8 to 12 minutes, until the fish flakes easily. Season with salt and pepper to taste and additional fresh lemon if needed.

The Facts: 100 calories; 1g fat; 0g saturated fat; 9g protein; 0g fiber

Poached Salmon with Cucumber-Chive Sauce

This recipe follows the poaching method of the previous recipe and is served with a creamy but light sauce. Use ¼ cup of the sauce per serving; you'll have some sauce left over.

Makes 2 servings

THE GOODS
2 4-ounce wild salmon fillets
1 ½ cups water
½ cup dry white wine

THE SAUCE
1 cup low-fat Greek yogurt
½ garlic clove, minced
½ cucumber, peeled and grated
2 teaspoons minced fresh chives (or substitute chopped fresh dill)
1 teaspoon lemon zest

THE BREAKDOWN
1. Fill a large skillet or frying pan with water and wine and arrange fillets so that they're completely covered by liquid, adding more wine if needed.
2. Bring liquid to a boil over medium-high heat.
3. Reduce the heat, cover the pan, and simmer for about 8 to 12 minutes until the fish flakes easily.
4. Combine the sauce ingredients in a medium bowl and mix well. Spoon over the poached salmon.

The Facts: 200 calories; 6g fat; 2g saturated fat; 32g protein; 0g fiber

Poached Eggs with Roasted Tomatoes and Grilled Garlic Toast

This is a great brunch or breakfast dish that turns eggs into something a little more fancy-gourmet. If you want to increase the number of servings, increase all ingredients except the vinegar.

Makes 1 serving

THE GOODS
　　1 thick slice country sourdough or whole wheat bread, toasted
　　　　and cut in half
　　1 teaspoon extra-virgin olive oil
　　1 garlic clove, cut in half
　　¾ cup Slow-Roasted Tomatoes (see page 219; you can make the
　　　　tomatoes a few days ahead and reheat them when ready to use)
　　½ teaspoon white vinegar
　　2 eggs
　　Salt and freshly ground pepper

THE BREAKDOWN
　　1. Heat a grill pan or skillet to make garlic toast. Brush the bread
　　　　halves with olive oil and rub with the cut side of the garlic.
　　　　Grill the bread garlic side down for 2 to 3 minutes, until slight
　　　　grill marks are made or the bread is lightly browned.
　　2. Fill a large, heavy saucepan with 1 ½ inches water and the vin-
　　　　egar (the vinegar helps keep the egg whites intact for a more
　　　　picture-perfect poached egg). Bring the water to a simmer.
　　3. Break one egg into a small bowl or ramekin and carefully slide
　　　　it into the simmering water. Repeat with the second egg, leav-
　　　　ing room between them in the saucepan. Poach for about 3
　　　　minutes for the yolks to remain runny or 1 to 2 minutes lon-
　　　　ger for a firmer yolk.
　　4. Arrange the toast halves on a plate and top each with warm
　　　　roasted tomatoes. Remove the eggs with a slotted spoon and
　　　　place atop the tomatoes. Sprinkle with salt and pepper to
　　　　taste.

The Facts: 340 calories; 18g fat; 4.5g saturated fat; 17g protein; 3g fiber

VARIATION: *To take this dish up another notch, sprinkle 2 or 3
teaspoons Parmesan shavings over the tomatoes. To make the dish
even more simple and speedy, skip the grill pan and toast the bread
in a toaster.

Poached Eggs with Asparagus, Parmesan, and Pepper

This is a super-simple meal that looks gorgeously colorful and elegant on a plate. If you want to increase the number of servings, increase all ingredients except the vinegar.

Makes 1 serving

THE GOODS

    3 stalks asparagus, ends snapped off and cut in half
    1 teaspoon olive oil
    ½ teaspoon white vinegar
    2 eggs
    2 tablespoons freshly shaved or grated Parmesan
    Salt and freshly ground pepper

THE BREAKDOWN

1. Steam the asparagus halves for 2 to 3 minutes, until al dente, and arrange nicely in the middle of your plate. Drizzle with the olive oil.
2. Fill a large, heavy saucepan with 1 ½ inches water and the vinegar. Bring the water to a simmer. Break one egg into a small bowl or ramekin and carefully slide it into the simmering water. Repeat with the second egg, leaving room between them in the saucepan. Poach for about 3 minutes for the yolks to remain runny or 1 to 2 minutes longer for a firmer yolk.
3. Remove the eggs with a slotted spoon and place atop the asparagus. Sprinkle the Parmesan shavings over the eggs and season with salt and pepper to taste. Serve with 1 slice of toasted multigrain, whole wheat, or exceptionally good Italian country bread.

The Facts: 250 calories; 17g fat; 6g saturated fat; 18g protein; 1g fiber

VARIATION: *If you have premade or homemade pesto sauce lying around, try a small dollop, 1 to 2 teaspoons, over the eggs. Or swap the asparagus for sautéed mushrooms with a teeny drizzle of truffle oil, about ¼ teaspoon (it's strong!). You can find truffle oil at your local gourmet market or online. It can be a bit pricey, but will last you a while.

Souped Up

Mom's Minestrone Soup

This might be my favorite soup or, rather, stew of all time (excluding my mom's famous split pea soup). I adapted this soup from my mom's old recipe—basically, I throw a ton of vegetables in along with kidney and white cannellini beans, tomatoes, a little vino, and a good Parmesan rind (the key to a richer flavor; remove the rind when the soup's done cooking). The soup tends to get more "stewy" after a day or two when all the flavors meld—that's when you know it's really ready to eat. You can't go wrong with a good, thick pot full of flavorful seasonal veggies!

THE GOODS

2 tablespoons extra-virgin olive oil
2 to 3 garlic cloves, minced
1 15-ounce can red kidney beans, drained and rinsed
1 15-ounce can white cannellini beans, drained and rinsed
1 small yellow onion, diced
3 to 4 carrots, chopped
2 to 3 celery stalks, chopped
1 to 2 zucchini, chopped
1 small bunch kale or spinach (optional)
2 baby red potatoes, cut into small chunks
1 28-ounce can whole tomatoes (I'm a big fan of San Marzano)
2 to 3 cups low-sodium chicken or vegetable stock (depending on how big your pot is and how much you want to make)
Salt and freshly ground black pepper
1 Parmesan cheese rind
2 bay leaves
½ cup whole wheat (or white) elbow pasta
½ cup dry red wine or sherry
Parmesan or Pecorino Romano cheese for grating

THE BREAKDOWN

1. In a large stockpot, heat the olive oil over medium-high heat. Add the garlic and cook for about 30 seconds.

2. Add the beans, mash them a little with a potato masher, and cook for about 2 minutes. Add the onion, carrot, celery, zucchini, kale, potatoes, tomatoes, and stock and season with salt and pepper. Add the Parmesan rind and bay leaves. Bring to a boil, then reduce the heat and simmer for 45 to 50 minutes.

3. Add the pasta and wine and cook for another 10 to 15 minutes. Remove the bay leaves and Parmesan rind and serve with grated Parmesan or Pecorino Romano.

The Facts: 300 calories; 6g fat; 1g saturated fat; 13g protein; 12g fiber

Tuscan White Bean and Escarole Soup

Perfect for chilly nights when you want something cozy, warm, and light. The white beans are rich in fiber and will fill you up fast while the escarole packs in vitamins A and K and folic acid.

Makes 6 servings

THE GOODS

1 ½ tablespoons extra-virgin olive oil
2 to 3 small garlic cloves, minced
3 cups low-sodium chicken broth or vegetable broth
2 cup carrots, coarsely chopped
2 cups grape tomatoes, halved
1 16-ounce can cannellini beans
1 teaspoon Italian dried herbs (such as basil and oregano)
Salt and freshly ground black pepper
1 head escarole, stem cut off and cut into 3- to 4-inch strips
Freshly grated Pecorino Romano or Parmesan cheese (2 tablespoons per serving)

THE BREAKDOWN

1. In a large saucepan, heat the olive oil over medium heat. Add the garlic and sauté for 1 minute. Add the broth, increase the heat to high, and bring to a boil.
2. Add the carrots and cook for 3 minutes. Reduce the heat to medium, add the tomatoes and cannellini beans, and cook for 4 to 5 minutes, until soft.
3. Add the Italian herbs and season with salt and pepper. Add the escarole and stir lightly until wilted. Simmer for 20-25 minutes. Mix the soup.
4. Serve with Pecorino Romano or Parmesan cheese sprinkled on top.

The Facts: 190 calories; 8g fat; 2g saturated fat; 12g protein; 8g fiber

VARIATION: *For another quick dish using cannellini or other white beans, try stewing them. Heat 1 tablespoon extra-virgin olive oil in a large saucepan, add 1 to 2 tablespoons diced shallot, and sauté for 2 minutes. Add 2 cups white beans, 2 cups chopped fresh tomatoes, 1 tablespoon minced fresh rosemary, ½ cup low-sodium chicken broth, and ⅓ cup white wine. Season with salt and pepper to taste and simmer over medium-low heat for about 20 minutes.

Your Mama's Chicken (or Turkey) Soup

Makes 6 to 8 servings

THE GOODS

1 small whole chicken (ideally free-range or organic), about 3 pounds
2 small yellow onions, chopped
3 to 4 carrots, chopped (leave the skin on for extra fiber and to save time on peeling)
3 to 4 celery stalks, chopped
Salt and freshly ground black pepper
½ cup brown rice (optional)
½ cup chopped leeks, white parts only

THE BREAKDOWN
1. Get out a massively large pot (like a good-size pasta pot), wash the chicken, and plop it in the pot. Fill up the pot to cover the chicken, about three quarters of the way to the top.
2. Add the onions, carrots, and celery and season with salt and pepper.
3. Bring to a boil over high heat, then reduce the heat to medium-low and simmer for about 1 hour, or until the chicken is fully cooked.
4. Turn the heat off, take the chicken out, cool slightly, and skin it, removing the white meat (and a little dark if you like) from the breast, thighs, and wings. Dump the meat back in the pot. Add the rice, if using, and leeks and simmer for another 30 to 40 minutes, until the rice is fully cooked and soft to the bite.

The Facts: 190 calories; 2g fat; 0.5g saturated fat; 24g protein; 2g fiber

VARIATION: *If you're jumping ahead and have already roasted up a nice chicken or turkey as explained in the following chapter and you've got a bare-bones carcass and some leftover meat lying around, you can easily make a quick soup—this is a great time saver and you're able to use the entire chicken or turkey—very green of you! Just leave out the initial step of boiling the chicken first. Plop the carcass, onion, carrot, celery, and seasonings in and then add a quart of low-sodium chicken broth and 1 to 3 cups of water, toss in the leeks and rice if using, and you're souped up and ready to go. Bring to a boil and then simmer for about an hour or so. Obviously, toss out the carcass before serving—not too appetizing.

Salt Licked—While we're on the topic of soups, let's do a rundown of the canned stuff to make a quick exposé of some hidden sources of sodium. Excess sodium in foods can translate directly to water retention, dehydration, and bloating, making you feel as though you gained a few extra pounds instead of losing them, not to mention the fact that a sodium-soaked diet poses problems for high blood pressure and heart disease down the line. Unfortunately, our consumption of salt isn't decreasing. Recent research found that by 2000, men were consuming 48 percent more sodium than they were in the 1970s and women, 69 percent more. Most Americans are consuming double that. Feel constantly bloated and parched? Well, now you know why! Using a bit of salt in cooking or a minuscule touch of it over meals is one thing, but added sodium in packaged foods puts you in the weight-loss danger zone. Here are the biggest sodium offenders that you'll find on grocery shelves:

— Frozen dinners, packaged snacks, canned tomato sauces, cold cuts, bottled dressings, and canned soups, to name a few. Canned soups are among the most notorious offenders. They're convenient to keep in your cabinets—hearty and filling for a quick, light meal—but they're often loaded up with more than 1000 milligrams of sodium or more per serving (that's almost half your daily recommended amount, all in an 8-ounce cup of soup!). Your goal is to come under 2300 milligrams of sodium per day, or about 1 teaspoon of salt. Strive to keep sodium to a minimum with canned, packaged, and frozen foods. You might be surprised with what you find. Even a basic item like a Thomas' bagel has 20 percent of your daily recommended amount of sodium, and a bowl of raisin bran has 17 percent. Your take-home rule of thumb: Shoot for 500 milligrams (600 milligrams tops) of sodium or less per item and serving, regardless of what it is.

> *Cheater's Secret:* Rather than racking your brain looking at labels, look for soups labeled "low-sodium" that contain no more than 140 milligrams of sodium. Try to choose brands that contain basic, whole ingredients (no high-fructose corn syrup necessary!) such as Amy's Organic, Pacific, Walnut Acres, and Imagine.

Refresher Course—Key Goals from Weeks 1 to 3

❑ Resize portions—3 to 5 ounces protein, ½ to 1 cup rice/pasta/grain, 1 cup/piece fruit, 1 to 3 cups veggies/salad (aim to cut total portions by 15 to 25 percent and set your plate up as: ½ fruits/vegetables, ¼ lean protein, ¼ healthy, complex carbs).

❑ Eat 2 servings of fruit per day; aim to have vegetables with lunch AND dinner.

❑ Drink 1½ to 2 liters of water per day.

❑ Don't skip meals—you'll lower your calorie-burn capability!

❑ Cheat it up each week with one or two indulgent meals (order what you wish, but still consider portions) and one or two treats (between 200 and 300 calories each).

❑ Exercise at least three or four days this week.

❑ Cut your alcohol intake per week by at least 25 percent.

❑ Food journaling . . . DO IT!

❑ Bring three to five basic office staples to work for snacks and emergencies.

❑ Re-plate and re-portion takeout and delivery food. Aim for half to three quarters of the to-go container.

❑ Watch portions like a hawk at restaurants, and leave at least five bites on the plate, if not a quarter to half. If the bread isn't awesome, lose it.

❑ Cut artificial sweeteners in half—aim for 1 to 2 packets per day (or less!) and keep weaning down.

Clean Up and Keep Cheating: Stop Stress Eating Without Depriving Yourself and Make a Comeback After Overdoing It

"Every day is a comeback. Wake up swinging."

–Kafi

WEEK 4 GOALS

- Check yourself! Look back at your food journals from Weeks 1 to 3—have you hit all the goals like a rock star? Check them off one by one. Accountability and consistency are key ingredients to your success and the sustainability of healthy eating habits and maintaining a healthy weight.
- Stop stress or emotional eating and make a list. Write out all your trigger foods that do not need to be in the house.
- If you've stalled on the scale, do a mini detox for your digestive system: For three to five days, boost fruit and veggie intake by 25 percent (make them the focus of every meal), and skip alcohol, coffee, dairy (except yogurt), and wheat products.
- Keep on food journaling. Highlight or circle any "extras" that have crept up throughout the week (such as random sweets, fistfuls of pretzels/chips, and extra snacks, cocktails or glasses of wine).
- Put everything on a plate! Look before you bite so you don't end up eating 400 empty calories without realizing it. For snacks, use a salad-size plate or even a smaller saucer.
- Support strong bones and a gorgeous figure by getting 3 servings of calcium daily from foods like yogurt, cheese, edamame, soy, rice, or skim milk. If you're not a fan of dairy or are lactose-intolerant, consider taking a supplement.
- Kick artificial sweeteners out the door for good. If you can't go Splenda-free 100 percent just yet, work your way down to ½ to 1 packet a day.

The Plan

Welcome to Week 4—you're officially hitting the halfway mark. Too bad, you may be hitting a bit of a wall (hey, this book isn't all sunshine and roses—this is real life, ladies). Work stinks this week, you're exhausted after too many late evening social obligations and too many early morning workouts at the gym, you're struggling to get to the grocery store, you feel like you've stalled out on the scale, and all you want to do is drown in a sea of chocolate, french fries, and champagne. Go ahead and scream. Balancing the demands of life and attempting to lose weight while maintaining your sanity is frustrating and exhausting at times. No worries, this week will help keep your head above water and avert the threat of a looming life crisis or weight loss plateau. Get psyched—as you've come to expect, here's a look at the week ahead.

A Look at the Week Ahead:

Look Back at Your Food Journals
Look at the first three weeks and evaluate how you're doing. Check off all the goals you've successfully incorporated into your daily/weekly routine. Do you feel like you're stressed and have hit a snag? If the scale isn't budging or you've had a rough couple of days, we're taking things up a notch with a mini "detox," detailed on page 195.

Stop Eating Out of Stress, Boredom, Depression, or Anxiety!
Write out your stress and emotional-eating foods that need to be tossed in the trash and write down what habits have been helping you lose the excess poundage. Recognizing and reminding yourself that your body (and your jeans) likes smaller portions (of awesome food), feels more energized and less bloated with 1 ½ to 2 liters of water daily, and loves a clean, kicking digestive system with lots of fruits and veggies, makes an incredible difference in your ability to implement the Cheater's goals and sustain your weight loss and great eating habits for the long haul.

Eat More Fruits and Veggies to Get Over the Hump
If you've hit a small plateau weight-wise, it's time for a midway cleanup for three to five days with more fruits and veggies (citrus in particular to release any excess water weight) and some lean protein and healthy complex carbs. Kick out items that can be bloating, like alcohol, coffee, dairy (except yogurt) and wheat-based products, like breads and pastas, for a few days to give your digestive system a break! (Dairy and wheat/gluten-based foods are more allergenic for a lot of us and may cause consistent low-level digestive stress.) You'll come out revived and back to your fighting weight afterward. Read on for your exact blueprint, but the general rule is: fruits—go from 1 to 2 a day to 2 to 3; vegetables—go from 25 to 50 percent of lunches and dinners to 50 to 75 percent.

Keep on Food Journaling
Paying extra attention to the little details in life (and in your diet) can make or break any goal. Highlight "extras" (like too many handfuls of M&M'S or pretzels, extraneous cocktails, or heavy meals) that may have weaseled their way in without you realizing it and might be causing a small derailment. Pinpoint how frequently (or not) they're coming into the picture and if they're causing you to stall out from achieving your goals at full steam.

Put Everything on a Plate
Particularly snacks and little extras here and there. Eating out of the bag or container is a recipe for disaster and excess calories. Twelve Doritos on a plate turns into forty grabbing from the bag. This often explains why the scale is stuck or you're not feeling as trim as you'd like. See ALL that you're eating before you dive in and build parameters and portions around it.

Get Your Calcium
Conduct some due diligence on your daily calcium intake. Are you getting your 3 servings from foods like yogurt, cheese, edamame and other soy products, rice, or skim milk? If not, consider taking a supplement.

Scale Down Your Sweeteners Even More
Artificial sweeteners and Splenda should be history by now. Decrease your sugar and carb cravings by switching to straight-up no sweetener or a natural one like sugar in the raw or agave nectar, 1 teaspoon per serving. If giving up Splenda is like giving up cigarettes, wean down to ½ to 1 packet a day and kick the habit by Week 7 or 8.

Go to page 178 for the Week 4 sample menu.

Week 4 — Cheater's Shopping List:

- ❑ Vegetables: 3 to 5 (or more) for the week: 4 plum tomatoes, 1 pint cherry tomatoes, 1 avocado, lettuce, 1 pound Brussels sprouts, 1 cucumber, carrots
- ❑ Fruit: 2 to 4 types (or more), your pick (enough to get you through 5 to 7 days, 2 servings a day): berrries, bananas, pineapple, grapes
- ❑ Protein: 1 pound chicken breasts, 1 4-ounce salmon fillet, 1 4-pound roasting chicken, eggs
- ❑ Healthy carbs: 1 pound fingerling potatoes, 1 sweet potato, 1 parsnip, whole grain cereal (more than 5 grams fiber, less than 7 grams sugar), all-natural granola (less than 10 grams sugar), whole wheat pita, whole wheat English muffins
- ❑ Dairy/calcium: Parmesan cheese, 3 to 4 low-fat plain yogurts or cottage cheese, skim or soy milk
- ❑ Other: walnuts, cashews, almonds, dried cranberries, ground flaxseed meal
- ❑ Fresh herbs and spices: garlic, thyme, rosemary, truffle salt
- ❑ Seasonings and oils: apricot preserves, lemon
- ❑ Snack stuff and staples: granola bars (more than 3 grams fiber, like Kashi TLC), hummus (if you don't already have it)
- ❑ Dessert/treat: all-natural/organic ice cream/frozen yogurt (like Stonyfield Farms or Häagen-Dazs Five), dark chocolate squares/bar, ingredients for The Cheater's Cookie (page 366)

See page 182 for "Week 4: Your Weekly Food Journal."

Week 4: Sample—Say Good-bye to Stress Eating

based on 1400-1600 calories

Week 4:	Monday	Tuesday	Wednesday
BREAKFAST 300-400 calories 7-9:30 a.m.	Start the week off right—HIT THE GYM 1 slice whole grain toast with 1 tablespoon organic peanut butter and banana slices Thank goodness you got a decent breakfast in at home because your life just blew up in your face between your relationship, work deadlines, and too many e-mails about your friend's wedding. It's going to be a tough day/week ahead. . . .	1 cup high-fiber cereal (more than 5 grams fiber) with 1 cup strawberries and skim or low-fat soy milk	½ cup 2% cottage cheese with 1 cup sliced berries or melon, and 2 teaspoons ground flaxseed or 1 table-spoon chopped walnuts
SNACK About 100 calories 10-11 a.m. (If you're not hungry, SKIP IT!)	Iced soy or skim latte	Skip it, you're too stressed to eat. Try a cup of green or herbal tea to relax a little.	Skip it
LUNCH 400-550 calories 12-2 p.m.	Salad from home 3 ounces grilled chicken with greens, cherry tomatoes, cucumbers, and 2 tablespoons homemade Caesar dressing (page 129) 1 cup homemade Toasted Whole Wheat Pita Chips (page 116) (prep dressing and pita chips the night before)	Office cafeteria, because sometimes work is crazy and you have to make the best of it. ½ chicken salad sandwich on multigrain bread, side salad, and an orange or some watermelon	Business lunch Navigate the menu as best you can. Go for chicken, fish, or an entrée salad like tuna Niçoise
SNACK 100-200 calories 3-5 p.m.	ACK! It's 6 p.m. and you didn't have time for a snack. STARVING. Preempt eating everything in the fridge when you get home by snagging a single slice of cheese and apple slices as soon as you walk in the door. Plan your pre-dinner snack ahead of time.	Horribly stressful, busy day. No time to breathe and you want to drown in something salty, sweet, crunchy and snacky. 10 to 12 honey whole wheat pretzels with 1 tablespoon peanut butter	Just got reamed out by your boss, awesome. Go for a breather coffee break. Skip the caramel latte with whipped cream and huge Rice Krispie treat. Instead, order a tall skim mocha and a brownie bite cookie and you'll still hit your ideal calorie target. Sneaky!

Thursday	Friday	Saturday	Sunday
Breakfast sandwich from home . . . because you woke up in dire need of a bagel, but are going the Cheater's route to handle stress scrambled eggs (I whole egg + I white) with 2 tomato slices and 2 pieces turkey bacon or I slice cheese on a whole wheat English muffin	3-mile run before work—get in an extra workout this week to alleviate stress and clear your head! I cup high-fiber cereal (more than 5 grams fiber) with I cup strawberries and/or blueberries with skim or low-fat soy milk	HIT THE GYM Banana or I cup pineapple chunks before the gym 6 ounces yogurt with berries and ¼ cup granola (like Bear Naked or Feed; look for 10 grams sugar or less per serving)	SLEEP LATE, it's Sunday! Take a yoga or Pilates class or get another run in if it's been a super-stressful week
I piece whole fruit or I cup grapes (back on track post-breakfast and feeling much better)	Laughing Cow wheel and I whole grain cracker	Skip it	Skip it
Make-your-own salad You know the drill . . . 1. mixed greens, spinach, or arugula 2. some type of protein 3. whatever veggies or fruits you wish to add 4. a sprinkle of I or 2 of the following: cheese, dried fruit, nuts, olives and/or avocado 5. I to 2 tablespoons vinaigrette or olive oil/lemon	Lunch out with coworkers; keep in mind you're doing dinner out the next two nights. ½ of an 8-ounce turkey burger, plain or with I slice cheese, lettuce, and tomato. Skip the fries; grab a pickle and side salad.	Hummus and avocado whole wheat pita with lettuce and tomato I serving Kettle Bakes Hickory Honey BBQ Potato Chips (if you're dying for some potato chips but they're dangerous to keep around, grab a single serving bag or portion them out, pack 'em up, and stash them out of sight)	Brunch out . . . After a crappy, emotional week, you just need some blueberry pancakes I large or 2 small blueberry pancakes (order whole wheat if they're an option) Side of low-fat yogurt and fresh berries (the protein and fat in the yogurt and fiber in the fruit will fill you up fast, unlike refined-carb pancakes)
½ cup homemade trail mix—¼ cup total of mixed almonds, cashews, raisins, dried cranberries, and dark chocolate chips plus ¼ cup Kashi Heart to Heart cereal or other multigrain cereal YOGA CLASS after work—de-stress yourself!	Office birthday ½ red velvet cupcake (if it's just mediocre, no need to finish it), small iced skim latte or an apple (balance out something sweet with something healthy and prevent that PM sugar crash). Thank goodness it's Friday. Go get a manicure and do something nice for yourself!	Running around town—grab the piece of fruit and a granola bar you stashed in your purse	Fresh cut veggies with ¼ cup hummus Bake Cheater's Cookies (page 366) to relax and distract yourself. Put all but 2 or 3 in the freezer or pack them up to bring to work on Monday. GO GROCERY SHOPPING TODAY!

Continued

Week 4:	Monday	Tuesday	Wednesday
DINNER 400-600 calories 7-8:30 p.m.	Long day—decompress and cook up a tasty meal for yourself. 4 ounces Broiled Salmon with Apricot-Mustard Glaze (page 218), I cup Roasted Root Vegetables (page 223), and I ½ cups steamed green beans	Go ahead and have a good cry, but don't dare bust out the ice cream container or peanut butter jar if you know they're potentially hazardous. Have a solid dinner first. If you're too drained to cook, order something healthful AND comforting. 2 cups spaghetti and meatballs from your neighborhood Italian restaurant (thankfully they have whole wheat spaghetti!) I cup pasta, I cup meatballs Side of broccoli rabe with garlic	Dead tired, go to sleep early after a light dinner. 4 ounces grilled chicken breast with Slow-Roasted Tomatoes (page 219) and a simple salad
SNACK 100-150 calories 8:30-9:30 p.m. (If you're not hungry, SKIP IT! Work in desserts and treats when you really want them and they're damn worth it!)	CHEAT TREAT #1: ½ cup Stonyfield Farms frozen yogurt or Häagen-Dazs Five ice cream (it's been an emotional day— portion it out first, then start spooning)		Fruit or skip it
WATER	2 liters	I liter—it's been a rough day	3 liters—extra to help work out that wine from last night
ALCOHOL/ OOPS!		¾ bottle of wine and an hour phone conversation with your best friend, oops!	
EXERCISE	Spin class at the gym		

Thursday	Friday	Saturday	Sunday
Sushi takeout: Miso soup and salad with ginger dressing (or 1 cup edamame) 1 roll of your choice (2 or 3 pieces sashimi if you think you'll still be hungry)	Thai takeout at friend's house: Split summer rolls or have tom yum soup or green papaya salad. Share grilled lemongrass chicken ½ cup jasmine rice	CHEAT MEAL #1 Dinner out at favorite neighborhood bistro: 4 ounces herb-crusted lamb with roasted vegetables and mashed potatoes (there's a lot of them, so aim for half. Why? Because you're dying for dessert!)	Make dinner and have leftovers for the next night: 4 ounces Rosemary-Garlic Roasted Chicken (page 216) 1 cup Roasted Brussels Sprouts (page 221) and 1 cup Roasted Fingerling Potatoes with Truffle Salt (page 224)
2 small squares dark chocolate (normally you would have done the whole bar—get individually wrapped squares or portion it and put it back)	See alcohol below	CHEAT TREAT #2: Share dessert—molten chocolate cake	CHEAT TREAT #3 1 Cheater's Cookie (page 366)—sooo good—and ½ cup skim or soy milk to get more calcium in for the day! (okay, it's been a ROUGH week, but you skipped one cheat-and-eat meal, so go ahead and have the extra treat—sometimes you just need it)
2 liters	2 liters	1 ½ liters	2 liters
	1 glass wine	2 glasses wine with dinner 1 vodka/soda	
Yoga	3 mile run/jog	60 minutes at gym	Yoga, Pilates, or a run

Week 4: Your Weekly Food Journal

Week 4:	Monday	Tuesday	Wednesday
BREAKFAST 300-400 calories *(Note your hunger level on a scale of 1 to 10 after each meal!)*			
SNACK About 100 calories *(If you're not hungry, skip it!)*			
LUNCH 400-550 calories			
SNACK 100-200 calories			
DINNER 400-600 calories			
SNACK 100-150 calories *(Work in desserts and treats when you really want them and they're damn worth it!)*			
WATER			
ALCOHOL/ OOPS!			
EXERCISE			

	Thursday	Friday	Saturday	Sunday

The Probability of a Plateau

I'm going to lay it all out on the table. In the whole grand scheme of revamping healthy eating habits and losing weight, reaching a plateau at some point is just about inevitable. You might not have changed a thing in your eating or exercise, but for some reason, the scale isn't budging and it's been a week or two . . . or sometimes even three or four. Does this mean you're doomed and all's lost? You've flatlined and can't figure out why. Is it time to throw in the towel and return to the "woe is me" damsel in despair role? Of course not—that's not how cheaters do things. Your body is simply re-adjusting itself to all the changes that are occurring—let it ride and it'll keep moving. Moderate, consistent weight loss (even ½ pound per week or 2 pounds per week) means it's coming off and is going to *stay off*. And remember, everyone is different and our metabolisms work according to their own calendar. It takes time to put the weight on, and it takes time to take it back off. As much as you don't want to hear it, patience and persistence are absolutely the key here. Our bodies may often come to a natural halting point for a few days, weeks, or even a month or two sometimes, whether it's after a five-, ten-, or forty-pound loss. I've seen this occur with countless women and men, though men tend to lose weight at a much faster pace thanks to genetics and hormones, lucky bastards.

The scale may get stuck for a few weeks and then out of nowhere another three to five pounds or more miraculously disappear. As much as we'd like to, we simply can't predict or control everything in our lives. So we're left to keep on going in order to move past that plateau.

There are, however, a few tricks to cheat the system and bust that barrier. Here are your cut-and-dry steps toward continued cheating and continued weight loss:

- **Variety in Your Food and Fitness Routine**—Variety keeps things spicy and saucy in every part of our lives. Eat the same three foods daily and bang out the same four-mile run a few times a week, and sure, you'll reach a natural slowdown. Your body enjoys a good challenge and varied workouts, and it requires an array of wholesome foods to get all the nutrients it needs to function at peak form. With your fitness regimen, change things up by adding a new exercise or yoga class, extending your workout time by just ten to fifteen minutes, or switching to interval or heart-rate training. With your food, do something different, like adding in new seasonal fruits and vegetables or a healthful complex carb or snack you love but that has fallen out of the rotation. Both of these simple adjustments can reignite your metabolism's fire and heat things up again.

• **Stop Stress and Emotional Eating**—There's something about stressful situations and the urgent, dire need to run for a stiff cocktail, a bar of chocolate, and a box of Cheez-Its (or whatever your sabotaging vice of choice is), ripping through it all so fast that you're left like a deer in headlights, dazed in a pile of orange crumbs and an empty liquor bottle. We've all been there before—medicating ourselves into oblivion with food for any number of reasons, or excuses, take your pick—your boss has chosen you as a personal punching bag, one stressful visit home just undid three years of therapy, a heart-hollowing breakup that came out of nowhere left you a dazed and confused wreck for weeks.

I honestly think stress eating and emotional eating are something passed down from female to female, like a twisted rite of passage. It never really makes us feel any better in the long run, nor does it resolve the blow-up confrontation you had with your boss or the breakup with your boyfriend, but there's something sickly soothing in the act of emotional and stressed-out munching. Sure, this may occur on occasion, a couple of days, a week, and then you realize it's not fun hiding under a blanket of food forever and you pop out of your funk. For countless other females, emotional eating and continuous binge eating behavior happens on a very frequent basis and is an extremely serious issue. These women are successful, strong, gorgeous, and so organized and regimented that one small shift in virtually anything can send them reeling in a downward, uncontrollable spiral of emotional eating.

If this might sound familiar to you, consider seeking the professional care of a therapist and/or a dietitian to bring underlying issues to light and break the cycle. It's not easy to confront, but emotional and binge eating can be 100 percent overcome. Life's just too short not to cheat, not to love every bite of food you take (or at least the vast majority of it), and not to treat your body with care, compassion, and confidence.

After all the chocolates and the Cheez-Its are finished, you're often left feeling worse than when you started, and guilty for "blowing it." You feel bloated, on sugar and carb overload, and it isn't pretty. The important thing is to get right back on the wagon and return to your healthful foundation, restock the fridge with your grocery staples, hit the gym to release some feel-good endorphins, or do something nice for yourself that doesn't involve food. Something to remember and ingrain in your head: No day is ever ruined. Lose the guilt; stuff happens. Just because you messed up at breakfast with a jelly donut does not provide an open invitation to an entire day of crummy eating habits. You did not just wreck an entire three weeks of work on one chocolate bar and some cocktails. That said, in order to squash a string of stress-eating episodes, your new Cheater's plan of action is to always, always get right back on the wagon at your next meal or snack and pick back up the healthful eating foundation you've established.

- **Stop the Drama! Know Your Triggers and Write Them Down**—Put the brakes on stress and emotional eating by getting to know exactly what situations or individuals provoke emotional and stress eating and what trigger foods you gravitate toward. Like connecting the link between you diving into a pint of fudge brownie ice cream every time after you've seen that old friend from high school who has turned incredibly condescending and makes you feel awful—why are you friends again? As painful and annoying as it sounds, writing triggers down helps you address them head-on and steer clear of having certain foods in the house or at the office. Remove all foods that are like suck-you-in sand traps—we all have a few.

- **Journal Your Thoughts**—Emotional journaling, or as I affectionately term it, "EmoJo," can be incredibly helpful and allow you to understand and deal with your personal stressors and anxiety triggers. Keep a chic little journal or jot it on some sticky notes, whatever works for you. Recognizing triggers brings us right back to the idea of making sure you have healthful snacks and food around and that you're able to recognize when you're stressed before all hell breaks loose. Think about all the positive changes you've been making and write those out as well. Know precisely the tactics, goals, and habits that are bringing you closer to feeling and looking the way you want. Revised portions, more fruits and vegetables at every meal, consistent meal and snack times, lots of water during the day, exercise three to six times a week . . . just to name a few.

CHEAT SHEET: The Nutritionist's Naughty Nibbles

I'm sharing my own personal triggers and go-to foods that I use on the occasional stressful day. I'm being honest with you so you can be honest with yourself. Write yours out and post them on the fridge or on your computer as a reminder of what to be watchful over. Notice the salty-sweet trend here—I'm a sucker for it.

- Ice cream (particularly mint chocolate chip, coffee, and hazelnut)
- Chips and salsa . . . and guacamole
- Red, white, rosé wine . . . I'm not too discriminating, as long as it's good
- Chocolate—dark, of course!
- French fries
- Chocolate-covered raisins
- Honey-wheat pretzels

Mindless Eating Makeover, Cheater's Style

Mindless eating—we've all gone down this rocky road before, often without even realizing it. You ripped open a bag of peanut M&M'S, intending to just have five, and an episode of *Grey's Anatomy* or *The Bachelor* later, somehow the entire bag has vanished. Oops. Another example goes back to that office candy dish that lures you every time you pass by . . . it's just a mini Milky Way, what harm's in that? If it's three or four times a month, not much . . . but three or four minis a day and we're talking an extra runaway 100 to 150 calories. Wondering where those extra five or six pounds came from over the year? You've found your culprit, and its name is "drive-by eating."

Whether you're unconsciously eating or eating out of utter boredom in front of the TV or at your computer, we're going to steer you away from runaway munching down a new sunlit path, turning the tables to a little-known concept called "mind*ful* eating." Notice the emphasis on "ful" here, and brand this phrase into your brain: *Turn off autopilot!* Think for a second about what the phrase means—for many of us, our bodies run constantly on autopilot: We eat certain foods because we think we're supposed to, because they're claimed to be healthy, but whether we really like them or not or whether they satisfy us is hard to distinguish sometimes. We eat the portions we're given, rather than the portions our body is telling us it needs.

CHEAT SHEET: How to Pull the Plug on Mindless Eating

- Eat at the table or sitting down, not standing up
- Focus on the tasty meal rather than zoning out to the TV
- Eat off a plate, not out of the bag, or the pot, or a container
- Set up a nice scene—ambiance helps you enjoy your food more and feel satisfied faster
- Take ten minutes to focus on the food whenever possible, not the Internet, a stack of work, your mail and bills, or the paper
- Plan out meals and snacks ahead of time if need be so there's no question of "what," "when," and "how much"

- **Make a Master List**—The Cheater's trick is to eat foods (and treats) that are distinctly satisfying to you—not your neighbor, your best friend, or your hairdresser. Pull out your handy list again, the Master List, if you will. In addition to recording the habits that are helping you shed pounds, write out the specific meals, snacks, and portion sizes that curb hunger and cravings fast. The options will be different for each one of us. Diving into a box of Wheat Thins knowing they're potential trouble and don't satisfy you is not going to do you any good. But taking note of that, and noting a portioned snack that *does* satisfy you (like an apple and 1 tablespoon of almond butter) helps you combat endless handfuls of Wheat Thins when they're next available. A few things on my own Master List include: running at least two to three times a week in addition to other types of exercise; an apple and a tablespoon of peanut butter or two whole grain crackers and an ounce of cheddar for an afternoon snack will totally put the brakes on my hunger and halt cravings; bagels, even half of a whole wheat one, just don't work for me regardless of what's on them because I feel a drop in blood sugar and am always hungry an hour later; two to three small squares of dark chocolate takes care of my sweet tooth every time and always leaves me smiling.

In addition to building out a Master List over time, it's also extraordinarily helpful not to keep mindless munchables around the house or your workspace if they're too hard to control. I'm thinking of things like cereal, nuts, peanut butter, yogurt-covered raisins—we all have our things. If these items do appear, turn the tables and make them mindful: Give them a purpose and a specific portion and incorporate them into a snack or meal that is satisfying. Cheat it up! Ten Wheat Thins with a Laughing Cow cheese, ten yogurt-covered raisins and ten nuts, one cup of cereal—only for breakfast and not snacking, one tablespoon of peanut butter spread on a slice of multigrain bread—not eaten out of the jar. Create an automatic stop sign for mindless eating, and when all else fails, know that if you can't stop with certain munchies . . . don't start!

Intuition? Yes, Trust Your Body!

One of the biggest pieces of advice I can offer you, possibly the most secretive Cheater's Secret is this: Listen to what your body is telling you. Intuitive eating is the key to staying healthy. We're so often caught up with calories, fat grams, carbohydrates, sugar versus no sugar—all the dieting minutia—that we forget about the bigger picture—how our body responds to certain foods, when it's hungry and when it's full. The fundamental, instinctive idea of actually trusting ourselves and our hunger cues goes right out the window. To tackle this problem and press the reset button, we're working to ramp up your diet with fresh, whole, real foods throughout these chapters (as you've hopefully noticed by now). Nothing too crazy, but real, fresh foods (not the diety fat-free or low-sugar stuff) serve to uncross all those wires in your body that have been sending messages to eat when you're *not* hungry for quite some time. By now, your body should hopefully start sensing when it's hungry and when it's full to a much greater degree—remember that it takes about fifteen to twenty minutes for your stomach to speak to your brain and cue satiety. You can directly feel how your body responds when you eat something that's spot-on and satisfying, healthful or not-so-healthful. This goes right back to the concept of eating meals and snacks that are distinctly filling for you and only you, because again, the more you're satisfied, the less you eat. Again, I call this the *satisfaction factor*. A prime example of this is a box of fat-free cookies. You can easily take down half a box and 500 calories and still not actually be satisfied. Now try the Cheater's version: Find a little joy and satisfaction in one SMALL full-fat, fresh-baked chocolate chip cookie. You just saved at least 300 calories and you shut the door on that sweet-tooth craving. Done and done.

You're successfully cheating the system by reprogramming your brain and stomach to feel and think again—so get in the cockpit, you're the pilot steering this damn plane. Unfortunately, programming yourself isn't an easy task, but the more cognizant you are around mealtimes, the easier it'll become, the smaller your portions will end up being, and the more satisfying food will be. As part of your goal list for this week, check in with yourself at least once a day at a meal and be present and mindful when you're chowing down. Your trusty food diary is an invaluable tool in mindful eating, so keep journaling!

Let's Get It On: Ambiance and Presentation Are Everything When It Comes to Beating Mindless Eating

There's something to be said for enhancing the mood at mealtimes. Cue the Barry White and Marvin Gaye tunes, please. In all seriousness, though, ambiance can make a drastic difference in how much you eat and how much you enjoy your meal. Think about the setting and location of where you typically eat an evening meal. Are you standing up in your kitchen, hovered over the counter attempting to scarf down food at the speed of light because you're so hungry? Or are you multitasking, trying to do fifty things at once while attempting to "enjoy" a meal? At the office stressed out like a basket case taking bite after bite without even tasting what's on your plate or, rather, in the takeout container? Glued to the TV at night and somehow polishing off double the amount of food you were intending to eat? The environment in which you eat and the presentation of your food is surprisingly important. Focus on your food—taste it. I know that sounds utterly silly, but it's true—your brain can only focus on so many things at once. *Take the time to take pleasure in your food.* Turn the TV off, maybe light a candle or two, sit down at a table rather than stand or sit on your couch, and make sure that you're coming home to a decently clean living space. Eliminating stress and clutter impacts your environment, which, in turn, can impact your food choices, eating speed, and portions.

When it comes to presentation, I'm an ardent supporter of making food look gorgeous and appetizing. If you're still skeptical about filling up on smaller portions, try swapping to a smaller plate or bowl that's got a super-cool design or pretty pattern. Don't just slop your food down—arrange it nicely, explore the inner Top Chef in you that's dying to break free. What would Tom Colicchio or Padma Lakshmi have to say if they judged you on your plate presentation? Trust me and try it out a few times—it works and you'll be much happier and more satisfied at the end of a meal.

Too Much of a Good Thing: Fix Your Fridge and Pantry to Squash Overstimulation and Overeating

Continuing down the line on the mind*ful* eating train, let's take a quick pit stop in the land of variety. I mentioned earlier in the chapter that variety is indeed a key component to a healthful, balanced, colorful diet. But where we can sometimes hit a snag is when the variety of food options becomes overwhelming and we end up wanting to eat everything in our cabinets. It's like going to the grocery store and overdoing it, bringing your groceries home and feeling compelled to taste-test a little bit of everything. Or hitting up an all-you-can-eat buffet and immediately going into overdrive, overstimulation mode . . . four plates, three desserts, and a massive stomachache and food coma later. Some people couldn't care less and aren't fazed in the least by a plethora of options in their pantry and fridge or at a restaurant. If, however, you are more likely to break into three different types of nuts, and taste each type of yogurt and cereal you just purchased within ten minutes of getting home from the supermarket, let's take a step back and reevaluate things for a second. The last thing we want to do is set you up for a crash-and-burn episode in your own kitchen. Two quick scenarios:

a) "Are you hungry?" "No, but this yogurt and granola looks so darn good, let me just taste it." Sorry, save it for later—at a real meal or snack time when you're truly hungry. Put the groceries away and book it out of the kitchen.

b) Take two: "Are you hungry?" "Yes, I'm famished." Okay, before you open the floodgates and are faced with a spread that could feed a small country, breathe, assess the situation and your options, build your ideal plate in your head, focusing on mini portions so you can taste a variety of foods, and then execute and conquer. Pick a meal or snack with "satisfaction factor," such as 1 ounce of cheese, 2 whole grain crackers, 1 handful of grapes, and 3 olives . . . and put it on a plate! There you go, lots of tastes with appropriate portions and a shot of protein, fiber, and healthy carbs to quell your hunger.

Cheater's Secret: Keep that staple grocery list on hand and build intelligently off it, like the clever Cheater that you are. Know what foods are tough to keep around. Again, for moi, it's ice cream . . . If I buy three flavors, I may need to try them all while I'm taking them out of the shopping bag and putting them into the freezer. Not a pretty picture, so I buy one or two flavors at a time and make sure to work one serving into my day as a specific treat or dessert.

Give Food a Home and Eat What You Want

If you have a fear of particular foods for whatever reason (it's been drilled into your brain that mangos are sugary vessels of evil, for example) or you're afraid to bring peanut butter into the house (for fear of eating the entire jar in one fell swoop), take a challenge to overcome your phobia. **Give food a home.** Yeah, it's a funny statement, but it's totally true. We touched on it earlier, but it's worth coming back to. Build a place within your day or your week to work in certain foods that you formerly filed away in the "forbidden" category. Back to our peanut butter example. Rather than just having the peanut butter jar open and available at all times, give peanut butter a specific use—so you know it's primarily for your favorite whole grain toast, PB, and banana breakfast, or you pair a tablespoon of it with some apple slices for an afternoon snack. If runaway nighttime snacking can get the best of you sometimes and you know that PB can be tricky to portion, its time is then in the morning or afternoon—off-limits in the evening.

Another example, for all you chocolate fiends. Can't live without chocolate on a daily basis? Rather than just leaving an open chocolate bar out for the taking, give a square or two a specific place within your day—like coupling one or two small squares with a yogurt or a skim latte for an afternoon snack or designating it as the final touch to complete your evening. Same thing with cereal. Assign it to serve as a meal, morning only, not a snack or a box that's open 24-7 fresh for the taking. Hominess is goodness, kiss fear and guilt bye-bye.

Dazed and Confused: The Stress and Sleep Connection to Weight Gain

Too much stress and too little sleep. Sound familiar? If so, it might be contributing to your clothes not properly fitting. And no, it's not likely that the dry cleaners shrunk every single sweater or pair of pants you own. You can clearly see the outward effects of stress and the lack of sleep. Your skin's a wreck, your eyes are eternally bloodshot and glazed over, you feel like a zombie and can barely move your legs when you walk, and let's not even discuss the situation that's occurring with your hair.

Here's what's going down on the inside. When you're consistently stressed out, your stress hormone, cortisol, jumps and can impact appetite and blood sugar levels. And if that's not nasty enough, extra weight tends to flock to your abdominal area. The feared and loathed "muffin top" strikes again. Not getting enough shut-eye can also put on the pounds. Research finds that getting less than 7 ½ hours of sound sleep can affect hunger and satiety hormones, your hunger hormone (ghrelin) increases, and your satiety hormone (leptin) drops and you can end up storing more fat. One study found that women who slept less than five hours a night were 30 percent more likely to gain thirty or more pounds a year than those who hit the sack for longer. When the alarm clock goes off, most American women have only gotten about 6 ½ hours of sleep, and that just doesn't cut it. When you're constantly exhausted or running on half a tank, you'll likely start craving simple carbohydrates and sugar for a boost of energy—visions of doughnuts, bagels, candy, diet soda, chocolate, and creamy coffee drinks start dancing around in your head. In actuality, all you really need is more sleep. So start snoozing to lose, ladies, and figure out your magic number, whether it's seven or eight hours. Watch caffeine and alcohol intake before bed, as they can prevent deep, sound sleep. Kick the caffeine around 3 to 4 p.m. and know your limits with the bottle.

Picking It Up When You've Reached a Plateau: How to Jump-start Weight Loss

What to do when you overdo it: Recovering from a tough workweek, too many parties, drinking binges, vacations, and holiday eating

Okay, back to the more hands-on stuff. I figure you've had your fill with psychology and physiology class for the week. When clients I've worked with hit the skids—whether they've reached a plateau, have trouble transitioning back to a normal routine after a long vacation, get sidetracked by a super-stressful deadline, started a new fitness routine and are overeating, can't snap out of summertime party-and-drink mode, are recovering from an over-the-top bachelorette party, spent a four-day weekend away eating super-rich food at every meal, are thrown off by a horrendous cold, or just feel like they need a boost—we bring out the big guns and refocus on the bare-bones basics. I've affectionately termed it "lean, clean, and green" eating. Think of it like you're taking your car in for a tune-up, or going in for a long-overdue bikini wax or haircut. I'm not talking about some crazy juice fast, extreme deprivation detox, or lemonade cleanse, we're simply giving your body a break for a few days—your digestive system has won an all-expense-paid relaxing trip to the spa. "Lean, clean, and green" can help reboot your metabolism, kick any major unexpected sugar cravings, undo excess water retention, get things running smoothly in the bathroom, and give your system a rest from too much sugar, alcohol, or heavy eating.

Here it is, all unwrapped and laid out. This natural, gentler detox is really only meant to be done for three to five days or up to a week, otherwise you're right back on the boring "diety" train. You might find it useful to bring it back out every so often after a string of party-hard weekends, the holiday season, or a "down in the dumps" week of emotional-stress eating. While you're going "lean, clean, and green," make sure you're drinking sufficient water, at least 2 liters a day. When your water intake runs a little dry, dehydration sets in and your energy levels plummet. In addition, there's a greater chance you'll wind up eating more, mistaking actual thirst for hunger. Another potential contributor to your plateau. The plan below and the calendar on page 200 map out the mini detox and illustrate what three days' worth of meals and snacks might look like. As you'll notice, it's not vastly different from what you're already doing, just cleaned up a notch or two.

CHEAT SHEET: Detoxifying, De-bloating Foods

- Apples
- Asparagus
- Broccoli
- Carrots
- Ginger
- Olive oil
- Quinoa
- Watermelon
- Sweet potatoes
- Artichokes
- Avocados
- Beets
- Brown rice
- Citrus fruits
- Lettuce and dark leafy greens (arugula, watercress, spinach)
- Onions and garlic

The Blueprint—"Lean, Clean, and Green"

Disclaimer: The meal and snack suggestions below are examples. You've got the freedom to swap ingredients or create similar meals and snacks according to your taste buds.

What's In: Citrus fruits, including lemons, oranges, grapefruits, and clementines, asparagus, beets, watermelon, artichokes, green tea, and parsley all act as gentle, natural diuretics and help squeeze out any extra weight you might be holding on to. Water, 2 to 3 liters a day: Say good-bye to a bloated belly.

What's Out: Foods that are more allergenic or may cause bloating or digestive backup—white sugar (cookies, candy, cakes), alcohol, a whole lot of starchy wheat products (pasta, white rice, white bread), soy (only if it tends to give you digestive issues and gas), dairy in high doses (try working with just yogurt, which contains healthy digestive bacteria, but leave cheese, milk, and butter out for a few days), artificial sweeteners (that's a given, though).

Liquid Assets
- Start the day off with 1 cup of hot water and the juice of ½ fresh lemon—this combo can really kick-start sluggish digestion. Lemon and citrus is acidic—it's like an astringent. You can clean your sink with lemon . . . we're just giving your digestive system a light cleansing.
- As much herbal or green tea as you want throughout the day
- 2 to 3 liters of water throughout the day . . . preferably some with lemon slices in it
- 1 cup of coffee max during the day (I know better than to yank your coffee out completely—I'd prefer not to receive death threats), but if you can do without it, you should

Breakfast Options
- Start off with citrus—½ grapefruit, 1 orange, 2 clementines, and choose something from the following options (depending on where you are, your workout schedule, etc.)

  a) 2 hard-boiled or poached eggs or 1 egg and 2 whites scrambled with veggies (like asparagus, spinach/tomato, mushroom, etc.) and 1 slice whole grain toast or fruit salad
  b) plain low-fat yogurt with berries or fresh fruit
  c) 1 slice whole grain toast and 1 tablespoon peanut or almond butter and apple or banana slices or fruit salad

A.M. Snack Options
- Piece of fresh fruit (another opportunity to get in some citrus)
- 10 to 15 baby carrots or fresh cut veggies with 2 tablespoons hummus

- 8 to 12 unsalted nuts (almonds, cashews, pecans, etc.)
- 2 Wasa or whole grain crackers and 1 Laughing Cow cheese or 1 tablespoon goat cheese (we're working with minimal dairy, but I snuck a little in there so you don't go bonkers)

Lunch Options

- Grilled chicken breast, tuna, or salmon with mixed greens/arugula/spinach and fresh veggies of your choice (asparagus, beets, artichoke hearts, avocado, broccoli, etc.) and ½ cup quinoa or brown rice (if desired) with olive oil and fresh lemon juice or balsamic vinegar, or a vinaigrette
- 1 cup veggie- or bean-based soup and 2 or 3 fresh roasted turkey, hummus, and avocado roll-ups (1 thin slice avocado rolled up in each turkey slice with a thin smear of hummus, and roll it up!) and 1 cup fresh cut veggies or a side salad
- 1 sushi roll and miso soup/salad or 1 cup edamame (about half an order)
- 2 cups steamed or lightly sautéed veggies, grilled chicken, and ½ cup black beans/brown rice
- ½ grilled chicken, Italian tuna, avocado/hummus or fresh turkey wrap (whole grain wrap with more than 3 grams of fiber) with a piece of fruit or a side salad

P.M. Snack Options

- Any options from a.m. snack
- Apple with 1 tablespoon peanut, almond, or cashew butter
- Fresh veggies with ¼ cup guacamole
- 2 to 3 multigrain crackers with 2 to 3 thin slices of avocado
- 1 fruit-nut bar (like Larabar, Clif Nectar Bar, or Kind Bar)
- Yogurt with berries
- 1 cup edamame

Dinner Options

- Grilled/broiled chicken or fish with steamed vegetables or salad and small baked or roasted sweet potato/potato or squash (or ½ cup brown rice, whole wheat couscous, or quinoa)

- Sushi/sashimi—2 cucumber wrapped (naruto) rolls and miso soup or salad or soup/salad and sashimi platter
- Turkey burger or grilled portobello mushroom with asparagus and mixed green salad
- Omelet with 1 egg and 1 to 2 whites with your pick of veggies and fresh herbs, plus a side salad (add 1 small potato or sweet potato if you're still hungry)

Evening Snack Options
- No wine, beer, or alcohol for five to seven days! I know, it sucks.
- Fresh or frozen fruit
- Glass of low-fat soy, rice, or almond milk
- 1 to 2 small squares of dark chocolate—once or twice over the week IF you need it

> **Cheater's Secret:** Citrus fruit may help you shed weight a little faster and curb your appetite. Research has found that citrus, particularly grapefruit, may help reduce insulin levels to manage blood sugar and promote weight loss. Study participants lost an average of 3.6 pounds and up to 10 pounds over 12 weeks when having half a grapefruit with meals. Obviously, you're not going to eat grapefruit for breakfast, lunch, and dinner (can we say "fad diet"!?), but when grapefruit and other citrus fruits are in season during the winter, try incorporating half a grapefruit with your yogurt or eggs at breakfast or an orange and ten almonds for an afternoon snack. You should be downing at least two fruits a day by now, so this shouldn't be too difficult a task!

Sugar-Sweet Sunshine

Now that you've effectively recharged your battery and are feeling back on track, let's take a moment to discuss a few of the things that may have thrown you off kilter in the first place. Sugar, and its artificial cousins, is literally everywhere.

Here's a good shocker: The average American consumes nearly

Week 4: Three-Day Detox Blueprint

Week 4:	Day 1	Day 2	Day 3
BREAKFAST	Hot water with lemon 2 poached eggs with 4 or 5 steamed asparagus spears 1 slice whole grain toast	Hot water with lemon ½ grapefruit 6 ounces plain low-fat yogurt with 1 cup fresh berries	Hot water with lemon 1 slice whole grain bread with peanut butter and banana
SNACK	1 orange	Cup of ginger peach green tea	2 clementines
LUNCH	Grilled chicken salad with artichoke hearts, tomatoes, and 1 tablespoon sunflower seeds with 1 tablespoon lemon vinaigrette	½ whole grain wrap (more than 3 grams fiber) with ¼ cup hummus, 3 slices avocado, lettuce, tomato, and red bell pepper 1 clementine	Salad with lentils, beets, and asparagus with olive oil and lemon juice ½ cup whole wheat couscous on the side
SNACK	1 cup edamame	15 pecans or walnuts	Apple with 1 tablespoon almond butter
DINNER	4 ounces broiled cod or tilapia with lemon and thyme Steamed broccoli Small baked sweet potato or ½ cup brown rice	Miso soup 2 cucumber-wrapped rolls	Scrambled Eggs or Omelet with Sautéed Mushrooms and Herbs (page 62) Side salad
SNACK	Skip it	2 pieces dark chocolate	½ grapefruit or 1 cup raspberries
WATER	2 ½ liters	3 liters	3 liters
EXERCISE	45 to 60 minutes	Yoga class	3 to 6 mile jog outside
ALCOHOL/ OOPS!	SKIP IT!	SKIP IT!	SKIP IT!

100 pounds of sugar per year—those small five-pound bags of sugar at the grocery store . . . we're talking twenty of them. That's insane. And what's more insane is that the majority of the sugar we're consuming doesn't even come from straight-up white grainy sugar, it comes from added sugars and cheaper corn sweeteners like high-fructose corn syrup found in food and beverage products. Soft drinks alone comprise nearly 33 percent of added sugars for many Americans, candy 16 percent. In all, we're taking in 17 percent more added sugars and sweeteners than in 1970. Our daily recommended value for sugar intake hovers around 8 teaspoons, as laid out by the USDA's 2005 Dietary Guidelines, but many of us take in a whole lot more than that—32 teaspoons (or about 500 calories), to be exact. What's all that boil down to? Having excess sugar means having excess calories, and that can cause weight gain. Drop the majority of sodas, mindless candy munching, coffee syrups and drinks, sugary-sweet fruit yogurts and bottled smoothies, sweetened salad dressings, and sauces in your daily diet and say good-bye to up to fifty pounds in a year—yeah, fifty pounds! In addition, a diet high in refined sugars can impact your health—from increased risk of diabetes to heart disease. Not to frighten you, but you'd be pretty surprised to find out where hidden sources of sugar lie, so here's a quick rundown.

Low-fat fruit yogurt (6 teaspoons sugar)
Ketchup, 2 tablespoons (2 teaspoons sugar)
Golden Grahams breakfast cereal, 1 cup (2 ½ teaspoons sugar)
Kellogg's Raisin Bran Crunch breakfast cereal, 1 cup (5 teaspoons sugar)
Stonyfield Farms Banana Berry Yogurt Smoothie, 10 ounces (9 ½ teaspoons sugar)
Starbucks Frappuccino Bottled Coffee Drink, 9 ½ ounces (8 teaspoons)
Jarred tomato pasta sauce, ½ cup (2 ½ teaspoons sugar)
Reduced-fat peanut butter, 2 tablespoons (1 teaspoon sugar)
Fat-free honey Dijon salad dressing, 2 tablespoons (2 teaspoons sugar)
Big Gulp, 32 ounce/1 liter soda (27 teaspoons sugar!)

**CHEAT SHEET: Sugar Bombs,
Words to Look for on Labels**

- Agave syrup
- Brown rice syrup
- Brown sugar
- Confectioners'/powdered sugar
- Corn syrup
- Dextrose
- Evaporated cane juice
- Fructose
- Glucose
- High-fructose corn syrup
- Honey
- Lactose (dairy products naturally contain sugar from lactose—which is absolutely fine!)
- Maltose
- Maltodextrin
- Malt syrup/barley malt
- Maple syrup
- Molasses
- Sucrose
- Turbinado sugar

It adds up fast, doesn't it? So is sugar completely off-limits? Definitely not in this book. You've already set yourself up for success by consuming mostly real, fresh, single-ingredient foods—no added sugars there. Natural sugar in food is another story, and is perfectly okay. Sugar contained naturally in fruits, vegetables, and dairy products get the green light—yes, you can have higher sugar fruits like pineapple, mango, and banana without guilt. If nature produced it, it's most likely pretty darn good for us and won't send the scale climbing.

As for white or brown sugar, use it in moderation. One teaspoon of sugar is 16 calories. So when I use a packet of sugar in the raw in my coffee most mornings, I can handle it—it's not the end of the world and I'm smart about where other sources of sugar are coming into my diet the rest of the day. For more natural sweeteners like honey, molasses, maple syrup, and agave nectar, the same thing applies. Use a small drizzle, about 1 to 2 teaspoons (not a quarter of the bottle) and you're good to go. Do, however, try to scout out excess added sugar on food labels, and if sugar (or any of its nicknames) are one of the first three ingredients, try to skip it—ingredients are listed in order of quantity on labels. And if there are multiple types of sugar tucked into the middle section of the ingredient list, it's probably still a smart call to leave it on the shelf. All that sugar can add up to a lot.

For treats that contain sugar or are sweetened, you know the deal—scaled-back sizes, once or twice a week. If you're dying for a brownie or small scoop of real ice cream, have it, but utilize your revamped Cheater portions of really great quality goodies. Remember, you're shooting for the best of the best, it's not worth settling for anything else, and you'll end up eating far less. Have one scoop of real ice cream rather than two or half or a third of the brownie if it's extra large, about half the size of your BlackBerry or iPhone. You're working with much more manageable portions now and you're not digging into sweets and treats every day, so they truly become an indulgence.

CHEAT SHEET: A Day's Worth of Sugar

What my sugar intake, added and natural, looks like on an average day:

- Small coffee with 1 tablespoon whole milk and 1 packet of raw sugar (1 teaspoon sugar added)
- Fresh fruit with yogurt for breakfast (no sugar added)
- Grilled chicken salad with homemade vinaigrette for lunch (no sugar added)
- Piece of cheese and a peach for snack (no sugar added)
- Grilled shrimp with roasted zucchini and tomatoes and orzo salad for dinner (no sugar added)
- 2 squares dark chocolate for dessert (2 teaspoons sugar added)

Total daily added sugar: 3 teaspoons

Cheater's Secret: Low-fat and fat-free items often have more sugar and carbohydrates added to them to replace flavor and mouthfeel. This goes back to my whole salad dressing and fat-free cookie theory—get the full-fat stuff and you'll fill up faster on a smaller amount, eat fewer overall calories, and be way more satisfied in the long run.

Cracking Down on Corn Syrup

If you're not really sure what the hell high-fructose corn syrup (HFCS) is, you're certainly not alone. A quick and dirty definition: It's a man-made derivative of corn and cornstarch. It was developed in the 1970s as a much cheaper type of sweetener than regular sugar. For quite some time, high-fructose corn syrup was blamed in part for the nation's obesity crisis. However, to date, research does not show that HFCS contributes specifically to weight gain any more than regular sugar does. But HFCS is typically found in processed foods—and the amount of those items many Americans eat can contribute to weight gain and obesity. Either way, as a general rule, I'd steer clear of items that contain HFCS on the ingredients list, as it's typically a red flag indicating that an item isn't very nutritious. You'll find corn syrup in virtually everything, which explains why our consumption of it has skyrocketed 373 percent since 1970. Where you generally won't find items containing HFCS are in stores like Whole Foods, Trader Joe's, Wild Oats, and health food stores.

Axing Artificial Sweeteners

Get ready, because a lot of you won't like what you're about to read. Your daily diet soda, the "light" strawberry yogurt you love so much, your coveted sugar-free frozen yogurt and chocolate-covered protein bars . . . they all got to go, see ya. Here's why: In my personal experience working with clients and in all the research that's out thus far, there's really not much, if anything, to gain from having something artificially as opposed to naturally sweetened. I tend to feel, and many of my clients can attest to, that consuming a lot of artificial sweeteners or sugar substitutes in your diet raises your flavor palate when it comes to sweetness. Artificial sweeteners are so sweet that they essentially desensitize your taste buds' ability to understand what something naturally sweet is supposed to taste like. So if you're a sugar-free fiend and were to bite into a luscious, juicy peach, you might not be able to distinguish how incredibly, naturally sweet it really is. "Oh, it's a good peach" rather than "Oh my god, this peach is amazing!"

Skeptical? As you read earlier, just one packet of Splenda, the yellow stuff, is 600 times sweeter than one packet of regular sugar. And because sweeteners are so overly sweet but don't contain any calories, our bodies don't register what is actually consumed. Sweeteners are sort of tricking the body—unfortunately, only to crave more sweet things and carby foods, and not to be satisfied. Back to the example of the good ol' chocolate chip cookie. You have one real-deal, oozing with chocolate, chocolate chip cookie and your body recognizes what it's getting. One small, really rich cookie and you're done. Not so much the case with a larger sugar-free, fat-free chocolate chip cookie that tastes something like sweetened sawdust and just leaves you wanting two more because your body doesn't register the fake fillers and sweeteners and you're not satisfied in the least. So in the end, you may end up consuming more calories than you really bargained for. I'd rather have a single fresh, warm gooey cookie, butter, sugar, and all, wouldn't you?

CHEAT SHEET: Sorting Out Sweeteners

Here's what to look for on labels to identify artificial sweeteners and sugar substitutes.

- Acesulfame K (Sunett, Sweet One)
- Aspartame (Equal, NutraSweet)
- Isomalt
- Malitol
- Mannitol
- Neotame
- Saccharin (Sweet'N Low)
- Sorbitol
- Sucralose (Splenda)
- Xylitol

Research is backing up this theory, finding that artificial sweeteners may contribute to weight gain or alter metabolism. One University of Texas study actually found that for every diet soda you drink per day, there's a 41 percent greater risk of being overweight. Not to mention we're still not sure of the long-term health effects of artificial sweeteners. What we do know is that the fake stuff can wreak havoc on our digestive systems. I don't know about you, but I like to avoid bathroom trauma at all costs. Artificial sweeteners and sugar alcohols are prone to speeding up digestion, exacerbating diarrhea, and having a laxative effect (read: nothing's worse than making a mad dash for the bathroom, god forbid you're stuck on the highway or your only option is a Port-a-John). Sugar alcohols are an altered form of carbohydrates (neither wholly sugar nor alcohol) that are used in sugar-free products to add a sweet taste, flavor, texture, and bulk. They're not completely metabolized or absorbed in our digestive systems. To be blunt, they basically hang out and ferment in your large intestine until excretion, which is not an appetizing fact. If you've got a sensitive stomach, sweeteners and sugar alcohols can be fairly fierce diuretics and can often cause bloating, stomach cramping, and not-so-girlish gas. All in all, not a winning situation. Your favorite skinny jeans will likely be much easier to zip up when you don't have to deal with the blasted bloat from one too many pieces of sugar-free gum or cans of diet soda.

So do both of us a favor, ditch the sweeteners—cold turkey, or at least continue weaning off them. Move down to ½ packet of Splenda in your coffee and then eventually to none or a packet of sugar in the raw, trade in the three packs of gum you're chomping a day for a few Altoids, swap the "light" yogurt and the sugar-free oatmeal for the real stuff. You'll not only aid the weight loss process but you'll also be able to taste actual real food again!

"Nature-Made" Sweeteners

Sweeteners made from the South American herb stevia, with brand names such as SweetLeaf, Rebiana, PureVia, and Truvia, have bombarded the market in the past few years as Mother Nature's version of a more natural sweetener. Recently approved by the FDA, they're nearly calorie-free at 11 calories per packet, are free of carbohydrates, and don't spike blood sugar levels, which makes them a nice, more natural option for diabetics and those who are blood sugar sensitive. Here's the one catch, though—they're almost 300 times sweeter than sugar. Which makes me a bit skeptical in terms of the whole flavor palate thing and keeping your sweet taste buds at steady, normal levels. It's one thing to sprinkle a little nature-made sweetener here and there, but when you start adding sweetener, artificial or natural, to countless products on the market, the amounts used can go off the charts . . . and then you're back to the same dilemma of toning down your sweet palate and carb cravings.

Nectar of the Gods, Agave

Agave nectar might sound a bit odd or health food store-ish, but it's another natural sweetener that's a nice blood-sugar-friendly alternative to sugar. Agave nectar is a natural sweetener made from the agave cactus. It looks like honey but has a sweeter taste and doesn't impact blood sugar as readily as honey and sugar do. It's a great choice for diabetics or individuals who are blood sugar sensitive. Aim for about a teaspoon or less if you're adding it to tea, coffee, yogurt, etc. Agave does contain calories, about 20 per teaspoon, and it does have carbohydrates, unlike stevia. But flavorwise, it's fairly close to sugar and its consistency can work well for baking. And who knew that when agave ferments, it's used to make tequila? So if you're looking for a slightly healthier margarita on the rocks, sweeten it with agave rather than sugar and you've got an instant chic, haute cocktail. More to come on your alcohol-loving tendencies in the next chapter.

> *Cheater's Secret:* Start with the basics and sweeten whatever it is yourself, like yogurt and coffee, because I guarantee you'll use much less sugar, stevia, honey, or agave nectar than any mass-market food manufacturer.

Femme Fatale: Keep Cheating AND Get All Your Necessary Nutrients

You're back in action and it's showing as you finish out Week 4. We've tackled much of the basic food stuff thus far, but what about all the pill popping you hear so much about? Should you be taking vitamins, supplements, herbs, protein powders? Sometimes I feel like walking into a vitamin shop is just asking to be overwhelmed and overserved. Ladies, don't be duped by the clerk at the vitamin store any longer—you don't need to run up $300 a month on supplements to feel your best each day. There are indeed certain nutrients we should pay attention to as females, as our needs differ slightly from our male counterparts. I'm a big proponent of "food first"—ideally you're getting all you need from your diet, which you typically are as a cheater. Obviously, life or a minor health concern gets in the way sometimes, in which case a basic women's one-a-day multivitamin is a smart insurance policy. As for female-specific nutrients, we're going to cheat it up again and cut straight to the three biggies, the "triumvirate," if you want to name them: calcium, iron, and folic acid. Eating consistently in the cheating fashion, you can rest assured that you're generally getting enough of every vitamin and mineral your body requires. (If you're pregnant or planning to become pregnant, you'll likely want to take precautionary measures and take a prenatal vitamin. Definitely make sure to speak with your physician or OB/GYN.)

Boning Up on *Calcium*

My mother's been drilling into me the importance of getting enough calcium for as long as I can remember. She's loveably over the top sometimes, but she's also usually absolutely right. Women in particular need to stock up on calcium to build and maintain bone density and prevent osteoporosis and its precursor, osteopenia, bone loss that affects millions of American women and can pose major health risk and cause bone fractures and height shrinkage in old age. I always like bad news first, so here it goes: We've only got till the age of about twenty-five to build bone density, then we're just left to maintain it. The good news: There are plenty of ways to stockpile and maintain calcium—whether through calcium-rich foods, a basic calcium and vitamin D supplement, and weight-bearing exercise (killer as they may be, those sweat-fest body conditioning classes are good for multiple reasons). Nutrients are generally best absorbed when they come from food (see the sidebar for a list of calcium-rich foods). Aim for about three servings of a calcium-rich food per day and you're golden—skim, Lactaid, or soy milk with whole grain cereal at breakfast, a slice of cheese on your sandwich at lunch, and a low-fat yogurt as a snack. Mission accomplished, so don't bother trying to add up milligrams.

CHEAT SHEET: Calcium-Rich Foods

Aim for 3 servings a day and you're golden.

- Milk, Lactaid, soy/rice/almond/hemp milk (yes, hemp milk—don't get any crazy ideas!)
- Yogurt, kefir, cottage cheese, cheese
- Almonds, dark leafy greens, broccoli, canned salmon (the bones have calcium)
- Tofu, edamame

Daily Calcium Requirements
Ages 19 to 50: 1000 milligrams
Over 50: 1200 to 1500 milligrams

CHEAT SHEET: Best Sources of Calcium

Food Item	Portion	Milligrams Calcium
Plain low-fat yogurt	I cup (8 ounces)	415
Salmon with bones	3 ounces	345
Sardines	3 ounces	345
Skim and low-fat milk	I cup (8 ounces)	300
Soy/rice/almond milk	I cup (8 ounces)	300
Fortified orange juice	I cup (8 ounces)	300
Total cereal	I cup	300
Cheese	I ounce	272

Tofu—most brands	3 to 4 ounces	200-400
Light ice cream	½ cup	200
Almonds	2 ounces	150
Blackstrap molasses	1 tablespoon	137
Spinach (cooked)	½ cup	130
Bok choy (cooked)	½ cup	126
Black beans	1 cup	120
Kale (cooked)	½ cup	103
Oysters	1 cup	90
Edamame	½ cup	80
2% cottage cheese	½ cup (4 ounces)	77

If you're not able to get your calcium through food on a daily basis, it's definitely worthwhile to consider a supplement, one that's paired with vitamin D, which aids calcium absorption—look for calcium citrate or calcium carbonate on the label.

Up through menopause, you're shooting for 1000 milligrams per day; postmenopause and during pregnancy, your daily recommended value bumps to 1200 milligrams per day. Most supplements come 500 milligrams per pill—take one pill at a time with meals for maximum absorption.

Iron Woman

Iron is essential in helping red blood cells carry oxygen to our cells, which in real-world speak means that it keeps our energy levels going strong. Lucky us, women often lose iron each month with our menstrual cycle. Losing a little too much, or being on the low side, can cause fatigue, anemia in more extreme cases, or, if you're like many women, you might notice increased cravings for iron-rich foods like red meat. If that's the case, listen to your body and eat some lean meat! For a CliffsNotes breakdown of iron, there are two types, animal-based and plant-based. Animal-based iron, coming most readily from sources like red meat, poultry, and fish, is most effectively absorbed. Iron from plant sources, like leafy greens and beans, is a little trickier, so if you're a vegetarian or vegan, you may want to consider taking an iron supplement or try to pair up vitamin C–rich foods when eating plant-based foods, as they aid absorption.

CHEAT SHEET: Iron-Rich Foods

Daily Iron Requirements

Premenopause: 18 milligrams a day
Preggers: 27 milligrams a day
Postmenopausal: 8 milligrams a day

Food Item	Portion	Milligrams Iron
Oysters	3 ounces	13.2
Liver	3 ounces	7.5
Prune juice	½ cup	5.2
Lean ground beef	3 ounces	3.0
Chicken	½ cup	3.0
Shrimp	3 ounces	2.6
Spinach	½ cup	2.4

CHEAT SHEET: Vitamin C–Rich Foods

Vitamin C is iron's soul sister to aid absorption
- Broccoli/cauliflower
- Brussels sprouts
- Cantaloupe
- Kale
- Kiwis
- Oranges
- Papaya
- Red bell peppers
- Strawberries
- Tomatoes

Flipping for *Folic Acid*

Folic acid is that ever-important nutrient that helps prevent birth defects and lowers risk of heart disease. You may have heard it called folate, which is folic acid found naturally in foods. Your goal is about 400 micrograms per day, and you've got plenty of foods to choose from: dark leafy greens like spinach and kale, asparagus, lentils, chickpeas and kidney beans, nuts. For all you baby mamas, your prenatal vitamin will cover you for folic acid so the food stuff can serve as an important backup.

CHEAT SHEET: Folate-Rich Foods

Premenopause: 400 micrograms a day
Preggers: 600 micrograms a day

Food Item	Portion	Micrograms Folate
Fortified cereal	1 cup	400
Cooked spinach	1/2 cup	100
White beans	1/2 cup	90
Asparagus	4 spears	85
Broccoli	1/2 cup	50
Avocado	1/2 cup	45
Peanuts	1 ounce	40

The Crown Jewels: Omega-3s—Fish Oil and Flaxseed

You all know by now that I'm not about to tout a ton of supplements, but I do think there are two worth a good mention. An omega-3 fish oil supplement has all the healthful fats you'll find in fatty fish like salmon, tuna, halibut, and sardines, sans the fishy taste or smell. These fats are pretty much a nutritional gold mine—they're great for a number of purposes, including fending off heart disease, lowering cholesterol, reducing signs of aging, and alleviating depression and mood imbalance. I'll often recommend an omega-3 fish oil supplement for these reasons as well as for helping to alleviate constipation and chronic stomach issues such as irritable bowel syndrome, as the healthy fat reduces inflammation, and I find from those I've worked with that it sort of smooths things out in your digestive system, acting as a soothing lubricant. If you're going with fish oil, look for capsules that have a lemon or citrus coating or natural flavoring . . . nobody wants to deal with gagging fish burps.

Flaxseed is a vegan source of healthy omega-3 fat that can have a ton of benefit for a variety of reasons. Similar to fish oil, flaxseed is heart-healthy and decreases inflammation. To reap the rewards, flaxseed needs to be in the oil form or ground into a meal, which looks like wheat germ. If you eat the seeds whole, they'll just go right through you, literally. The oil can go bad quickly, so keep it in a dry, dark place. The ground stuff has a nice dose of fiber, and I've found that for those with constipation, it's a great natural way of getting things moving again. Toss 1 to 2 tablespoons into your morning cereal, yogurt, oatmeal, or smoothie.

The Story on Soy . . . And Other Vegetarian Protein Sources

Soy has received a lot of attention the past few years. To eat or not to eat, what's the deal? Like with so many things, it's got its own share of pluses and minuses. Plus: Soy is a complete source of vegetarian protein and is rich in calcium and antioxidants. Soy is also high in fiber and healthy omega-3 fats, which help lower heart disease risk and high cholesterol and protect against certain types of cancer. It's versatile and comes in a number of different shapes and sizes, including tofu, soy milk, edamame, soy flour, soy yogurt, and tempeh. Minus: Soy is often touted as a "wonder food," an easy way to boost protein intake and satiety, and processed soy is found in any number of energy bars, cereals, smoothies, hot dogs, burgers, cheese, "unchicken" nuggets, cookies, chips, and ice cream—all in the name of health, right? Yet again, we return to the argument of whole foods versus more processed or adulterated foods. My vote's clearly in the corner of real, whole foods and it stands the same with soy. More highly processed soy products may also take a toll on sensitive stomachs, causing excessive bloating and gas, so watch your intake if you're prone to tooting. Bottom line, stick to soy as it was intended, in the least processed forms possible.

Wondering about other healthy sources of vegetarian and vegan protein? There are plenty to choose from—beans and legumes, nuts and nut butters, and quinoa. Quinoa, along with soybeans, is one of the few vegetarian protein sources that is a complete protein— meaning that it contains all the necessary compounds (amino acids) that make up a true protein source, like eggs, poultry, meat, fish, and dairy. Quinoa's a nutrient-packed, gluten-free whole grain that hails from South America and has a deliciously nutty aroma.

Summing It Up to Conquer Stress and Ward Off a Plateau

Take a breather—there was a lot to get through in the first section of this chapter. So what's the big take-home message? Focus your thoughts on stress and emotional eating, and how to successfully get around it or get through it without unraveling your hard work thus far. Cheat your way to toppling stress by yet again playing smarter. Have specific tactics laid out and ready to deploy when things get hairy and stress or emotions pick up and your rock-solid eating habits take a downturn. Here is a quick summary of three cheating tactics to beat the stress and keep you moving forward.

Cheat and Beat #1: Step away from the food and find another outlet to handle stress. Hit the gym once or twice more this week, or make your standard workout more intense. Physical activity releases endorphins to help boost your mood, clear your mind, and manage the stress that much better. Other nonfood tactics to try and include: Treat yourself and get a massage or manicure, invest in a frivolous magazine (*US Weekly* or your favorite fashion mag comes to mind) and step out of reality for a little while, go for a walk or to the movies with a friend—I know it sounds cheesy, but we just want to get you out of the house to release and reboot yourself.

Cheat and Beat #2: If you've got to stress-eat on occasion, work it into your week and keep portions on target. I admit, sometimes getting a manicure or immersing yourself in *US Weekly* just doesn't do the job, and a delectable plate of french fries and a cheeseburger or a scrumptious red velvet cupcake from your beloved neighborhood bakery is all you can think about to battle a stressful or emotional situation. Time to cheat it up and work that meal or treat into your overall week. Plug it in as one of your two *cheat and eat* meals or treats. Savor it, love it, get the stress off your shoulders, and get right back to your healthy staples at the very next meal or snack.

Cheat and Beat #3: Whip out your list of foods to have at home and foods to keep far out of sight. Write them down and post them up where you can see them. I've included two sample lists—one showing foods that could do some serious damage if kept at home (not all of these may apply to you; feel free to insert your own red flag items). The other list illustrates some basic staples that should already be in your fridge or pantry, serving to build your healthy foundation whether you're at home, on the go, or at work.

CHEAT SHEET: Stress-Eating Foods to Boot Out of the House

- Snacky salty little crackers like Wheat Thins, Triscuits, Kashi TLC Crackers, Cheez-Its
- Yogurt- or chocolate-covered raisins or nuts, mini candies
- Cereal, if you're prone to mindless munching out of the box
- Ice cream, if you eat from the container or can't stop after a single serving
- Tortilla chips or potato chips
- Insert other munchy foods that might do you in:

    _____

    _____

CHEAT SHEET: Super-Basic Staples to Stay on the Wagon

- Low-fat plain yogurt or cottage cheese
- At least 2 fruits and 2 or 3 vegetables
- 1 or 2 or more types of cheese for snacking and cooking (1 ounce per serving)
- All-natural peanut, almond, or other nut butter (no eating from the jar!)
- Whole grain bread or wraps
- 1 or 2 lean proteins for the week, like chicken breast, shrimp, and tofu
- Eggs
- Low-fat or skim milk or soy milk

Take Out Your Stress by Turning On the Oven

Another fantastic, cheatable way of addressing stress is to actually get in the kitchen and cook! Cooking up a healthfully delicious dish or trying a new recipe is a great way to alleviate stress and set your mind on something productive. Even baking treats—for a specific purpose or person—can be really relaxing for a lot of us. The key here, of course, is not to eat half the dish out of the pot or nibble your way through the cooking or baking process. Make the recipe or dish all the way through, and plate it or save it for a later date or your next meal.

To help you beat stress by way of the kitchen, let's tackle your oven and try out some comforting dishes that require broiling and roasting, two simple, healthy cooking methods that use direct dry heat. If you broil something, you're cooking it under a grill, with heat coming from above. Most ovens will have a specific "broil" setting on the knob.

Broilers are fantastic for cooking meats, fish, poultry, and heartier veggies, or for lightly browning the tops of dishes. Roasting also involves high direct heat, whereby food is cooked uncovered to create a golden-brown surface and lock in the flavor and moisture of more tender cuts of meat and poultry. Roasting is similar to baking, but the heat is cranked up just slightly. The dry heat doesn't require too much oil or fat, and all you've really got to do is arrange your ingredients on a baking sheet or in a roasting pan and you're ready to go—there's no major babysitting involved, which leaves you more time for the zillion other things you've got to do. We're starting with just the bare bones, with dishes like roasted vegetables, including tomatoes, zucchini, red peppers, and Brussels sprouts, and a classic roasted chicken. One major caveat here: Be extra careful not to overcook foods when broiling or roasting or your meal could end up charred to death, so dry it might be mistaken for a lethal weapon.

Rosemary-Garlic Roasted Chicken

This is one of my favorite recipes on a fall or winter Sunday afternoon. Making roasted chicken and turkey often seems daunting to a lot of us, but it's actually one of the most straightforward dishes you can prepare. Season the bird, pop it into the oven, walk away, and let it cook until done. That's it. And it looks gorgeous on the table . . . an easy, impressive entrée to serve up at a dinner party or for the holidays. An easy rule of thumb is to allot one pound of meat per person, as you've got to factor in the weight of the bones/carcass. A 3- to 4-pound whole chicken serves 4 people; a 10-pound turkey serves about 8 to 10 people.

Makes 4 servings

THE GOODS
1 3- to 4-pound organic, free-range chicken
2 tablespoons unsalted butter, at room temperature
2 garlic cloves, minced
2 tablespoons minced fresh rosemary (or a mixture of fresh herbs, like rosemary, thyme, and sage)
Salt and freshly ground pepper
2 celery stalks, chopped
1 small onion, chopped
3 carrots, chopped
1 cup low-sodium chicken broth

THE BREAKDOWN
1. Preheat the oven to 425°F. Clean and rinse the chicken and pat dry.
2. In a small bowl, mix together the butter, garlic, and rosemary.
3. Tie the chicken legs together with kitchen string and rub three quarters of the butter mixture under the skin of the chicken directly on the flesh. Rub the remaining butter on the top and bottom of the breast and season with salt and pepper.
4. Place the celery, onion, carrots, and chicken broth in the bottom of a roasting pan. Place the chicken in the pan on a roasting rack, breast side up.
5. Roast for about 1 ½ hours, until the juices run clear when the chicken is pricked. Baste with pan juices every 20 minutes or so. Check the temperature between the thigh and the leg—an instant-read thermometer should read 180°F.
6. Remove the chicken from the roasting pan, carve, and serve with some of the roasted vegetables.

The Facts: 200 calories; 7g fat; 4g saturated fat; 23g protein; 2g fiber

Broiled Salmon with Apricot-Mustard Glaze

Makes 2 servings

THE GOODS
  2 4-ounce salmon or sea bass fillets
  Salt and freshly ground black pepper
  2 tablespoons apricot preserves
  1 tablespoon Dijon mustard

THE BREAKDOWN
  1. Preheat the broiler. Season each salmon fillet with salt and pepper.
  2. In a small bowl, mix together the preserves and mustard. Brush over each fish fillet.
  3. Place the fish (skin side down for the salmon) on a baking sheet covered with aluminum foil. Broil about 6 inches from the heat source for 6 to 7 minutes, until cooked through and browned.

The Facts: 190 calories; 4g fat; 0.5g saturated fat; 23g protein; 0g fiber

VARIATION: *If you want to do something a little different, add a pecan crust to the fish. Combine 3 tablespoons finely chopped pecans, 3 tablespoons whole wheat breadcrumbs, and 1 teaspoon minced thyme. Brush the salmon with the apricot-mustard glaze and cover each fillet with the pecan topping. Bake the salmon at 400°F for 20 minutes instead of broiling.

VARIATION: *You could also swap the fish for chicken breasts or thighs—just cook a little longer, 14 to 16 minutes 6 inches from the broiler. Or get creative and swap out the apricot-mustard glaze for another marinade or topping. A few tasty ideas include:

- Homemade or store-bought pesto—Spoon 2 teaspoons pesto atop each fillet (great for salmon, tuna, white flaky fish, and chicken)
- Balsamic vinegar, honey, garlic, red pepper flakes—Marinate the fish at least 15 to 30 minutes with a mixture of 3 tablespoons balsamic vinegar, 2 teaspoons honey, 1 smashed garlic clove, and ¼ teaspoon red pepper flakes (great for salmon, tuna, meatier white fish like sea bass and cod, chicken, and pork)
- Lemon and fresh herbs—Marinate the fish for 30 minutes with a mixture of 2 tablespoons fresh lemon juice, 1 tablespoon olive oil, 1 teaspoon fresh chopped herbs, such as basil, thyme, or rosemary, ¼ teaspoon salt, ¼ teaspoon freshly ground pepper, and 1 smashed garlic clove, if desired (great for salmon, tuna, white flaky fish, chicken, and pork)
- Miso glaze—Combine 2 tablespoons brown sugar or honey, 2 tablespoons water, 1 ½ tablespoons low-sodium soy sauce, and 1 tablespoon miso paste and heat in a small saucepan. Cool and marinate the fish for at least 15 to 30 minutes. Serve with chopped scallion for garnish. (Miso is a fermented Japanese soybean paste. You can find it your local grocery or Asian market. White miso paste has the mildest flavor, and is great for salmon, tuna, sea bass, cod, and chicken.)

Slow-Roasted Tomatoes with Garlic and Thyme

Slow-roasted tomatoes are quite possibly one of the best things you'll ever put in your mouth. Okay, maybe that's exaggerating a bit, but they're delicious. They're juicy, flavorful, and so versatile—a perfect topping for chicken, fish, or bruschetta, a great addition to pasta and panini, and the base for any number of easy, elegant appetizers. Well-prepared as you are, you can make roasted tomatoes ahead and store them for a couple of days in the fridge.

THE GOODS

2 to 3 pounds plum or vine-ripened tomatoes, or 1 to 2 pints
   cherry tomatoes
1 to 2 tablespoons extra-virgin olive oil
2 garlic cloves, minced
2 teaspoons fresh thyme leaves (or simply toss in a few sprigs)
Salt

THE BREAKDOWN

1. Preheat the oven to 350°F.
2. Depending on what you're pairing them with and your preference, either cut tomatoes in half or make a small X down
   one side just to pierce the top of the skin.
3. Place the tomatoes in a large bowl and drizzle with the olive
   oil. Add the garlic and thyme, season with salt, and toss to
   coat evenly.
4. Roast on a parchment-lined baking sheet for 45 to 60 minutes.

The Facts: 60 calories; 23g fat; 3.5g saturated fat; 10g protein; 14g fiber

VARIATION: *For even slower-roasted, super-succulent tomatoes, roast at a lower heat—250°F for 3 to 4 hours.

Roasted Zucchini, Summer Squash, and Grape Tomatoes

*Yet another incredibly easy, healthful option for getting your veggies in
and incorporating some healthy fat into your diet (love the olive oil).
There's something about roasted zucchini and yellow squash and juicy
baby tomatoes that's utterly delicious. I think you'll agree. Go plain
with just a drizzle of olive oil and some sea salt and fresh garlic or dress
it up with some feta cheese and toasted pine nuts, a touch of basil or
thyme, or sprinkle with some grated Parmesan and fresh pepper before
putting into the oven.*

Makes 6 to 8 servings

THE GOODS AND THE BREAKDOWN
1. Preheat the oven to 400°F.
2. Take 2 medium zucchini and 2 medium yellow/summer squash, trim the ends, and cut into spears or diagonal strips or rounds about 1 inch thick.
3. Place the zucchini and squash, along with 1 pint of whole grape tomatoes, in a large bowl and drizzle with 3 tablespoons extra-virgin olive oil. Toss in 3 or 4 smashed garlic cloves (press down on the whole clove with your large chef's knife to smash or crack it). Sprinkle the veggies with salt and pepper to taste and mix.
4. Transfer your veggies to one or two baking sheets and roast for about 10 to 15 minutes, until lightly browned and soft.

The Facts: 80 calories; 6g fat; 1g saturated fat; 2g protein; 2g fiber

Roasted Brussels Sprouts with Balsamic-Glazed Pecans

The steps in this recipe are similar to those in the previous recipe. We're just swapping in some cancer-crushing cruciferous vegetables and turning up the heat slightly (note of caution: Be careful how many you eat if you're prone to gas).

Makes 6 servings

THE GOODS
1 pound Brussels sprouts, ends trimmed (cut the sprouts in half if they're medium to large or leave whole if they're small)
1 tablespoon extra-virgin olive oil
Salt to taste
2 tablespoons balsamic vinegar
1 teaspoon honey
¼ cup chopped toasted pecans

THE BREAKDOWN

1. Preheat the oven to 450°F.
2. Place the Brussels sprouts in a large bowl. Toss with the olive oil and season with salt.
3. Transfer to a baking sheet and roast for 20 to 25 minutes, until the leaves are browned. About halfway through, shake the pan to keep the sprouts from sticking.
4. In a small saucepan, simmer the balsamic vinegar with the honey for about 5 minutes to reduce a little. Pour the reduction over the pecans and stir to coat. Toss the glazed pecans with the sprouts.

The Facts: 100 calories; 6g fat; 0.5g saturated fat; 3g protein; 3g fiber

VARIATION: *Do something different and swap the Brussels sprouts for a whole head of cauliflower. Drizzle with 2 tablespoons olive oil, sprinkle with salt, and roast for 60 to 75 minutes.

Ridiculously Easy Roasted Red Peppers

THE GOODS AND THE BREAKDOWN

1. Preheat the oven to 450°F.
2. Cut 2 or 3 red peppers in half lengthwise and remove the seeds. Lightly grease a baking sheet with olive oil and place the peppers cut-side-down on the sheet.
3. Roast for 30 to 35 minutes, until the skin starts to blister and blacken. Turn every 10 minutes or so as they brown. Remove from the oven and place in a brown paper bag or in a bowl and cover with a plate—this helps loosen the skin so you can easily rub it off. Allow the peppers to cool for about 20 minutes. Peel or rub off the skin—it should come right off. Cut the peppers into thin strips or pieces.

The Facts: 15 calories; 0.5g fat; 0g saturated fat; 0g protein; 1g fiber

VARIATION: *Looking for an easier way out? Hold the pepper with metal tongs and place directly on a gas stove burner on a high flame. Continue turning to cook evenly. Cook until the skin blisters and blackens all over. Continue with placing the peppers in a brown bag or bowl. If you're prone to accidents, however, you might opt for the less hazardous oven option. We'd prefer not to have to call the fire department due to a kitchen mishap.

VARIATION: *Use roasted red peppers as a topping for poultry, fish, or burgers, on a sandwich or in a salad, or puree into a dip with olive oil or hummus. Check out the Roasted Red Pepper and Feta Dip on page 259.

Roasted Root Vegetables

Makes 8 to 10 servings

THE GOODS

1 pound sweet potatoes, cut into small chunks
1 pound parsnips, cut into small chunks
1 pound carrots, cut into 1-inch slices
1 pound red or yellow beets, quartered
2 small onions, quartered
6 garlic cloves
2 tablespoons chopped fresh rosemary
1 tablespoon chopped fresh thyme
Salt and freshly ground black pepper
¼ cup extra-virgin olive oil

THE BREAKDOWN

1. Preheat the oven to 425°F.
2. Combine the vegetables in a large bowl with the garlic, fresh herbs, and salt and pepper to taste.
3. Spread the vegetable mixture on two baking sheets brushed with olive oil or olive oil spray. Brush the vegetables with the olive oil.

4. Roast for 20 to 25 minutes, turn or shake the vegetables, and roast for another 20 to 25 minutes, until browned and tender.

The Facts: 170 calories; 6g fat; 1g saturated fat; 3g protein; 6g fiber

Roasted Fingerling Potatoes with Truffle Salt

These potatoes are ridiculously tasty and a great way to make a side dish a little fancier with the addition of truffle salt. You can find truffle salt at your local specialty food store or at Whole Foods. It's got a very strong flavor, so a small pinch goes a long way.

Makes 4 servings

THE GOODS

12 to 14 medium fingerling potatoes, or 20 to 25 baby fingerlings
1 ½ tablespoons extra-virgin olive oil
Salt and freshly ground black pepper
Truffle salt for dusting

THE BREAKDOWN

1. Preheat the oven to 425°F.
2. Place the potatoes in a large bowl and drizzle with the olive oil. Season with a tiny touch of regular salt and pepper to taste. Evenly distribute on a baking sheet and roast for 25 to 30 minutes, stirring midway through. Remove from the oven and dust with truffle salt, ¼ to ½ teaspoon, and serve.

The Facts: 190 calories; 4.5g fat; 0.5g saturated fat; 4g protein; 4g fiber

Gimme Some Meat! Lean and Mean Meats

Cheater's Secret: Keep your eye out for the grade and cut of meat when perusing the meat counter. Select cuts are generally your leanest options, whereas Prime and Choice are going to be more heavily marbled and fatty.

	Calories (per 3 ounces)	Total Fat	Saturated Fat
BEEF			
Tenderloin/filet mignon	129	5.5 grams	2 grams
Flank steak/London broil	120	4.6 grams	1.75 grams
95% Lean ground beef	105	4 grams	1.8 grams
Eye round roast	104	3 grams	1 gram
Top round roast	114	3.5 grams	1 gram
Top sirloin	98	2.8 grams	1 gram
LAMB			
Leg	112	4 grams	1.5 grams
Loin chop	113	4 grams	1.5 grams
BISON/BUFFALO			
Extra-lean burger	105	3 grams	1 gram
Top sirloin steak	103	2 grams	.8 gram
VEAL			
93% lean ground veal	122	5.75 grams	2 grams
Shank	92	2.4 grams	0.5 gram
PORK			
Chop, loin	125	7 grams	2.7 grams
CHICKEN			
Thigh, skinless	101	3 grams	1 gram
Leg, skinless	102	3 grams	1 gram
Breast, skinless, boneless	93	1 gram	0 grams
TURKEY			
Turkey breast, white meat	98	1 gram	0 grams
Ground turkey, 99% lean	90	1 gram	0 grams

Refresher Course—Key Goals from Weeks 1 to 4

❑ Resize portions—3 to 5 ounces protein, ½ to 1 cup rice/pasta/grain, 1 cup/piece fruit, 1 to 3 cups veggies/salad (aim to cut total portions by 15 to 25 percent and set your plate up as: ½ fruits/vegetables, ¼ lean protein, ¼ healthy, complex carbs).

❑ Eat 2 servings of fruit per day; aim to have vegetables with lunch AND dinner.

❑ Drink 1 ½ to 2 liters of water per day.

❑ Don't skip meals—you'll lower your calorie-burn capability!

❑ Cheat it up each week with one or two indulgent meals (order what you wish, but still consider portions) and one or two treats (between 200 and 300 calories each)

❑ Exercise at least three or four days this week. If stressed or emotional, add in an extra day or a relaxing yoga class to clear your head.

❑ Cut your alcohol intake per week by at least 25 percent.

❑ Food journaling . . . DO IT!

❑ Bring three to five basic office staples to work for snacks and emergencies.

❑ Re-plate and re-portion takeout and delivery food. Aim for half to three quarters of the to-go container.

❑ Watch portions like a hawk at restaurants, and leave at least 5 bites on the plate, if not a quarter to half. If the bread isn't awesome, lose it.

❑ Put all snacks and meals on a plate to halt mindless eating.

❑ If you hit a plateau, jump-start your metabolism again: For three to five days, boost fruit and veggie intake by 25 percent (make them the focus of every meal), and skip alcohol, coffee, dairy (except yogurt), and wheat products.

❑ Artificial sweeteners should be completely kicked to the curb by now. If not, bring intake down to ½ packet per day.

CHAPTER 5—WEEK 5

Boozing It Up with Brains

"The best hangover cure I've managed to come up with is being pregnant. No drinking, period."

—Danielle

WEEK 5 GOALS

- Continue cutting back alcohol intake by 25 percent and set a goal number of drinks to divvy up throughout the week as you wish, two, four, six, or eight total over a given week, and make them good to the last drop.
- Keep charging forward and sketch out ahead of time what your weekend ideally looks like in terms of meals, snacks, and drinks.
- Snap back from a long weekend by restocking your fridge before the binge with the basics both at home and at work.
- Plan your recovery day meals with healthy hangover alternatives (see pages 247 to 253 for ideas)
- Strong-arm your exercise routine to account for a few extra drinks and calories consumed. Add an extra day of activity, increase your time or intensity, or change things up—try a new class, like spinning or kickboxing, do something outdoors, or stretch out, relax, and tone those muscles with a Pilates or yoga class.

The Plan for Boozing and Schmoozing

Welcome to Week 5. You've cleared the potential stressful or emotional hump of last week—little bumps in the road are bound to happen sometimes. Life's full of challenges, and eating and drinking smartly is certainly among them sometimes, particularly when you're faced with countless food decisions (possibly hundreds) each and every day! Hey, you learn along the way what works for you, and hitting those bumps often makes food and drink that much more exciting, vibrant, and laughable, because you're constantly progressing and building healthy, delicious habits. None of us is perfect, I most definitely have my fair share of "oopses," and to be honest, I relish in them—isn't that what cheating's all about? Those moments of slippage keep me on my toes and keep me aware of the fact that my body really appreciates good-quality, well-prepared food (whether it's healthy or, in smaller quantities, not-so-healthy) and an unbelievable glass of wine or a well-made cocktail on occasion. Feed yourself junk, feel like junk.

By now, you should be moving along nicely, hitting (or just about hitting) double digits on the scale. You'll likely notice a distinct difference in how your clothes fit and how you feel overall. Sometimes the scale (and our metabolism) makes no sense. It's not budging, but you feel phenomenal and you're fitting back into clothes you haven't worn in three years. Your question: What gives? My answer: Who cares? What's on the scale is just a number! I realize that's quite easy to say, but it's true. Sometimes agonizing over a specific number is pointless and a complete and utter time-suck. Like I've been encouraging all along, focus on how your body feels—it's often way more telling than any scale ever will be.

Okay, so let's get down to business now that you've "detoxed" your way back to feeling like you can take on the world and whatever it chucks at you. We've all had those weeks that are so crazy you just can't wait for the weekend to unwind . . . and to think it's only Monday. (Place massive glass of wine in hand, ASAP. Please!) The weekend's the perfect time to take a breather, clear your head, put things in perspective, and push ahead with your healthy eating and cooking goals. It's also the perfect time to cheat it up, indulge, de-stress, and have some serious fun . . . while still handling food-and-drink-flowing situations with poise.

A Look at the Week Ahead:

Continue to Drink Less
As you've been doing, reduce alcohol intake by 25 percent and set a total goal number of drinks for the entire week. You might find it more effective to pick one weekday and one to two weekend days to sip one or two drinks each night and leave it at that.

Plan Your Weekends
Plan ahead for the weekend. What's on tap for your social calendar? Build your weekend food AND drink plan to give you some general guidelines to work with. If you've got a big night out ahead of you, skip the Bloody Mary at brunch and forgo the afternoon cookie treat. Keep your weekend in balance just as you do with your workweek.

Stock Up on Go-To Healthy Staples
Be sure to have some healthy basics still in the fridge when the weekend rolls around. This way, you'll actually have something decent to eat rather than having to go out every meal, and you're able to stay on track the day after a big boozing session.

The Best Hangover Remedy
Tend to a hangover with healthier meal options. Not to worry, they're still damn delicious and will help get you past the nausea and headache (see pages 247 to 253 for ideas). And if you're in for a heavy weekend of drinking, do a little extra at the gym the week before to compensate a little for the extra calories you'll be imbibing. Kick it up a notch and do something different or exercise a little longer, fifteen to thirty minutes.

Week 5: Sample—Party Planning
based on 1400-1600 calories

Week 5:	Monday	Tuesday	Wednesday
BREAKFAST 300-400 calories 7-9:30 a.m.	1 cup (½ cup dry) plain oatmeal (like McCann's) with cinnamon, ¼ cup diced apples, and 1 tablespoon chopped walnuts	HIT THE GYM Banana pre-workout 1 egg plus 1 egg white scrambled with 1 to 2 tablespoons feta or goat cheese and veggies of choice (like tomatoes and spinach or mushrooms and zucchini) 1 slice whole grain toast	1 cup high-fiber cereal (more than 5 grams fiber) with 1 cup strawberries (or a serving of fruit) and skim or low-fat soy milk
SNACK About 100 calories 10-11 a.m.	Skip it Cup of green or herbal tea	10 roasted cashews	½ cup cottage cheese
LUNCH 400-550 calories 12-2 p.m.	Open-faced tuna melt (1 slice whole grain toast with ¾ cup low-fat tuna salad and 1 slice melted cheddar or Gruyère cheese) Side salad or an apple	Sushi at work Miso soup and salad Spicy tuna roll (Remember the low-sodium soy sauce!)	Brown bag peanut butter and banana sandwich on whole grain bread and a string cheese or low-fat yogurt
SNACK 100-200 calories 3-5p.m.	Fruit-nut bar (like Clif Nectar or Kind) stashed at your desk	Small skim latte and 1 or 2 whole wheat fig bars (like Newman's Own)	1 apple and 10 cashews HIT THE GYM—evening body conditioning or boxing class

Thursday	Friday	Saturday	Sunday
2 whole grain waffles (like Van's Multigrain or Kashi Golean) with 1 cup berries and 1 tablespoon maple syrup	6 ounces low-fat plain yogurt with ¼ cup granola and sliced strawberry or diced mango	SLEEP LATE, then tackle hangover! 2 or 3 small homemade whole wheat pancakes (page 249) with banana slices, 2 tablespoons chopped pecans, and 1 tablespoon maple syrup plus 2 pieces turkey or veggie bacon	4 to 6 mile jog/run Pre-run: 1 small nectarine and ½ whole wheat English muffin with peanut butter
1 pear	Skip it—the granola filled you up at breakfast	Water with lemon or Mango-Peach Iced Tea (page 267) Keep hydrating!	
Make-your-own salad You know the drill . . . 1. mixed greens, spinach, or arugula 2. some type of protein 3. whatever veggies or fruits you wish to add 4. a sprinkle of 1 or 2 of the following: cheese, dried fruit, nuts, olives, and/or avocado 5. 1 to 2 tablespoons vinaigrette or olive oil and lemon	Catered work lunch, make it work to your advantage ½ grilled chicken, tomato, mozzarella, and pesto panini with a side salad OR 1 piece of pizza (try to get some veggies on there) and a big ol' side salad	Light lunch on the go: Greek salad with 2 ounces grilled shrimp or a hard-boiled egg (tomato, cucumbers, olives, 2 tablespoons feta, and red onion) plus 2 tablespoons red wine vinaigrette OR Watermelon-Feta Salad (page 120) plus ½ cup chickpeas	CHEAT MEAL #1: Sunday afternoon football watching (and drinking) 2 buffalo wings with 2 teaspoons blue cheese and celery or 5 nachos ½ veggie burger or grilled chicken sandwich Share an order of fries— they're too good at your local pub to resist 2 light beers
0% or 2% Fage Greek yogurt with honey and 2 teaspoons pistachios Yoga or Pilates class after work	⅓ cup trail mix	HIT THE GYM, then the GROCERY STORE! Lots of water and a little sweating, your hangover's done and gone!	Grab a seltzer with lime in between your beers to pace yourself on a Sunday afternoon!

Continued

Week 5:	Monday	Tuesday	Wednesday
DINNER 400-600 calories 7-8:30 p.m.	1 ½ cups veggie chili (like Amy's Organic) with 2 tablespoons shredded cheddar cheese and 1 tablespoon light sour cream Side salad or 1 to 2 cups steamed or fresh veggies	Girls' night at out local Latin place with the BEST mojitos Share the famous roasted corn 4 ounces grilled tuna with mango salsa ¾ cup black beans and rice	4 ounces Moroccan Lamb Meatballs with Lemon-Mint Yogurt Sauce (page 262) 2 cups Roasted Zucchini, Summer Squash, and Grape Tomatoes (page 220)
SNACK 100-150 calories 8:30-9:30 p.m. (If you're not hungry, SKIP IT! Work in desserts and treats when you really want them and they're damn worth it!)	Fruit or nada, you've got mojitos coming tomorrow night—think ahead!		2 squares of dark chocolate
WATER	1 ½ liters	2 liters	2 liters
ALCOHOL/ OOPS!		2 mojitos (it was supposed to be 1, but they're too darn good)	
EXERCISE		60 minutes	Body conditioning or boxing class

Thursday	Friday	Saturday	Sunday
CHEAT MEAL #2: Date night Watch the wine intake, tipsy girl! Make it one of your fun meals for the week. Share an appetizer and be mindful of entrée portions.	Super-easy meal after work, prep for a long night out 1 cup whole wheat pasta with 3 to 5 ounces shrimp sautéed with 2 teaspoons olive oil, 1 garlic clove, ¼ cup chopped sun-dried tomatoes, and ¾ cup canned artichoke hearts. Sprinkle with 2 tablespoons grated Parmesan cheese. 2 cups arugula or mixed greens with 2 teaspoons olive oil and fresh lemon juice.	Friend's cocktail party 1. Scope the scene first 2. Build a plate in your head 3. Armed and ready to eat 1 chicken skewer, 2 meat-balls, 1 spinach-feta phyllo thingy (delish!), bunch of fresh veggies with 1 table-spoon dip, 2 crackers with Brie, 3 strawberries 2 glasses of champagne (okay, so we went just over the 6 drink mark, but you paced yourself, at a cocktail party nonetheless. Swap a "treat" for an extra 2 drinks and keep cheating.)	Sober up and make Sunday dinner for you and your roomie or significant other 1 ½ cups Chicken with Mushrooms and Red Wine Sauce (page 160) 1 Steamed Artichoke with 1 tablespoon Garlic and Lemon Sauce (page 45)
		CHEAT TREAT #1 2 Bite-Size Bebè Brownies (page 263)	2 Chic Chocolate-Covered Strawberries (page 264)
1 ½ liters	2 liters	Extra water to beat your hangover—3 liters	2 liters
2 glasses wine	Drinks out with your girls! 2 vodka-sodas and 1 glass of Prosecco	2 glasses champagne	2 light beers (at 11 drinks, you're a little on the high side this week—keep next week on the low end)
Yoga or Pilates		Quickie 30 to 45 minute sweat-fest	4 to 6 mile run/jog

Week 5: Your Weekly Food Journal

Week 5:	Monday	Tuesday	Wednesday
BREAKFAST 300 to 400 calories *(Note your hunger level on a scale of 1 to 10 after each meal!)*			
SNACK About 100 calories *(If you're not hungry, skip it!)*			
LUNCH 400 to 550 calories			
SNACK 100 to 200 calories			
DINNER 400 to 600 calories			
SNACK 100 to 150 calories *(Work in desserts and treats when you really want them and they're damn worth it!)*			
WATER			
ALCOHOL/ OOPS!			
EXERCISE			

Thursday	Friday	Saturday	Sunday

Week 5—Cheater's Shopping List:

❑ Vegetables: 3 to 5 (or more) for the week: 3 tomatoes, 1 pint cherry tomatoes, 1 cucumber, arugula, spinach, 1 onion, zucchini, 2 artichokes, mushrooms

❑ Fruit: 2 to 4 types or more, your pick (enough to get you through 5 to 7 days, 2 servings a day): apples, bananas, strawberries, pears, watermelon

❑ Protein: 1 pound chicken breasts, 4 ounces shrimp, 1 pound ground lamb, eggs, 1 can tuna, turkey/veggie bacon

❑ Healthy carbs: whole grain cereal (more than 5 grams fiber, less than 7 grams sugar), whole grain bread, whole wheat pasta, whole wheat pancake mix

❑ Dairy/calcium: feta cheese, cheddar cheese, string cheese, 3 or 4 low-fat plain yogurts or cottage cheese, skim or soy milk

❑ Other: kalamata olives, dates, 1 can artichoke hearts, sun-dried tomatoes, 1 can veggie chili (like Amy's), pecans

❑ Seasonings and spices: mint, cumin, coriander, 1 lemon

❑ Snacks and staples: all-natural granola and/or fruit-nut bars (like Kind, Larabar, Clif Nectar), pistachios, whole wheat fig bars

❑ Dessert/treat: strawberries, dark chocolate squares/bar

Weekend Prep

Just as you've been doing since day one, take a look at what your weekend has in store for you so you're able to plan accordingly. Write one or two heavier eating/drinking meals into your food journal ahead of time so you don't end up with a string of four or five wrecking-ball evenings. Think about what's on the agenda. Do you have friends coming into town or your best friend's birthday bash on Saturday night? Meeting friends to watch an afternoon football or basketball game at your neighborhood pub (which likely means early afternoon drinking), or are you hosting a blow-out house party? Going out for a ridiculous meal at the new restaurant you've been dying to try or grabbing brunch with your girlfriends where the mimosas just don't stop?

Plot out your social commitments and where you want to allot a more indulgent meal or a few extra drinks on a particular day or night. Clearly we can't plan for everything in life, but having a baseline idea of what your week might look like can really help alleviate the stress and potential caloric disaster of one too many nights out. Test out working with an ideal number of drinks per week and distribute them accordingly depending on what events and soirees are on your calendar. As you're already doing, choose the appropriate number, and shoot for at least 25 percent less than what you're currently sipping. So if you're averaging ten or twelve drinks a week (or more), let's revise that to six or eight, a more realistic target for weight loss, and fewer hangovers. If you're not a big drinker and typically have five or six drinks a week, bring it down a notch to three or four. And if you're coming in at just two or three, you're good to go, no major concerns. Imbibe and enjoy. If you foresee an extremely social week of drinking ahead of you, consider swapping your two *cheat and eat* treats or desserts for an extra two or three drinks. That's some genius cheating right there. This is, after all, the diet you can drink on.

Under the Influence: The Down-Low on Alcohol

I'm the first to admit, I love a good glass of wine, a refreshing cocktail, or a frothy beer. I certainly wouldn't go so far as tagging myself as a "boozehound," but I do like a solid drink—I went to college in the South, I think it was bred into me. What's the deal with alcohol and weight? It's not the devil, but it can and will pack on excess poundage if you're not careful. If you can't get rid of that spare tire around your middle section, look no further than the wineglass in front of you. I know, it's precisely what you didn't want to hear, but it's incredible how quickly alcohol calories can add up. Your average 5-ounce glass of wine comes out to about 110 to 120 calories. Same thing for a 12-ounce light beer and a 1.5-ounce shot of liquor. On the downside, alcohol's converted directly into sugar and tends to make a cozy home right around our waistline. Hence the endearing term "beer gut."

Curb the drinking and you'll undoubtedly see a shift in your weight as well as in your sleeping patterns, energy levels, and digestive system. If you've ever woken up after a long night out feeling bloated and gassy and can't hold down any form of food, you know what I'm talking about.

On the upside, there are a lot of good things associated with alcohol. There's a cheating silver lining in just about everything! As you've likely heard, red wine is loaded with antioxidants and helps reduce risk of heart disease and high blood pressure and can slightly raise "good" HDL cholesterol—if you're consuming one glass per day for women, one to two glasses for men. This is where we get the "French paradox" theory—many French drink wine daily, but their diet tends to be higher in "less healthy" saturated fats (read: Brie and triple-cream cheeses) and yet somehow they have a much lower risk of heart disease than Americans. They're obviously on to something with red and white wine. Studies show that the antioxidant compound resveratrol, found in red grape skins and red wine, and tyrosol, found in white wine, seem to be the keys to wine's heart-health benefits. Preliminary research shows that the resveratrol in red wine may also help fight fat cell development and hamper fat storage. Additional research notes that the flavonoids (antioxidants) in wine may boost cognitive function, reducing risk of Alzheimer's, and that moderate wine drinkers (one glass per day for women, two for men) tend to have higher levels of heart-healthy omega-3 fats. And finally, to the delight of all of you beer drinkers, specific types of brew, particularly darker porters and stouts like Guinness, are also rich in disease-fighting antioxidants and may help lower cholesterol and cancer risk, thanks to barley and hops.

See, we managed to fit in your beloved pinot noir, pale ale, or vodka–club soda. But before you drink up, let's discuss which alcoholic beverages will take you further in terms of calorie smarts and taste. Would you rather have one strawberry daiquiri or three mojitos? Maybe it depends on the day, but check out the stats in the next section so you can do some alcoholic damage control.

Cheater's Secret: Keep at least three of five weekday nights bone dry. Sure, a glass of wine with dinner each night can be perfectly healthful, but if you're looking for easy ways to shave off calories, skipping a drink is a no-brainer. Again, 100 calories per glass of wine: 100 extra calories per day is about ten extra pounds a year.

Get Your Drink On

Cheers! Before you throw back a drink or three, here are a few handy rules of thumb to keep in mind.

- **Manage the Mixer**—You've likely read this a zillion times, but sugary sweet mixers and juices like tonic water, soda, cranberry juice, sour mix, and fruity, creamy "girly" drinks like piña coladas and apple martinis are caloric disasters on ice just waiting to be sucked down. Sugary mixers and juices can easily add on an extra 100 to 300 calories to your preferred drink—which may turn a single drink into the caloric equivalent of a small meal! I realize it sounds pretty grim, and by no means would I ever eternally banish any drink from touching your lips, but just consider the frequency and occasions that you're having richer, calorie-laden drinks. If you're basking in the sun on the beach in Costa Rica or Brazil on vacation, yeah, a piña colada or tropical drink is a must-have once or twice over the course of three or four days. Or if you're at your family's annual holiday party and it's tradition to have a glass of your uncle's infamous eggnog or your cousin's killer White Russian, absolutely start sipping (one to two glasses, not five).

- **Revise Your Standard Order**—On an average week, however, consider where your alcohol calories are coming from and tweak things to make them work to your cheating advantage. For instance, if vodka-cranberry is your standard go-to order at the bar, start with one and then switch to a lighter version . . . ordering a vodka and club soda or seltzer with a splash of cranberry and a lime. Same flavor and concept, a whole lot less sugar and calories (there's zilch in club soda and seltzer). Otherwise, opt for a flavored vodka or other type of liquor . . . a citrus or raspberry flavored vodka, for example, with seltzer water and a lime wedge. More flavor, fewer calories and sugar. And if you're a die-hard devotee of sweeter drinks and fancy cocktails and can't go without them, cheat it up and again trade in your *cheat and eat* dessert calories for an extra two or three drinks over a week. Sneaky, but you end up with your desired alcohol in the end.

- **Space It Out and Cut Corners When Drinking for the Long Haul**—Whether you're planning to attend an all-day beach party, a wedding reception that kicks off at 2 p.m., a Saturday brunch that flows into dinner, or you're simply bracing for a particularly long night out, there are those situations that require a whole lot of drinks over a whole lot of hours, which generally translates to a whole lot of calories. Here are some quick cheating tactics to make the best of it and still have a great time:

  ◆ If you've got a long evening ahead of you at your local bar and are obsessed with beer that's heavier and more caloric (basically most beers on the list that aren't tagged "light"), start with one or two real-deal beers and then switch it up to a "light" brand, like Amstel, Corona, Heineken, or Coors Light, to save a few calories, typically about 50 per serving.

  ◆ Summertime day drinking is the perfect occasion to reach for a spritzer, half white or rosé wine and half seltzer or club soda. It's refreshing, half the calories, and somewhat hydrating at the same time!

  ◆ Extend your stay at the bar and make your drinks last longer by having a glass of water or seltzer between each alcoholic beverage. Staying hydrated keeps you from feeling horrendous the following morning and keeps alcohol calories in check. And if you just want to be out but aren't up for a night of boozing, keeping a bubbly glass of seltzer and lime in your hand is a great call. No one will know it's missing the vodka.

Cheater's Secret: If you're having a frozen margarita or frozen drink, have one small glass and be done. Frozen margaritas and fruity drinks can quickly blow calories and sugar out of the water (400 calories and beyond), in part because they're typically made with sugary bottled mixes and because they're generally served in enormous glasses the size of your head. If you love them, stick to a small one—one—and switch to a lighter drink, if any, like a glass of wine or a light beer afterward. Better yet, get your margarita on the rocks made from scratch (with or without a touch of salt) and skip the excess sugar from bottled mixes. And if you're

CHEAT SHEET: Budgeting Your Booze

Item	Size	Calories
Seltzer water with lemon or lime	8 ounces	0!
Champagne/Prosecco	5 ounces	98
Light beer	12 ounces	105
Shot of liquor (vodka, gin, bourbon, whiskey, rum, tequila, etc.)	1.5 ounces	110
Vodka and club soda	8.5 ounces	110
White wine	5 ounces	114
Red wine	5 ounces	115
Bloody Mary	10 ounces	125
Martini	2.2 ounces	135
Mojito	3.5 ounces	149
Beer	12 ounces	155
Kamikaze shot	3 ounces	180
Rum and Coke	8.5 ounces	182
Vodka and tonic	8.5 ounces	183
Gin and tonic	7 ounces	189
Screwdriver (vodka and OJ)	7 ounces	208
Cosmopolitan	4 ounces	213
Vodka and cranberry	8.5 ounces	217
Apple martini	4 ounces	235
Long Island iced tea	8.5 ounces	276
Piña colada	8 ounces	303
Margarita on the rocks	6 ounces	327
Amaretto sour	6 ounces	421
Strawberry daiquiri	8 ounces	421
Frozen margarita	8 ounces	500

CHEAT SHEET: Beverage Breakdown

Item	Size	Calories	Sugar
Starbucks, Mocha Frappuccino with whipped cream	Grande, 16 ounces	380	47 grams
Better Bet: Starbucks Iced Skim Café Mocha	Tall, 12 ounces	130	20 grams
Starbucks Vanilla Latte with 2% milk	Grande, 16 ounces	250	34 grams
Better Bet: Starbucks Skim Latte with cinnamon	Grande, 16 ounces	130	18 grams
Jamba Juice Strawberry Surf Rider	Original, 24 ounces	480	105 grams
Naked Juices/Smoothies Berry Blast	Bottle, 15.2 ounces	260	52 grams
Better Bet: Jamba Juice Bright Eyed and Blueberry	Small, 12 ounces	200	33 grams
Vitamin Water, Energy Tropical Citrus or Revive Fruit Punch	Bottle, 20 ounces	130	33 grams
Better Bet: Hint Water (natural flavors like Mango Grapefruit and Raspberry-Lime)	Bottle, 16 ounces	0	0
Snapple Peach Iced Tea	Bottle, 16 ounces	200	48 grams
Lipton Iced Brisk Lemon Iced Tea	Bottle, 20 ounces	325	81 grams
Better Bet: Teas' Tea (or any unsweetened iced tea)	Bottle, 16.9 ounces	0	0
Soda (Coke, ginger ale, Dr Pepper) (Hello, high-fructose corn syrup!)	Bottle, 20 ounces	239	66 grams
Better Bet: Flavored seltzer or sparkling water or plain with lemon or lime	Bottle, 16 ounces	0	0
Better Bet: GuS Grown-up Soda or Fizzie Lizzie (if it's got to be soda on occasion; these don't contain high-fructose corn syrup)	Bottle, 12 ounces	90 to 98	24 grams
Orange juice (or any juice, ideally it's 100% juice)	Carton, 16 ounces	217	43 grams
Better Bet: Freshly squeezed OJ or other juice	½ cup (4 ounces)	57	10.5 grams
Better Bet: ½ OJ and ½ seltzer (a spritzer!)	1 cup (8 ounces)	57	10.5 grams
Red Bull or Rockstar Energy Drink	Can, 16 ounces	227/276	55/61 grams
WAY Better Bet: WATER!!!	Unlimited	0	0

looking to get the most of out your drink (and a feel-good buzz), frozen drinks from a machine often run super-short on the alcohol. When you're shelling out $8 to $12 per drink, I'm all about getting the most for your money!

Cheater's Secret: Remember that many restaurants overpour wine. I love that restaurants and wine bars are usually overly generous with their wine pours, but it's easy to forget that a single serving of wine is just 5 ounces rather than the typical 8- to 10-ounce pour they're serving you. Do the math and that's nearly double the calories. Sip slowly, take your time to savor the vino, and make that glass last a little longer because there's a good probability it's closer to two servings than just one.

Liquid Sugar: Other Empty-Calorie Beverages

While we're on the topic of drinks, I figured I'd take a quick detour to discuss some calorie-soaked nonalcoholic beverages that might creep their way into your day more frequently. We're working strategically here—if you're sipping on a Frappuccino or vitamin-enhanced water every now and then, no big deal, but if you're downing one or more daily, that's an easy item to have less frequently, shave off a good 100 to 300 calories, and shed some pounds without missing too much. Take a look at where extra liquid calories and sugar might be making their way into your diet (remember that 8 teaspoons, or 32 grams, of added sugar is your daily recommended value). See "Cheat Sheet Beverage Breakdown on the opposite page for reference.

Kiss Cottonmouth Good-bye: Handling a Hangover . . . Healthfully

You don't recall much of last night, but you're damn sure of one thing—you've awoken with a miserable, head-splitting hangover. Admit it, we've all been there on occasion (even nutritionists). The morning after an "out-till-3 a.m., late-night pizza-eating" bender of an evening and you know the standard scenario . . . the warm sun's streaming through your billowy Pottery Barn curtains, you peel your comforter back with all your might, and struggle to open your weary, bloodshot eyes. "What the hell did I do last night? Where am I? Crap, what time is it? Did I sleep the day away?" A frantic look to your right—sigh of relief, you're in your own bed. A darted look to your left—double sigh of relief, there's no stranger lying beside you. Time to get up and deal with the thick layer of cotton in your mouth and the jackhammer that's pounding in your head. We're beginning this journey at rock bottom and boldly moving upward to the jackpot goal of reviving you from last night's haze with some healthful first aid for your hangover from hell. Damn those last two tequila shots at 3 a.m.!

Let's take a moment to break down the anatomy of a hangover. Why does your body feel like it could lie on the couch all day long in a near-comatose state, and how can you nurse yourself back to normalcy? It's plain and simple; your body's exhausted and majorly dehydrated and it's screaming, literally, for the vitamins and minerals it's been depleted of (thank you, Mr. Dirty Martini #3).

Hangovers rear their ugly heads due to a number of physiological factors affecting the brain and bodily organs, particularly the liver and kidney. The body views alcohol as a toxic threat, and does its best to metabolize it and excrete it from our systems. Thanks to the diuretic effects of alcohol, our poor kidneys are gushing water at light speed, sending alcohol and water out in urine. Yes, this is what happens after you "break the seal." Other pleasant hangover symptoms like diarrhea, vomiting, sweating, an upset stomach, and inflammation can cause additional water loss along with weakness, light-headedness, headaches, and the inability to sleep well. Alcohol overindulgence can also cause low blood sugar, or hypoglycemia, which again leads to weakness and lethargy. And last, all that water loss causes electrolyte imbalance—our cells' potassium and sodium levels are totally out of whack without sufficient water. Think of your body's hangover cell as a shriveled-up prune—it's parched! The consumption of four drinks over the course of a night leads to the excretion of an entire quart of water, 32 ounces. So that basically leaves you out stranded in the desert, pining for some serious rehydration.

Cheater's Secret: Wonder why you can't drink like you used to in college? That's because our ability to metabolize alcohol (and beat out hangovers) decreases as we age. For females, we often see a drop-off around the age of twenty-five. Your college days of drinking at frat parties or clubs until the wee hours of the morning and waking up not feeling a thing are sadly over. Hey, at least you're a cheap date these days.

As genuine as your intentions might be to get right back on the "horse of health" and plow through your headache, shakiness, and nausea, most of us generally don't think to gravitate toward the healthful foods and beverages we really need to alleviate a hangover. It's usually a juicy cheeseburger and shoestring french fries and the biggest Diet Coke you can find—from the fountain, of course. In a conversation a few years back with my charming, intelligent, very social younger brother, he asked, "Is it really true that you're supposed to have grease after a big night of drinking to soak up the alcohol?" I'm not really sure where this myth originated, but I responded to him by asking, "Well, how do you normally feel after you've had a huge meal swimming in fat and grease—on an average day when you're *not* hung over?" "Like crap," he quickly responded. So why on earth do we think this type of meal would help cure a hangover when your body's already feeling utterly horrible?

Think about nutrient-rich combos instead the next time you need a morning pick-me-up to help put you on the path to hangover recovery. One possible option could be a super-easy egg scramble with tomato, spinach, and feta cheese with whole grain toast and a cup of fresh fruit salad and as much water as you can guzzle—shoot for two to three liters over the course of the day. A little protein, healthy fat, some complex carbohydrates for a quick blood sugar boost, and lots of water go a long way to nurse that hangover. Okay, I'll concede here—sometimes you just need some grease. It might not make you feel much better in the long run (or it may backfire on you—like one of my dearest friends who, in dire hung-over straights, beelined for Burger King before boarding a plane, only to puke her grease-stained meal back up in the airport bathroom), but for the first few bites, that grease is like utter heaven. So like the cheaters we are, let's compromise around the concept of balance here—part healthful, nutrient-rich meal to repair your torn-up insides, and part greasy-spoon indulgence. A grilled chicken sandwich with avocado and french fries, ideally half the portion if you're served a mountain of them. Better yet, swap them for sweet potato fries if you can get them. You've got all the components you need—lean protein to reboot your energy and metabolism, some healthy fat from the avocado to buck your inflamed intestines, and of course your fries. Guzzle down a few massive glasses of water and you're on your way to recovery.

> *Cheater's Secret:* Sweet potatoes rock out with antioxidants and may help minimize inflammation and your pounding headache. Remember, you're shooting for a fist-size portion, one small sweet tater or half of a large one. Or about a cup of fries. For speedy prep, fork them a few times, wrap in a paper towel, and microwave for 5 minutes. Otherwise, make baked fries and cut a sweet potato into rounds or thin wedges, brush with a tablespoon of olive oil, sprinkle with salt, pepper, garlic, and paprika, and bake at 400°F for 20 to 25 minutes, until crisp.

If neither of those meal suggestions will do and you're really in need of breakfast comfort food, dig into two small pancakes (if you have the option of whole grain or whole wheat, take it) topped with a cup of fresh berries, a drizzle of Vermont's finest maple syrup, and a side of low-fat plain or vanilla yogurt. Why not opt for the mouthwatering mountain of fluffy buttermilk pancakes drowning in syrup, you ask? Tasty as they are, they have a greater chance of leaving you in a coma on the couch afterward. Helping a hangover requires restoring your body with the vitamins, minerals, and water it's been depleted of. Whole grain pancakes pack in B vitamins and fiber, which help replenish energy levels and stabilize blood sugar levels, which have been temporarily kicked out of whack while your body attempts to process all that alcohol. The side of yogurt gives a nice dose of protein, calcium, and fruit and provides a quick burst of natural sugar, antioxidants, and water to quell your pounding head and help you rehydrate.

Indeed, traditional buttery, golden pancakes are delicious, but like most other items made with white refined flour, our bodies digest pancakes, waffles, and donuts very quickly. As you learned in Chapter 1, when we eat refined flour and sugar, our bodies break down these carbohydrates into glucose (the building blocks of energy), utilize the energy, our blood sugar spikes up, and our metabolism quickly peaks. Shortly afterward, again because refined foods are so easily digested, our blood sugar plummets and our energy levels are zapped. And then we're back to being tired and hungry again, not to mention still feeling like a train wreck because of the hangover. It's a vicious cycle, but fiber helps to halt it. Fiber-rich foods like whole grain flours (and pancakes), multigrain breads, fruits and vegetables, high-fiber cereals, and healthy grains like brown rice and whole wheat pasta and couscous all work to stabilize blood sugar and hunger and keep our metabolisms going along all day at a steady clip. In the end, if you're gonna do regular pancakes, waffles, or French toast, keep portions small (silver-dollar-size pancakes are perfect, or a slice of French toast) and pair them like we did above, with a side of yogurt and berries or a poached egg for some protein and a teensy bit of fat to keep blood sugar levels stable.

So to bridge all of this information together, I've provided a few easy recipes to help your hangover at home.

Egg Scramble with Tomato, Spinach, and Feta Cheese

Pair this delicious scramble with 1 or 2 slices seven grain or 100% whole wheat toast, or 1 whole wheat English muffin and/or 2 pieces turkey bacon or sausage and 1 cup fruit salad.

Makes 1 serving

THE GOODS
   1 teaspoon unsalted butter or olive oil
   1 whole egg and 2 egg whites (or 2 eggs)
   2 teaspoons low-fat or skim milk
   Salt
   Freshly ground black pepper

2 tablespoons crumbled feta cheese
½ cup diced tomato
½ cup fresh spinach or ⅓ cup frozen spinach, thawed and
  drained

THE BREAKDOWN

1. Melt the butter in an 8- or 10-inch nonstick skillet over medium heat.
2. In a small bowl, whisk together the eggs and whites, milk, a dash of salt, and pepper to taste. Add the feta, tomato, and spinach.
3. Add the egg mixture to the skillet and allow the eggs to start cooking slightly, about 30 seconds. Using a spatula or wooden spoon, push the edges toward the center of the pan and tilt as needed to allow for even cooking. Continue turning the eggs until completely cooked through but soft and fluffy, 1 to 2 minutes.

The Facts: 250 calories; 17g fat; 5g saturated fat; 18g protein; 2g fiber

---

EGG SCRAMBLE SUBSTITUTIONS . . .

1. Start with: 1 egg and 2 whites (or 2 eggs)

2. Pick your "poison"
- Add some cheese, if desired
- 2 tablespoons shredded cheddar cheese
- 2 tablespoons shredded Monterey Jack cheese
- 2 tablespoons crumbled feta cheese
- 2 tablespoons grated Parmesan or Pecorino Romano cheese
- 2 tablespoons goat cheese

3. Add 1 to 3 veggies (or go buck wild and throw in more!)
- ½ cup diced tomato
- ⅓ cup frozen spinach, thawed and drained, or ½ cup fresh spinach
- ½ cup sliced mushrooms
- 1 tablespoon diced onion or green onions

- ½ cup steamed chopped broccoli florets
- ½ cup chopped steamed asparagus
- ½ cup diced green, yellow, or red bell peppers
- ½ cup roasted red pepper strips

4. Add fun stuff and fresh herbs!
- ⅓ cup salsa or pico de gallo
- 1 to 2 tablespoons chopped jalapeños or other hot peppers
- ⅓ cup black beans
- 2 to 3 thin slices of avocado
- 1 to 2 teaspoons minced fresh basil, tarragon, cilantro, chives, or mint

Pancake Perfection

Inhale a mountain of steaming pancakes at your local diner and you might not feel so hot an hour later, but like any seemingly "indulgent" food, when prepared with good ingredients and served up in the right portions, pancakes can absolutely become part of a healthful, yummy meal. Get your comfort-food fix and keep things balanced by serving pancakes with a small side of yogurt and berries or an egg. The egg or yogurt add in some protein and keep your blood sugar and satiety rocking steady.

Makes 2 to 3 servings

THE GOODS
½ cup all-purpose flour
½ cup whole wheat flour
1 cup low-fat milk or buttermilk
1 teaspoon baking powder
½ teaspoon baking soda
2 tablespoons sugar
2 teaspoons vanilla extract
2 eggs
¼ teaspoon salt
Canola oil or melted butter for brushing

THE BREAKDOWN

1. In a large bowl, whisk together all the ingredients except the canola oil together until well blended. Add any filling of choice if desired (see below).
2. Heat a medium nonstick skillet and brush with canola oil or butter. Pour about 2 tablespoons batter into the skillet to make silver dollar pancakes (it will make 6 altogether) or about ¼ cup batter to make medium pancakes (it will make 3 or 4 altogether). Flip the pancakes when bubbles start to form at the top, about 1 ½ minutes, then cook until lightly golden on the underside. Repeat until all the batter is used.

The Facts: 250 calories; 4.5g fat; 1.5g saturated fat; 12g protein; 3g fiber

Cheater's Secret: Who knew *buttermilk* is actually very low in fat? It's a great, creamier, slightly richer addition to pancake batter or to dressings and marinades.

VARIATION: *For a heartier, higher-fiber pancake, try buckwheat flour, which packs in fiber and protein.

VARIATION: *Sweet shortcut—Use a whole grain or whole wheat pancake mix.

Pancake Filling and Topping Substitutions . . .

Step 1. Start with the basic pancake mix
Step 2. Pick your "poison"
Add or top with:

2 sliced bananas, ¼ cup chopped pecans or walnuts, 1 teaspoon ground cinnamon
1 cup fresh blueberries and/or sliced strawberries
¾ cup canned pumpkin, 1 teaspoon ground cinnamon, ½ teaspoon freshly grated nutmeg
1 cup diced apples, ¼ cup chopped walnuts, 1 ½ teaspoons ground cinnamon (for a quick warm topping, cook apples,

nuts, cinnamon, and 2 teaspoons sugar over medium heat until soft, 8 to 10 minutes)

¼ cup dark chocolate chips and 1 to 2 sliced bananas

1 to 2 sliced bananas, sautéed with 1 teaspoon butter, 1 tablespoon dark rum, 1 teaspoon dark brown sugar, and 2 tablespoons walnuts (use as a topping)

Berry syrup—Heat 2 cups mixed berries, like strawberries, blackberries, and blueberries, in a small saucepan with 2 teaspoons sugar and the juice of ¼ lemon. Cook over medium heat for 8 to 10 minutes, until a chunky sauce/syrup forms (use as a topping).

Pair it with: A dollop of plain low-fat yogurt and some additional fresh fruit on top of your short stack for a little boost of fiber, protein, and calcium to balance out those carbohydrates. Use a drizzle, 2 teaspoons or so, of real-deal maple syrup, molasses, or honey. Skip the sugar-free, fat-free stuff with all the additives and opt for Vermont's finest.

Making the Best of Brunch Out When You're Hung Over

If your night was just over the edge and turning on your stove simply just isn't an option, here's a good game plan for brunch at the neighborhood diner or the local hot spot you and your friends frequent.

1. Eggs Benedict (edited)—2 poached eggs on an English muffin (whole wheat if they have them); pop some spinach on there and make it Florentine for some extra B vitamins, folate, and fiber. Hollandaise sauce on the side, or skipped entirely (too many calories, too much saturated fat). Grab a side of turkey bacon (or 1 to 2 slices of regular bacon) if you're really craving it and try to swap greasy hash browns for a side of fruit salad or mixed greens. Snag a few bites of hash browns from your friend's plate if you must. Most places now have healthier options on the menu, like a side of fruit or turkey bacon. If you don't see what you're looking for, ASK . . . it's harmless!

2. A grilled chicken or portobello sandwich or a turkey burger or lean beef burger (remember your 4-ounce protein

portion—the burger's probably 8 ounces). Top it with some type of veggie, whether roasted red pepper, grilled onion, tomato, lettuce, or the works. Add a slice of cheese and/or 2 to 3 thin slices of avocado or a small dollop of guacamole—rich avocado boasts heart-healthy monounsaturated fats and does wonders to satisfy your craving for something "deliciously indulgent." Either skip the greasy fries and opt for a side of fruit salad—I promise you'll feel better—or order both if you must and have half of the fries. Again, that fruit's a hydrator, and you're pretty parched right now.

Cheater's Secret: If you thought avocado was off-limits because of its fat content, think again. Avocado brings a lot to the table— taste, texture, and healthy monounsaturated fats. Do keep in mind, however, that it's high in calories—sorry to disappoint you, but no free-for-all guacamole and chips. One whole avocado has about 300 calories and 27 grams of fat (only 4 of them are saturated, though!). One fourth of the avocado is equivalent to a single serving, about 75 calories. Think 3 to 4 thin slices. And if you were wondering, avocado's a fruit, not a vegetable!

3. Steak or grilled tofu or chicken salad with lots of deliciously fresh veggies. A salad for Sunday "hung-over brunch"? Remember, fruits and vegetables are loaded with vitamins and minerals and water to hydrate you and flush the alcohol out of your pores. Request a vinaigrette dressing or olive oil and vinegar. Heavy, creamy dressings like ranch and blue cheese have a time and a place in moderation, but this isn't one of them. Too high in saturated fat and calories, they're not the best complement to a cleansing, nutrient-dense salad and may just send that queasy stomach of yours running to the bathroom in upheaval. To add a cheating component to your meal of greens, order a side of fries or sweet potato fries and share it.

Sadly, there's no easy, magic-pill cure for hangovers, but a day of detoxing with fresh foods and lots of water will do wonders. Don't stress too much on the calories; otherwise you'll end up driving yourself crazy and feeling worse. Just try to keep things from landsliding from one less-than-healthful meal to the next. The most important thing is to keep a "bender evening" (or the occasional "bender weekend") isolated and head right back to your established healthful habits so you can keep moving forward, feeling and looking your best.

Cocktailed Consumption: Cheat and Eat at Parties with Nibbles, Snacks, and Sweets

In my opinion, weekend cocktails go best with some thoughtful nibblings. Whether you're hosting a pregame wine and cheese gathering or are attending a liquor-soaked cocktail party, we've got some chic, super-tasty appetizers for you to master with ease. Who knew you could put out such a deceptively gourmet spread. A few good-quality ingredients, simple preparation, and effortlessly perfect presentation is how you'll blow the crowd away, and you'll ensure that you're keeping things light, fresh, healthful, and, of course, indulgent. If you're the one hosting, you've got that much more of an upper hand because you're the one planning the menu and making most of the food. If I'm hosting something, I usually end up running around like a chicken with my head cut off prepping stuff and chatting with friends and guests and just enjoying the scene. Call me a dork sporting a hot apron (or just call me "Martha"), but I love playing host and entertaining. Regardless, you know how you prepared things and what went into them. Think about building a balanced, well-portioned plate in your mind ahead of time and then take action. Fill a small plate up once, getting some vegetables in there somehow, make a second round for three to four clutch nibbles, and you're good to go—it saves you room for an additional cocktail or a little sweet or two.

Create a Cheating Plan of Attack

If you're a partygoer, however, a table full of appetizers and desserts can be pretty daunting or overwhelming at times—stimulation overload when you're faced with a smorgasbord of snacks and you're not really sure what your plan of attack should be. Fear not, there's always a way to make food work for you. The great thing about cocktail parties is that the food portions tend to be teensy, so you're able to get in a whole lot of tastes and flavors without filling up too fast. But beware not to be deceived—just because the egg roll or fried coconut shrimp is small doesn't mean it's free of calories. Cheat the system with the following helpful tips:

Look first, then shoot—Peruse the smorgasbord, pick out a few (read: three or four) of your favorite appetizers or hors d'oeuvres (yes, even if one or two are fried or on the heavier side) and then balance out the remainder of your plate with lighter fare, like crudité— fresh fruit, veggies, and a bit of dip, a few small pieces of cheese, and a couple of crackers, maybe two or three pieces of sushi if it's available . . . you get the idea. If there are bowls of pretzels, nuts, or candy innocently placed throughout the room and you tend to have trouble keeping your hands out of them, remove yourself from trouble and step away. Don't even start with one handful if it's too hard to then stop. Cheat and save those extra calories for a drink or small dessert.

Hit the bar and then dessert—Notice how I had you beeline for the food first. You've now got something in your stomach to help buffer the effects of alcohol. One too many cocktails from the second you walk in the door and you know what happens to your defenses around the chips and dip. Forget it, you left your defenses in the dust after your second glass of Prosecco or champagne. Eat a little first, then head to the bar or drink table. Make dessert a separate part of the evening—save the best for last if you're a sweet fanatic. Rather than picking up a brownie bite or a mini cupcake with your appetizers, make a mental note of one or two little treats ahead of time and then section them off for later in the evening when you're really scouting out something sweet. Because you've already established your portion plan ahead of time, you'll do a better job of sticking to it, regardless of how many cocktails you've had.

Pace yourself—Pace yourself in terms of nibbling and drinking because calories can rack up rather quickly when you're just taking "bites" here and there. Refer back to your nightly goal for drinks, whether one, two, three, or four, depending on how the rest of your

CHEAT SHEET: Build Your Perfect Party Plate Without Going Overboard on Portions or Calories

- I cup crudité (3 asparagus spears, 4 red bell pepper strips, 2 pieces of broccoli), plus 2 tablespoons dip or hummus
- 2 crackers (whole wheat if available), plus 2 small pieces of cheese (equivalent to an ounce or a regular serving)
- I crostini with a topping
- 2 mini meatballs
- 2 or 3 heavier or fried apps, like spinach-feta bites, coconut shrimp, bacon-wrapped dates, or spring rolls
- 5 to 7 olives or salted nuts

Later for dessert:
- I to 2 mini treats, like brownie or blondie bites, chocolate-covered strawberries, mini cookies, chocolate truffles, mini fruit tartlets, or éclairs
- I cup or a few pieces fresh fruit

week panned out. And as obnoxious, though hopefully not condescending, as this is going to sound, engage in conversation and enjoy the party (away from the food table or the bar if it's helpful). If you're dealing with a passed hors d'oeuvres situation, the same pace-yourself theory applies.

Use the buddy system—Pair up with a fellow cheater and conquer the party together. With a partner in crime, you provide yourself some backup assistance and a checks and balances system if you end up having one too many cocktails and your judgment starts to wane. Check in with your buddy midway through the party, clink your glasses, and affirm success with food and drink and keep moving.

Make it pretty—Let's talk visuals for a second. The often-overlooked but invaluable art of plating and presentation, making your food look simply irresistible (we already know it's gonna taste incredible). What looks better, tastes better (at least you'd hope it does!). Invest in a few cool platters, plates, and serving bowls and I promise it'll change the whole look of your table.

Whatever you choose, get creative and have fun with the food you're putting out . . . your guests will definitely be appreciative!

> *Cheater's Secret:* A quick note on choosing fancy cheeses for your cheese platter, if you're doing one. My best advice, go to a decent cheese shop or a nice/gourmet grocery store and ask for assistance! I still get completely overwhelmed every time I walk up to the cheese counter, but the people behind the counter are there to help; they won't bite and will usually allow you to taste-test whatever cheeses you want. Make sure to mention a few key things about the party you're hosting: What's your budget (first and foremost, as some cheeses can be crazy expensive), does the party have a theme, how many people are coming, and are you looking to go gourmet or do you just want keep things tasty and simple? The cheese expert will likely lead you to a few different cheeses varying in texture (from soft, semisoft, to hard), flavor (rich, buttery, nutty, sharp, etc.), and type (goat, sheep, and cow). Pick a few, maybe even inquire about food and wine pairings, and you're good to go.

Cheating by the Bite—Festive Fare That's Healthy and Indulgent

Okay, let's get down to details. Here's a sampling of recipes for perfectly posh—and nutritious—appetizers and desserts to serve up when you're hosting a cocktail party, bridal or baby shower, wine and cheese preparty, or day of football watching.

Simple Antipasto Plate

Makes 10 to 14 servings

THE GOODS

⅓ to ½ pound each of 2 or 3 types of good-quality cheese, like Gouda Parrano, Brie, Boucheron or other goat cheese, aged cheddar, or Manchego

CHEAT SHEET: Classic Cocktail Party Sample Menu

Here are some suggestions for a healthfully chic spread:

- Crudité platter of fresh asparagus spears (blanched), red bell pepper strips, cauliflower, carrot sticks, marinated artichokes (store-bought), and zucchini spears with a light vegetable dip or Roasted Red Pepper and Feta Dip (see recipe, page 259)
- Spicy marinated olives and spiced mixed nuts
- Toasted garlic-herb pita chips
- Cheese, crackers, and fruit platter—pick two to four types of nice cheese that go well with the theme of your party and your budget; pair cheese with some fancy truffle honey, quince paste, or fig spread and fresh fruit like grapes, apple and pear slices, dried apricots, dates, or strawberries; pair a few types of crackers, like a basic table water cracker, a peppery or herbed cracker, and a whole grain pick or two
- Artichoke and White Bean Bruschetta (see recipe, page 258)
- Crostini with goat cheese, fig spread, and caramelized onions
- Asian BBQ Chicken Wings or Swanky Skewers (see recipe, page 261)
- Bite-Size Bebè Brownies (see recipe, page 263)
- Chic Chocolate-Covered Strawberries (see recipe, page 264)

2 cups mixed Greek, Italian, or Spanish olives

¼ pound each of 2 or 3 types of cured meats, like prosciutto, soppressata, or chorizo

4 cups fresh fruit, like melon slices, grapes, and berries

4 ounces quince paste or fig spread (available at some cheese shops, gourmet grocery stores, or Whole Foods)

½ box each of 2 or 3 types of crackers or crostini toasts (make at least one cracker whole grain or whole wheat)

THE BREAKDOWN

Arrange everything nicely on a platter, and you're done!

The Facts: 210 calories; 12g fat; 6g saturated fat; 13g protein; 1g fiber

Artichoke and White Bean Bruschetta

Makes 18 to 20 bruschetta (about 2 tablespoons dip per serving)

THE GOODS

1 14-ounce can artichoke hearts, drained, rinsed, and quartered
1 15-ounce can cannellini beans, drained and rinsed
1 ½ tablespoons extra-virgin olive oil, plus more for brushing
1 large garlic clove, minced
2 tablespoons chopped fresh parsley
¼ teaspoon red pepper flakes
1 tablespoon fresh lemon juice
¼ teaspoon salt, or to taste
Freshly ground black pepper
1 tablespoon fresh lemon zest, plus more for garnish
1 18-inch whole grain baguette, sliced into 18 to 20 ½-inch
   pieces

THE BREAKDOWN

1. Preheat the oven to 350°F.
2. Place all the ingredients up through the lemon juice into a food processor and puree, mixing well until desired consistency is reached, be it smooth or slightly chunky. Add the salt, pepper to taste, and lemon zest and mix well.
3. Place the baguette slices on a baking sheet and brush lightly with olive oil. Bake for 6 to 8 minutes, until toasted and lightly browned. Spread 1 to 2 tablespoons of dip on top of each bread slice and arrange on a serving platter. Garnish each toast with extra lemon zest if you like.

The Facts (per serving, 2 bruschetta): 200 calories; 8g fat; 1g saturated fat; 4g protein; 2g fiber

Roasted Red Pepper and Feta Dip

This is an addictive dip that packs in antioxidants and vitamin C from the peppers and some creamy richness from the feta. Pair it with fresh veggies or toasted whole wheat pita chips. If you like a little more spice, swap the red pepper flakes for ½ small jalapeño or roasted hot pepper.

Makes about 2 cups (2 tablespoons per serving)

THE GOODS

    2 red bell peppers, roasted and peeled (see page 222)
    2 tablespoons extra-virgin olive oil
    1 small garlic clove, peeled
    1 cup crumbled feta cheese
    1 tablespoon fresh lemon juice
    ½ teaspoon salt
    ¼ teaspoon red pepper flakes

THE BREAKDOWN

1. In a food processor, combine the roasted peppers, olive oil, garlic, feta, and lemon juice and puree until smooth.
2. Stir in the salt and red pepper flakes. Refrigerate until ready to serve.

The Facts: 50 calories; 4g fat; 1.5g saturated fat; 1g protein; 0g fiber

Butternut Squash Bruschetta with Pine Nuts and Sour Cherries

This recipe brings together great autumn flavors for an interesting, satisfying, and antioxidant-packed appetizer.

Makes 2 to 3 dozen bruschetta

THE GOODS

    1 medium-large butternut squash
    2 teaspoons extra-virgin olive oil, plus more for brushing

1 small yellow onion, diced
1 can cannellini beans (white beans), rinsed and drained
½ to ¾ cup low-sodium chicken broth or vegetable broth
2 sprigs fresh rosemary, chopped (1 to 2 tablespoons)
¼ cup pine nuts, toasted
1 cup sour cherries, jarred in natural juices and drained (available at Whole Foods or your local specialty foods store)
½ teaspoon salt
¾ cup freshly grated Parmesan or Pecorino Romano cheese
1 crusty French or whole wheat baguette

THE BREAKDOWN

1. Preheat oven to 350°F.
2. Cut the squash in half, brush with olive oil, and roast cut-side-down for 30 to 35 minutes, until about three quarters of the way done (still slightly hard but able to be cut). Remove from the oven and cool, then peel/cut the skin off and cut into small chunks.
3. Heat the olive oil in a deep skillet or saucepan on medium-high heat, add the onion, and sauté until translucent, about 5 minutes. Add the cannellini beans, squash, chicken broth, and rosemary. Reduce the heat to a simmer.
4. Add the pine nuts, cherries, salt, and Parmesan and cook until most of the broth evaporates and it becomes "stew-like"—the squash should be slightly mashed and slightly chunky.
5. Cut the baguette into slices about 1 inch thick. Arrange on a cookie sheet and brush lightly with olive oil. Toast in oven for 4 to 5 minutes, until crisp and lightly browned. Place a spoonful of squash mixture onto the bruschetta and arrange on a serving tray or plate.

The Facts: 100 calories; 2.5g fat; 0.5g saturated fat; 4g protein; 2g fiber

VARIATION: *I love this dish so much (as do my friends and family), that I often drop the bruschetta and serve it up as a side dish.

Game Day Asian BBQ Chicken Wings or Swanky Skewers

These wings are a coveted football game-day standby. Upon request, I make them every year for the Super Bowl, and they're actually an amazing, pretty darn healthful addition to the whole spread. People will love them so much they'll be indebted to you, begging for more. The recipe's a family secret and I'm sharing it with you, so keep it under wraps!

Makes about 12 servings, 4 to 5 wings each

THE GOODS

    4 to 5 pounds free-range/organic chicken wings
    1 ½ cups low-sodium soy sauce
    1 ⅛ cups hoisin sauce
    ¼ cup plum sauce
    3 scallions, minced
    6 large garlic cloves, minced
    ¼ cup cider vinegar
    ½ cup honey

THE BREAKDOWN

1. Rinse the wings and pat dry.
2. Combine all the remaining ingredients in a medium saucepan and bring to a boil over medium-high heat. Reduce the heat and simmer for 5 minutes. Remove from the heat and cool completely.
3. Place the wings in a storage container, pour the marinade over, and marinate for at least 4 to 6 hours, or overnight.
4. Preheat the oven to 375°F. Line two baking sheets with aluminum foil or use two roasting pans.
5. Distribute the wings on both pans, saving the excess marinade for basting. Bake, uncovered, for 1 to 1 ½ hours, basting every 20 minutes with the remaining marinade and turning the wings about halfway through to brown evenly. Cool, then serve.

The Facts: 180 calories; 2g fat; 0.5g saturated fat; 15g protein; 0g fiber

VARIATION: *To turn these suckers into cocktail party–appropriate swank skewers (no mess, a little prettier), just swap out the chicken wings for about 3 pounds skinless, boneless chicken breasts cut into 2-inch-wide strips or chicken tenders, or do half of the recipe with peeled and deveined shrimp. Marinate the chicken or shrimp, then when ready to bake, skewer the chicken strips or shrimp onto bamboo or wooden sticks (soak them in water for 5 minutes before). Skewer the chicken lengthwise, straight through, or alternate one side after the other to create a wavelike shape with the chicken. Skewer the shrimp 3 or 4 to a skewer in a C shape so they don't fall off. Preheat the broiler and broil the chicken 5 minutes on each side and the shrimp 2 to 3 minutes on each side, until golden brown, basting both with extra marinade halfway through and turning over.

Lamb Meatballs with Lemon-Mint Yogurt Sauce

These meatballs bring on a Middle Eastern flavor and are great for parties (serve them with toothpicks) or to make for a speedy dinner and serve with a fresh tomato, cucumber, and onion salad. I love the way the dates add just a touch of sweetness to the meatballs and take the taste up a notch.

Makes about 30 mini meatballs

THE GOODS
    1 pound ground lamb
    ¼ cup minced onion
    1 garlic clove, minced
    1 egg, beaten
    ½ cup whole wheat breadcrumbs
    1 teaspoon ground cumin
    1 teaspoon ground coriander
    8 dates, pitted and finely chopped

2 tablespoons minced fresh mint
½ teaspoon salt
¼ teaspoon freshly ground pepper

LEMON-MINT YOGURT SAUCE
16 ounces (2 cups) 2% Greek yogurt
¼ cup peeled and finely chopped cucumber
2 tablespoons minced fresh mint
½ teaspoon ground cumin
Juice of 1 lemon
2 teaspoons lemon zest

THE BREAKDOWN
1. Preheat the oven to 350°F.
2. Mix all the meatball ingredients together in a large bowl. Form into about 30 meatballs about 1 tablespoon each.
3. Place the meatballs on a baking sheet and bake for about 20 minutes, until lightly browned.
4. Mix together the ingredients for sauce and serve over the meatballs or alongside.

The Facts: 70 calories; 4.5g fat; 2g saturated fat; 4g protein; 0g fiber

VARIATION: *For a quick dish without turning the oven on, sauté the meatballs in a large skillet with 1 teaspoon olive oil for 12 to 15 minutes, until browned.

Bite-Size Bebè Brownies

Straight from the old-school Bronx kitchen of my grandmother Bebè, these brownies were a standby in my family's freezer when I was growing up. I've made them slightly more cheatable, cutting them to be bite-size, which makes them perfect for parties. They're super-rich and satisfying—one or two indulgent bites will do the trick when you're scavenging for a chocolate fix. You can add ¾ teaspoon instant espresso powder for a little kick if you like. And if you're baking for a big group, go ahead and double the recipe.

Makes 24 brownies

THE GOODS

6 ounces (about 1 cup) semisweet or dark chocolate chips (dark chocolate chips—70% cocao—will give you richer flavor, and they sneak in more antioxidants—brownies can be healthful in moderation!)

⅓ cup unsalted butter

2 eggs

½ cup sugar

½ cup all-purpose flour

½ teaspoon baking powder

Pinch of salt

1 to 1 ½ teaspoons vanilla extract

1 cup chopped walnuts

THE BREAKDOWN

1. Preheat the oven to 350°F and grease an 8-inch square pan.
2. Melt the chocolate chips and butter in a small metal bowl over simmering water. (This is called a double boiler; you can either purchase one or jimmy rig it like I do by placing a medium mixing bowl directly over a small to medium saucepan.)
3. In a large bowl, use an electric beater to beat the eggs with the sugar until blended. Stir in the flour, baking powder, and salt. Add the chocolate mixture and vanilla. Stir well and add the walnuts.
4. Pour the mixture into the prepared pan and bake for 20 to 25 minutes, or until a toothpick inserted in the center comes out crystal clean.

The Facts: 120 calories, 8g fat; 3g saturated fat; 2g protein; 0g fiber

Chic Chocolate-Covered Strawberries

A perfect example of bridging health and indulgence, chocolate-covered strawberries are unbelievably easy and always go fast when served. This

recipe is nothing new or exotic, but at about 50 calories apiece, go ahead and have two or three for a more frequent cheatable treat.

Makes about 20 strawberries

THE GOODS

6 ounces bittersweet or dark chocolate (look for 60% cacao or more), chopped, or ½ 11.5-ounce bag chocolate chips
1 pound strawberries (about 20)

THE BREAKDOWN

1. Set up a double boiler over barely simmering water, add the chocolate, and stir until melted and smooth. Remove the chocolate from the heat and dip each strawberry about half-way into the melted chocolate. Place on a cookie sheet lined with parchment or waxed paper.
2. Place in the fridge for about 30 minutes, until the chocolate sets. You can keep the strawberries refrigerated until the chocolate is set, about 30 minutes, or 5 minutes in the freezer.

The Facts (per strawberry): 50 calories; 3.5g fat; 2g saturated fat; lg protein; lg fiber

White Wine Peach Sangria

Makes 10 servings

THE GOODS

3 tablespoons Triple Sec or Cointreau
1 bottle dry Spanish white wine, such as Albariño, chilled
2 cups thinly sliced peaches
2 cups sliced strawberries or whole blueberries or raspberries
2 10-ounce bottles club soda, chilled
Lemon or lime slices (optional)
Mint sprigs (optional)

THE BREAKDOWN

1. Combine the Triple Sec, wine, and peach and strawberry slices and stir well. Cover and chill.
2. To serve, add the club soda and stir gently. Serve with lemon or lime slices and fresh mint sprigs, if you like.

The Facts: 120 calories; 0g fat; 0g saturated fat; 0g protein; 2g fiber

Lemonade Vodka Spritzers with Raspberry and Mint

Note of caution: These might be spritzers, but they can be deceiving . . . a little too good if you're not careful!

Makes about 10 servings

THE GOODS

⅔ cup sugar
1 ½ cups vodka
1 cup fresh lemon juice (from about 4 lemons)
1 ½ cups seltzer water or club soda
¾ cup fresh mint leaves
1 cup raspberries

THE BREAKDOWN

1. Combine the sugar, vodka, lemon juice, and seltzer in a large pitcher.
2. Muddle the mint and raspberries in a separate bowl and add to the pitcher. Shake the pitcher well and serve in glasses over ice.

The Facts: 140 calories; 0g fat; 0g saturated fat; 0g protein; 1g fiber

Mango-Peach Iced Tea

Makes 8 to 10 servings

THE GOODS

8 tea bags (black tea like English breakfast or Ceylon is perfect)
1 quart boiling water
1 ripe mango, peeled and chopped
1 peach, peeled and chopped
3 tablespoons agave nectar
Juice of 1 lemon
5 cups ice cubes, plus more for serving
Lemon slices for serving

THE BREAKDOWN

1. Place the tea bags in the boiling water and steep for about 8 minutes, then remove the tea bags and cool.
2. In a blender, puree the mango, peach, agave nectar, and lemon juice.
3. Add the ice and fruit puree to the tea and pour the tea into a pitcher. Serve in glasses filled with ice, and garnish with lemon slices.

The Facts: 45 calories; 0g fat; 0g saturated fat; 0g protein; lg fiber

Refresher Course—Key Goals from Weeks 1 to 5

❏ Resize portions—3 to 5 ounces protein, ½ to 1 cup rice/pasta/grain, 1 cup/piece fruit, 1 to 3 cups veggies/salad (aim to cut total portions by 15 to 25 percent and set your plate up as: ½ fruits/vegetables, ¼ lean protein, ¼ healthy, complex carbs).

❏ Eat 2 servings of fruit per day; aim to have vegetables with lunch AND dinner.

❏ Drink 1 ½ to 2 liters of water per day.

❑ Don't skip meals—you'll lower your calorie-burn capability!

❑ Cheat it up each week with one or two indulgent meals (order what you wish, but still consider portions) and one or two treats (between 200 and 300 calories each).

❑ Exercise at least three or four days this week—kick it up a notch if you have a heavy week of drinking and/or eating ahead.

❑ Cut your alcohol intake per week by at least 25 percent.

❑ Food journaling . . . DO IT!

❑ Bring three to five basic office staples to work for snacks and emergencies.

❑ Re-plate and re-portion takeout and delivery food. Aim for half to three quarters of the to-go container.

❑ Watch portions like a hawk at restaurants, and leave at least 5 bites on the plate, if not a quarter to half. If the bread isn't awesome, lose it.

❑ Put all snacks and meals on a plate to halt mindless eating.

❑ Artificial sweeteners should be completely kicked to the curb by now. If not, bring intake down to ½ packet per day.

❑ Get back on board with the basics after a long night out and a hangover.

Get Your Grocery Shopping Groove On: Shop Like a Pro and Love It

"Grocery shopping is like a sport. Master each aisle and come out in first place every time."

—Melissa

WEEK 6 GOALS

- Hit the grocery store and really learn the full lay of the land. Make a list and plan for the week ahead so you're always prepared and will never go hungry again!
- Double-check and/or edit your staple grocery list from Weeks 1 to 5.
- Make sure the foods you're buying have top-notch ingredient lists. If there are more than three to five ingredients you've never heard of, or that appear to be manhandled, leave the item on the shelf.
- Do a double take and make sure you're getting those veggies in at lunch AND dinner.
- Check yourself and make sure that water intake is plentiful, 1 ½ to 2 liters per day, and that your exercise goal is on target, at least three or four times a week. Find one or two small, sneaky ways to get even more active, like taking the stairs more often or walking rather than driving.
- You're kicking butt and taking names. Reward yourself at the end of the week . . . with something other than food!

The Plan

Welcome to the home stretch, ladies. By now you should be feeling the benefits of skimmed-down portion sizes, satisfying food, and a hell of a lot of water. You've hit the double-digit zone on the scale, and people around you are really noticing. Take a good peek at the goals outlined for this week and commit to them. Change takes time, and you're certainly well on your way after a month and a half. It's like you're now entering the second phase of a new, burgeoning relationship. The thrill and excitement is still there, but reality and consistency is setting in and really starting to stick. As goal #1 for this week reads, you're headed to the grocery store. We've managed to avoid spending too much time there for a while now, but I think you're fully ready and primed to peruse the abundant food selection with ease, confidence, and conviction. This chapter will help you see the grocery store in a slightly brighter light while also providing you with the tools necessary to stock and maintain a healthful, cheatable kitchen—you'll know what items you need, how often, and how much to purchase by the close of this chapter. In essence, we're taking all the mini grocery lists for each of the recipes you've read and tested in the previous chapters and are now putting all the pieces of the puzzle, and the bigger picture, together with a masterful well-stocked fridge and pantry as the end product.

A Look at the Week Ahead:

Take a Full-on Field Trip to Your Local Grocery Store
Make a list to plan for the week/weeks ahead. Peruse each and every aisle, get to know exactly what's available and where things are located, so future trips will be streamlined and expedited. You'll always be in and out in 20 minutes or less, barring a massively long line at checkout.

Take a Closer Look at Your Staple Grocery List
The one you've been building from Weeks 1 through 5. These are fundamental items that should always be in your fridge and pantry

regardless of what recipes or dishes you intend to make in a given week. Are there items that need to be removed or added? Your schedule and food preferences will influence your list. Maybe you tried a new spice that you want to use more often—add it in. Can't stand garlic? Try making milder shallots or leeks a staple. Like things super hot and spicy? Always keep fresh chiles or red pepper flakes around. Find that sweet potatoes or quinoa give you major energy during workouts? Two more items to put on your personal list. Revise the list and go shopping!

Check the Label
Pay some attention to ingredients lists and know what to look for and what to leave behind. If you can't pronounce or spell more than three to five ingredients, the item does not come home with you!

Mind Your Veggies
Sometimes the most basic habits can start slacking when we're not looking. Assess your daily vegetable intake, which should be quite high by now, and make sure they're showing up in meals or snacks at least twice a day.

Keep Hydrated
Check yourself and make sure that water intake is plentiful, 1 ½ to 2 liters per day and that your exercise goal is on target, at least three or four times a week. Find one or two small, sneaky ways to get even more active, like taking the stairs more often or walking rather than driving.

Stay the Course
Your cheating efforts are seriously paying off, but now is not the time to get cocky and nosedive deep into old ways (like bagels for breakfast daily or pizza for dinner three times a week). Give yourself a pat on the back with something aside from food . . . you're already having a ton of great meals and drinks during a given week. Maybe it's the new handbag or pair of shoes you've been eyeing, or a weekend away with friends, a massage, or session with a personal trainer. Go ahead, you deserve it.

Week 6: Sample—From Grocery Store to Kitchen

based on 1400-1600 calories

Week 6:	Monday	Tuesday	Wednesday
BREAKFAST 300-400 calories 7-9:30 a.m.	1 cup high fiber cereal (more than 5g fiber) with 1 cup strawberries (or a serving of fruit) with skim or low-fat soy milk	Quick breakfast smoothie with 6 ounce low-fat plain yogurt or skim/soy milk + ½ cup frozen blueberries and blackberries + ½ banana + 1 tablespoon ground flaxseed + 1 teaspoon agave nectar. Throw it all in the blender!	½ cup 2% cottage cheese with 1 cup fresh pineapple chunks and 2 teaspoons flaked coconut or 1 tablespoon chopped pecans/cashews
SNACK ~100 calories 10-11 a.m.	Skip it, not hungry	1-2 whole grain crackers (like Wasa) with almond butter or goat cheese	Iced coffee with 2 tablespoons whole milk!
LUNCH 400-550 calories 12-2 p.m.	Make-Your-Own Salad You know the drill . . . 1. mixed greens, spinach or arugula 2. some type of protein 3. whatever veggies or fruits you wish to add 4. a sprinkle of 1-2 of the following: cheese, dried fruit, nuts, olives, and/or avocado 5. 1-2 tablespoons vinaigrette dressing or olive oil/lemon	Make an extra chicken breast the night before for a quick chicken salad with a 6-inch whole wheat pita or in a whole grain wrap 1 cup diced chicken breast + 2 teaspoons mayo + 2 tablespoons each chopped grapes and celery + 2 teaspoons chopped pecans + salt and pepper to taste	Bring leftover soba noodles with grilled chicken, veggies, and peanut sauce for lunch
SNACK 100-200 calories 3-5 p.m.	granola bar or fruit-nut bar (like 18 Rabbits, Kashi TLC, or Larabar) HIT THE GYM—evening body conditioning or spin class	1 cup cherries and 10 pecans or almonds from your desk drawer	1 cup fresh veggies, 2 whole grain, 3 tablespoons hummus 3 mile run/jog after work or yoga/Pilates
DINNER 400-600 calories 7-8:30 p.m.	Soba Noodles with Grilled Chicken and Peanut Dressing (1 cup noodles, 3 ounces chicken, 1 cup veggies) (pg 311)	Long day, see what groceries are left in the fridge and use them! Make a simple omelet with whatever cheese and veggies you have in your fridge, and a side salad	CHEAT MEAL #1 Friend's birthday dinner Assortment of Spanish tapas/small plates The order's out of your control, but request at least 1 veggie-heavy dish and grilled shrimp or chicken skewers

Thursday	Friday	Saturday	Sunday
HIT THE GYM I cup (½ cup dry) plain oatmeal (like McCann's) with banana slices and 2 teaspoons maple syrup	Late to work Jet into Starbucks for the Egg White, Spinach & Feta Wrap (280 cals, 9g fat) or hit your local deli or the office cafeteria for I egg scrambled or hard-boiled, I slice whole grain toast and fruit	Swimming or tennis or biking outside I piece whole grain toast with 4 slices smoked salmon and I tablespoon reduced-fat cream cheese	SLEEP LATE, skip to brunch
I orange or peach	Skip it.	I cup fruit salad	
Sushi for lunch Seaweed or green salad, I roll and 2 pieces sashimi	Make-Your-Own Salad You know the drill . . . 1. mixed greens, spinach or arugula 2. some type of protein 3. whatever veggies or fruits you wish to add 4. a sprinkle of 1-2 of the following: cheese, dried fruit, nuts, olives, and/or avocado 5. 1-2 tablespoons vinaigrette dressing or olive oil/lemon	Open-faced whole wheat English muffin with 2 slices fresh mozzarella, 2-3 tomato slices and I teaspoon Basic Pesto (pg 310) popped into the toaster oven or toasted at 400°F for 5-7 minutes until cheese lightly browns Mini side salad	BRUNCH Breakfast burrito with eggs, black beans, cheese, salsa, and 2 tablespoons guacamole *If the burrito's enormous, aim for ½ to ¾!
Grab some edamame at lunch for a quick, protein-packed snack (about I to I ½ cups)	CHEAT TREAT #1 Frozen yogurt break with coworkers I small frozen yogurt with strawberries and I tablespoon graham crackers or chocolate chips	At the movies—share a small popcorn, sans the butter, or better yet, bring your own along with a bottle of flavored seltzer water. Or try my trick at the movies when water won't cut it—¾ soda water + ¼ sprite	Small skim hot chocolate or an iced skim mocha for some afternoon sweetness
3-ounce pork loin or grilled tofu with I ½ cups steamed broccoli and ¾ cup Curried Quinoa with Cashews and Currants (pg 312).	4-ounces grilled shrimp with lemon and garlic, I ½ cups steamed broccoli and ¾ cup Coconut Rice with Cilantro and Ginger (pg 313)	CHEAT MEAL #2 Indian restaurant Share tandoori vegetables (I cup) and your favorite heavier dish chicken tikka masala (about ⅔ cup), ½ cup basmati rice, ¼ cup raita yogurt sauce	I cup Whole Wheat Penne Pasta with I cup Spicy Italian Turkey Sausage, Eggplant, and Olives (pg 306) and 2 tablespoons Pecorino Romano cheese

Continued

Week 6:	Monday	Tuesday	Wednesday
SNACK 100-150 calories 8:30-9:30 p.m. (If you're not hungry SKIP IT! Work in desserts and treats when you really want them and they're damn worth it!)	I cup fresh mango slices	3 frozen banana bites drizzled with 2 teaspoons chocolate syrup and rolled coconut flakes	4 bites banana-caramel bread pudding
WATER	I.5 liters	2 liters	2 liters
ALCOHOL/ OOPS!			I glass sangria, I glass wine with dinner
EXERCISE	Gym		3 mile run or yoga/pilates

Week 6 — Cheater's Shopping List:

- ❑ Vegetables: 3 to 5 (or more) for the week: 2 tomatoes, red bell pepper, carrots, celery, broccoli, eggplant
- ❑ Fruit: 2 to 4 types (or more), your pick (enough to get you through 5 to 7 days, 2 servings a day): cherries, bananas, strawberries, pineapple, mango
- ❑ Protein: 1 pound chicken breasts, 4 ounces shrimp, 2 links turkey sausage, 3 ounces pork loin, 2 ounces smoked salmon, eggs
- ❑ Healthy carbs: whole grain cereal (more than 5 grams fiber, less than 7 grams sugar), whole grain bread, whole wheat English muffins, whole wheat penne, soba noodles, brown jasmine rice, quinoa
- ❑ Dairy/calcium: Parmesan cheese, fresh mozzarella, reduced-fat cream cheese, 3 to 4 low-fat plain yogurts or cottage cheese, skim or soy milk
- ❑ Other: mixed Greek/Italian olives, pine nuts, light coconut milk, currants
- ❑ Seasonings and spices: basil, garlic, ginger, curry powder, cilantro, 1 lemon
- ❑ Snack stuff and staples: hummus
- ❑ Dessert/treat: chocolate syrup, coconut flakes, banana, butterscotch chips (if they can't stay in the pantry without being devoured, skip them!)

Thursday	Friday	Saturday	Sunday
½ cup 0% or 2% Greek yogurt with 1 tablespoon butterscotch chips	Skip it	Skip it	CHEAT TREAT #2 1 more Cheater's Cookie leftover in your freezer with 4 ounces skim/soy/almond milk!
1.5 liters	2 liters	2 liters	2 liters
		2 beers with dinner	1 glass wine with dinner
Gym		Swimming, tennis, or biking	

Make a List and Man Your Grocery Carts . . .

Before we step through the doors of your nearest grocery store, take a moment to think about your week ahead and start some productive planning with a physical shopping list and potential weekly meal and snack plan. Maybe it's the handy sample calendar on the pages prior . . . or at least similar to it. I've mentioned the value of getting organized before, and I know it sounds silly, but game-planning for the coming week allows you to be prepared for whatever the work-week may pelt at your pretty little head. Having healthy meals and snacks already prepped on paper, or at least in your mind, gives you the ability to have control of what you're eating and it ensures that you'll actually enjoy it. Think about your week ahead—what social or work engagements do you have, will you be traveling, how many nights will you be home to cook a quick dinner or prepare an easy lunch for the next day? Deduce your week as best as possible. If you know you'll be home for dinner three nights, pick out three recipes to whip up. Or if you can't think that far in advance (I admit, I rarely do), stock your fridge and pantry with some basic mealtime staples, like those you'll find in the pages that follow. We're again talking about those ten to fifteen items, or a few more, that should be on hand at all times and can serve as the base components for some quick and easy no-brainer weeknight meals, running-out-the-door

Week 6: Your Weekly Food Journal

Week 6:	Monday	Tuesday	Wednesday
BREAKFAST 300-400 calories *(Note your hunger level on a scale of 40-100 after each meal!)*			
SNACK ~100 calories *(If you're not hungry, skip it!)*			
LUNCH 400-550 calories			
SNACK 100-200 calories			
DINNER 400-600 calories			
SNACK 100-150 calories *(Aim for at least 2 hours before bed!)*			
WATER			
ALCOHOL/ OOPS!			
EXERCISE			

Thursday	Friday	Saturday	Sunday

breakfasts, and grab-and-go snacks. Refer back to your preliminary staples list on pages 189 and 215 that you've already been working with for the past few weeks. Build out your weekly list again, adjust it if need be, and make it slightly more comprehensive for quick lunches and dinners. Breakfast and snacks should come easy by now. We're pulling your office staples, at-home staples, and your "stay-on-the-wagon" staples all together in the pages ahead. Later in the chapter, you'll also get the low-down on additional pantry and fridge essentials that are longer-lasting and round out a well-

---

CHEAT SHEET: Marissa's Personal Cheater Weekly Staples

2 to 4 fruits
❑ Peaches, berries, melon, apples, pears, bananas, etc.
I aim to purchase fruit when it's in season, so it always varies—you get more flavor and nutrients and it's usually cheaper! See page 330 for a quick guide to produce by season.

3 to 5 vegetables
❑ Arugula, spinach, or some type of lettuce, green beans, tomatoes, bell peppers, carrots, etc.—the seasonal rule applies here as well

2 to 4 whole grains/pastas/breads/starches/cereals
❑ Sweet potatoes, whole wheat or regular pasta, artisan-baked whole grain bread, granola

3 or 4 lean proteins for lunch and dinner
❑ Chicken breast, fresh fish fillet, chickpeas or cannellini beans, chunk light tuna (I prefer the Italian tuna packed in olive oil, as it's perfect to toss into salads—little dressing needed!)

2 to 4 spices, seasonings, and fresh herbs
❑ Lemons, garlic, basil, rosemary

2 or more dairy products/eggs/cheese
❑ Eggs, skim milk or unsweetened almond milk, low-fat plain yogurt, 2% cottage cheese (you either love it or hate it—I LOVE it!)
❑ Bonne Bell cheese wheels and cheddar or Marchego for snacking; Pecorino Romano and goat cheese for cooking and salads

2 or 3 healthy snacks for the week
❑ Fruit and nut bar, like Kind, and roasted nuts

1 or 2 indulgences
❑ For me, it's usually some type of dark chocolate bar (having a little chocolate around at all times is a necessity!)

CHEAT SHEET: Your Cheater's Weekly Staples

2 to 4 fruits
❑ _____

3 to 5 vegetables
❑ _____

2 to 4 whole grains/pastas/breads/starches/cereals
❑ _____

3 or 4 lean proteins for lunch and dinner
❑ _____

2 to 4 spices, seasonings, and fresh herbs
❑ _____

2 or more dairy products/eggs/cheese
❑ _____

2 or 3 healthy snacks for the week
❑ _____

1 or 2 indulgences
❑ _____

---

stocked kitchen—items like oils, spices, vinegars, and canned and frozen goods. Wondering what a few of my own personal staples are? Flip back a page and you'll find 'em . . . a nutritionist's little secrets exposed. Insert your own personal staples above.

Now that you've got your baseline grocery list out of the way, let's tackle the true task at hand. We all know that grocery shopping regardless of the day and time can be painful if you wander the aisles unsure of what you plan to take home. With your grocery list already in hand and a list of kitchen staples to stock up on, you'll whiz right through the aisles in no time flat. Acquaint yourself with your grocery store, get to know what's where, get to know the product selection, and get to know the hot dude behind the fish counter (he might smell a bit funky, but you'll end up with a little salmon or shrimp freebie every now and then!). Soon enough, you'll be racing through the store in no time flat, like dreamy Dale Jarrett at the Indy 500.

Shopping Tactic #1: The Perimeter

Always, always shop the perimeter of the grocery store first. The outer aisles are typically where you'll find fruits and veggies, fresh meats, poultry, fish, eggs, and dairy products. Embrace the motto "fresh is best," because in most cases, it really is. Frozen, packaged, and canned foods have their time and place, but fresh items should generally be the core of your daily diet. Pack in the fresh produce. Yes, your fridge may start to resemble a garden, and no, the stuff won't spoil if you plan and purchase wisely.

- **Fruit and Veggies**—To start, choose 2 to 4 fruits and 3 to 5 vegetables that you will work into your meals and snacks over the week. Get fruits you can take to the office and either store for a day or two at your desk, or if you have an office fridge from which goodies will not be stolen, even better.

  ◆ When it comes to the vitamins and minerals in fresh produce, hands down, they're great nutritional powerhouses, packed with antioxidants and nutrients to prevent disease, boost immunity, and give your skin a Grecian goddess–like glow, among a plethora of other benefits. Let's tackle fruit first. Contrary to many fruit-slamming diets of the past (no offense, Mr. Atkins and South Beach), fruit is our friend. If a food was put on this earth, that's a very good indication that it's meant to be eaten and is packed with goodness. Like I've mentioned before, some fruits, such as bananas, pineapples, mangos, and grapes, do contain slightly more sugar, but it's a natural source of sugar and complex carbs, which our body digests differently than refined, processed sugars. Full of water, fiber, and vitamins and minerals, fruit provides a quick boost of energy and satiety, adding some serious volume to fill you up without all the extra calories. At 75 calories per serving, one cup of fresh pineapple chunks isn't going to tip the scales. By now, you should be getting in the USDA's recommended 2 to 3 servings of fruit per day (one serving is one small/medium piece of whole fruit or one cup of diced melon/pineapple, grapes, or berries). If you're still a little fruit-fearing, set your daily goal initially at 1 to 2 servings and work up. You'll easily hit your daily fruit goal with just a single bowl of whole grain cereal (like Kashi Golean or bran flakes) and a cup of sliced bananas and strawberries for breakfast and a crispy, crunchy apple with a little natural peanut butter as an afternoon snack. Welcome back to the world of fruit. Leave the guilt at the door.

To complete your grocery checklist, choose 3 or 4 of your seasonal fruit favorites. Again, scoping out fruits and veggies that are in season is a great way to ensure lower price points, more nutrients, and way, way more taste and flavor. Try to buy enough fruit to last you through the week. If you find yourself fruitless and frazzled by Wednesday or Thursday, don't fret. You should be able to find basic fruit like bananas and apples at delis or fruit stands around your work or home.

For vegetables, choose 3 or more that you can use either in a salad or on their own in a simple dinner. Some sample picks could look like: one bag baby or regular carrots, 3 or 4 tomatoes (when they're in season), a head of broccoli, ½ pound sugar snap peas or snow peas, a bunch of asparagus, and a bunch of lettuce or greens. As a general rule of thumb, the darker a green leafy vegetable is, the more nutritious, so you can skip over the iceberg, which has very little nutritional value aside from water. As you know, your daily goal for veggies is about

4 to 6 servings (1 serving is 1 cup raw veggies and/or greens or ½ cup cooked). At this stage in the game, you're a pro at incorporating veggies at lunch and dinner, so you're pretty much guaranteed to reach your daily target. Throw in some vegetables at breakfast (spinach or mushrooms in an omelet, for instance) for some nutritional extra credit.

- **Dairy, Eggs, and Cheese**—Next up, work your way toward the dairy and refrigerated sections. Pop some organic eggs, skim or soy milk, a fresh hunk of Parmesan or Pecorino Romano cheese, and maybe a few organic, plain low-fat yogurts for breakfast or a snack into your basket and then move the troops out.

Cheater's Secret: Organic means that the item was raised or produced without the use of hormones or additives (more to come on organic versus conventional foods in the next chapter—find out when it's really worth spending the extra cash).

Cheater's Secret: Ditch the extra sugar and calories in fruit yogurts and opt for plain most of the time. Excess added sugars in products means extra calories that add up way too quickly. You'll save nearly 50 calories and more than 10 grams of sugar by switching. Try sweetening plain yogurt with fresh fruit and/or a teaspoon of honey instead.

- **Meat, Poultry, and Fish**—Swing by the meat and poultry section and grab a package of chicken breasts, preferably free-range or organic. Split that sucker up when you get home and separate the breasts into plastic storage bags. Raw chicken breasts may be refrigerated safely for up to one to two days or stored in the freezer for nine to twelve months. Let's say you've decided to shoot for salmon for tonight's dinner and chicken for tomorrow's. If there are two chicken breasts in the package, wrap one breast in a storage bag and place it in the freezer. Wrap the other breast in plastic wrap or store it in an airtight container and put it in the fridge. Keep in mind that your trusty serving size of meat, poultry, or fish is 3 to 5 ounces, which is about the size of your fist or a little larger than your BlackBerry or iPhone. Before you leave the meat section, throw some 95% or 97% lean ground beef or turkey into your cart for burgers or meatballs later in the week and grab precut turkey slices for lunches. Applegate Farms is a great brand for cold cuts, as it has no hormones, nitrates, gluten, or preservatives and it's pretty low on sodium (read: no bloating, flatter tummies). Check your grocer for other similar brands, or even better, freshly roasted sliced turkey cut straight off the bone. Yum . . . it's almost like Thanksgiving 365 days a year!

And last, but certainly not least, head over to the fish counter. Time for a little eye-batting flirtation with the hot seafood dude. Bring on some brain-boosting, satisfying wild salmon, "a quarter pound, please" (insert smile and flip hair here, as they'd usually rather cut a half pound). While you're flirting away, let's bait and tackle the topic of both mercury and healthy fats in fish for a moment.

Mercury Rising—You've heard a lot of talk and seen innumerable warnings from the Food and Drug Administration (FDA) regarding mercury levels in certain types of fish and the associated toxicity risks. There's a lot of misinformation out there about fish and mercury levels. Don't discredit all fish and shellfish just yet—there are plenty of healthful, low-mercury seafood choices that can and should make frequent appearances on your plate. Keep in mind that some types of fish contain more mercury than others, and these are the ones you'll want to steer clear of. Excess consumption of mercury may pose risks to women of childbearing age and to young children, causing damage to the developing brain and potentially causing learning deficiencies and delayed mental development. Mercury contamination can also cause muscle weakness, fatigue, headaches, and numbness. As recommended by the FDA, women and young children should aim to consume a maximum of one serving (6 ounces) of "high-mercury" fish per week. That's equivalent to one 6-ounce tuna steak, one can of albacore "white" tuna, or 1 serving of swordfish or sea bass. You can be more lenient with fish in the low to medium category, such as chunk light tuna, shrimp, and salmon, consuming up to 12 ounces, or 2 to 3 servings, per week. Overall, expectant and new mothers and young children should limit mercury consumption as much as possible. Check out www .thefishlist.org and www.oceansalive.org for a detailed listing of the mercury levels in fish and shellfish.

CHEAT SHEET: Minding Mercury

Fish High in Mercury
Tuna (ahi, yellowfin, bluefin, albacore)
Shark, lobster, swordfish, orange roughy

Fish with Low to Medium Amounts of Mercury
Canned chunk light tuna
Salmon (choose wild whenever possible)
Catfish, cod, flounder, halibut, shrimp
King mackerel, tilefish, Chilean sea bass

Fishing for Good Fats—Now that we've conquered the mercury dilemma, why should you choose to eat fish? Low in calories and high in heart-healthy omega-3 fatty acids, many fish boast a wealth of health benefits you don't want to pass up. Again, omega-3 fatty acids are healthy polyunsaturated fats and come in a variety of forms, docosahexaenoic acid (DHA), eicosapentaenoic acid (EPA), and alpha-linoleic acid (ALA). These fats are *essential* to our diet, meaning that our bodies

CHEAT SHEET: Seafood Sampler
(per 3-ounce serving)

Type	Calories	Fat	Saturated Fat	Protein	Cholesterol	Mercury Content
Halibut	119	2.5 grams	0 grams	22 grams	35 milligrams	.252 ug/g
Salmon (Sockeye)	185	9 grams	1.6 grams	23 grams	74 milligrams	.014 ug/g
Scallops (6 large)	75	.5 grams	0 grams	16 grams	28 milligrams	.050 ug/g
Shrimp (6 large)	84	1 gram	0 grams	18 grams	166 milligrams	ND
Snapper	109	1.5 grams	0 grams	22 grams	40 milligrams	.189 ug/g
Swordfish	130	4 grams	1 gram	21 grams	40 milligrams	.976 ug/g
Tilapia	96	1.7 grams	0 grams	20 grams	50 milligrams	.010 ug/g
Tuna (fresh)	92	1 gram	0 grams	20 grams	38 milligrams	.383—.625 ug/g

can't produce them on their own, so instead we need to get them from food sources. Foods high in omega-3 fatty acids promote cardiovascular health and cognitive function, aid digestion, enhance mood, decrease blood pressure and inflammation, and aid prenatal and postnatal neurological and vision development. Numerous research studies have also assessed the effectiveness of omega-3 fatty acids in the treatment of depression and attention deficit disorder (ADHD).

Cold-water fatty fish such as wild Alaskan salmon, wild canned pink or sockeye salmon, mackerel, oysters, herring, sardines, and albacore tuna lead the pack when it comes to omega-3s, and they also happen to be low in environmental contaminants. The American Heart Association recommends that individuals consume at least two 6-ounce servings of fish rich in omega-3 fatty acids per week to make the most of their health benefits. Other plant-based, vegetarian foods abundant in omega-3s include canola and flaxseed oil, walnuts, avocado, and ground flaxseed.

Wild Child: When and Why to Go Wild—If you've caught on that I'm emphasizing wild fish, there's good reason for it. The next time you're standing in front of the fish counter, take a good, long look at the wild salmon in comparison to farmed salmon. You might notice that the farmed fillets are a little more shiny and oily to the eye and paler in color than the wild ones. Wild fish are grown and caught in their natural environment, lakes, rivers, and oceans, as opposed to farmed fish, which are raised in man-made conditions. Farm-raised fish are frequently found to contain higher levels of contaminating toxins that are present in their feed. Farming practices can also alter the taste and color of fish. Farmed salmon, for instance, are generally paler pink, have a more distinct fishy flavor, and are slightly fattier than their wild counterparts. Because of their close quarters, they don't have the opportunity to move around freely and are actually more gray than pink (they're often injected with coloring to achieve that salmon color we're used to, which is a little gross—I'd prefer to keep injections of any kind to a bare minimum in my food). The downfall is that wild fish and seafood may be accompanied by a higher price tag, but if you look for wild salmon during peak season, May through September, or when there's a sale, you'll get a decent price break. The same goes for other types of wild fish and seafood. Watch for Pacific wild salmon when possible—that's the good stuff. As for the term "previously frozen" on fish and seafood, you'll always get much better flavor and texture from fresh fish, but nutrient-wise, they're right on par with each other.

Overboard and Overfished—If you haven't really given a thought to overfishing before, you might consider it next time you're purchasing or ordering fish. The issue of overfishing can take a pretty serious toll on the environment and our ecological systems, and it encourages the growth of fish and seafood farms, which, as we found above, isn't always ideal. In the spirit of greening your food intake, take a quick look at some options that are more eco-friendly and those that aren't so much. Among the *least* eco-friendly fish choices are orange roughy, Chilean sea bass, and swordfish. As for the *most* eco-friendly fish choices, catfish, halibut (Pacific), mussels, tilapia, scallops, striped bass, and salmon (Alaskan, wild) are among your best bets. A number of environmental organizations and ecology advocacy groups have compiled helpful lists and wallet guides to aid consumers in making seafood choices. The Environmental Defense organization has a user-friendly wallet guide available at www.thefishlist .org and a buying guide for seafood at www.oceansalive.org/ eat.cfm. And leave it to Apple to offer an iPhone application called "Seafood Watch," where you'll get the latest sustainable suggestions at your fingertips. No iPhone? You could always dial up FishPhone (I'm dead serious). Text 30644 and type in FISH, followed by the name of the fish you want to purchase. You'll receive an eco-conscious response with a "green" or "not so green" answer so you can choose your fish intelligently and ethically at the same time. It's a pretty awesome tool when you're staring at the fish counter or at a restaurant menu wondering what to order.

Overall, fish and seafood are great additions to work into your meal planning. A few helpful pieces of advice . . . be inquisitive and ask what fish is most fresh, confirm that a particular type of salmon or tuna is definitely wild or was raised in reputable conditions, or that those plump-looking scallops are indeed fresh rather than previously frozen. If you happen to be in a coastal area, opt for seafood and fish that's abundant and local—this helps to guarantee a higher degree of freshness and flavor, and you'll be contributing to the local economy at the same time.

With all that said and done, one 4-ounce piece of wild salmon is in your care and the cuteness of the fish dude is officially confirmed. Move on and save some eyelash batting for another day.

CHEAT SHEET: Eco-Friendly Fish List

Seafood Watch and the Monterey Bay Aquarium have denoted these fish as "super green" healthy choices as all are low in contaminants and mercury, contain the daily minimum recommendation of omega-3 fats, and are environmentally friendly. Other "healthy choices" are also low in contaminants but contain slightly lower amounts of omega-3s.

Super Green Fish—Best Catches	Other Healthy Fish—Best Catches
Albacore tuna (pole-caught from the U.S. or British Columbia)	Artic char
Mussels	Bay scallops
Oysters	Crayfish
Pacific Sardines	Dungeness crab (wild-caught from California, Oregon, or Washington)
Shrimp (wild-caught from Oregon)	Squid (wild-caught from the Atlantic)
Rainbow trout	Pacific cod (line-caught from the Alaska)
Salmon (wild-caught from Alaska)	
Spot prawns (wild-caught from British Columbia)	

Shopping Tactic #2: Tackle the Inner Aisles with Ease

Nervous about what's lurking in aisle 4—the snack aisle where chips, chocolate, and cookies are beautifully, sometimes sinfully, bountiful? If aisle 4 is too daunting and brings back bad childhood nightmares . . . *don't go down that aisle*! See, there's a free piece of advice from your nutritionist/therapist you didn't have to shell out major bucks for. If snacky snacks are going to be devoured in no time, hold off until you feel more in control and more comfortable with having them around the house—just as we learned with stress eating and mindless munching. Remember, they're called treats for a reason. Indulgence in moderation is the key, as it allows you to relish in cheating that much more. So bottom line, it's decidedly all right to tackle the grocery store in stages, ease into it like a fine wine, or go full-throttle ahead for all you competitive overachievers. Either way, it's a win-win situation. If you've achieved inner Zen and are at one with aisle 4, go ahead and hit it up. Think about snacks for the week and a healthy treat or two to have in your cupboard at home, fruit-nut or granola bars like Kashi or Nature Valley or Larabar for when you're on the go, some cinnamon graham crackers to pair with natural peanut butter for an energizing afternoon snack, Nutella spread and banana slices for a more pleasure-seeking snack, or a *really* good brand of dark chocolate for those dire moments of need.

> *Cheater's Secret:* Yes, dark chocolate does have health benefits, but keep it to 50 to 75 calories a day so your waistline doesn't expand. A recent research study published in the *Journal of the American Medical Association* found that the antioxidants in dark chocolate help lower blood pressure with just 30 calories worth of chocolate a day. Sadly for you chocolate lovers, that doesn't give you license to scarf down a chocolate bar a day. Max out at 50 to 75 calories, that's about the size of 1 large square or 2 small squares in a chocolate bar. Hey, 50 calories or not, it's still chocolate—I'll take the mini bite and say thanks. Other studies show that dark chocolate can help prevent heart disease and insulin resistance that occurs with diabetes. Look for brands with 65% or more cacao so you can garner the health benefits. Try good-quality brands like Bonnat, Dagoba, Green & Blacks, sweetriot, Mast Brothers, Equal Exchange, Ghirardelli, and Valrhona (good quality means good flavor and rich taste, which means you'll eat less and enjoy it more!). Aim for 2 small squares for some guiltless decadence.

Back to business—take a look at your grocery list and determine what other items you need. Low-sodium soy sauce for the salmon you want to prepare tonight, check; recycled napkins, check (we're thinking green here, so show some love to Mother Earth and her trees, please); unsalted almonds (raw or roasted is totally cool), check; a nice loaf of 100% whole wheat or seven grain bread firm enough that you can't smush with one fist, brown rice, double check; high fiber whole grain cereal, check. Wait a sec. Let's take a step back and decipher the previous laundry list.

The Slippery Sodium Slope—First, why low-sodium for the soy sauce? We've touched on this before, but for a speedy refresher course, low-sodium products are always a fantastic choice when available—they cut back on excess sodium that's often found in processed foods, condiments, lunch meats, canned soups, and frozen prepared foods. A consistently high intake of salt in our diets can cause dehydration, bloating, and water retention and may increase the risk of high blood pressure, hypertension, and cardiovascular disease. Low-sodium labels indicate that the product contains no more than 140 milligrams sodium per serving. Again, a smart rule of thumb for canned soups and frozen foods when checking out the nutrition label is to look for 500 milligrams of sodium or below per serving.

Cheat with Flavor: The Spice-Satiety Factor—You've hit the spice aisle and are a bit overwhelmed. When you're looking to infuse a dish with automatic flavor or heat or that extra wow factor without any excess fat or calories, there's really no need to look further than herbs and spices—it's a win-win situation. And what's even more brilliant is something called the "spice-satiety factor." Research shows that spices and seasoning actually influence our brain's ability to regulate appetite. The more flavorfully spiced or aromatic a dish is, the more satisfied we are and the less we physically need to eat. Satisfaction comes fast when you spice things up in the kitchen . . . or in the bedroom if you have a dirty mind and want to go that route. In addition, the more spice or herbs you use, the less fat, butter, oil, or cream you need as a flavoring agent. And there go a couple hundred calories in your next meal right there.

Cheater's Secret: Many spices and fresh herbs are also excellent sources of antioxidants and help reduce risk of cancer, Alzheimer's, high blood pressure, high cholesterol, diabetes, and other diseases—cinnamon, cumin, curry, oregano, thyme, rosemary, ginger, garlic, chiles, and turmeric, to name a few.

CHEAT SHEET: Basic Spice and Herb Groupings

Indian—cardamom, curry, turmeric, coriander, chiles, fennel, tamarind, cumin

Asian—chiles, star anise, sesame seeds, peppercorns, five-spice powder, ginger, cilantro, basil, lemongrass, Kaffir lime leaf

Middle Eastern—cumin, anise, caraway, cinnamon, nutmeg, turmeric, cardamom, allspice

Mediterranean—saffron, paprika, cumin, rosemary, oregano, basil, bay leaves, fennel, garlic

Latin—cumin, chiles, oregano, annatto, cilantro, garlic

Savory-sweet—nutmeg, cinnamon, cloves, vanilla

Basic seasoning—rosemary, thyme, sage, tarragon, garlic, lemon

---

Spice and Metabolism—There's lots of talk about fiery spices, metabolism, and weight. "Chiles will boost your metabolism through the roof—eat them by the bushel." Uhhh, yeah ... a slight exaggeration that might inflict some serious physical pain, but spicier foods and a compound called capsaicin in chiles can actually bump metabolism up a notch and burn fat a wee bit faster. Ever wonder why you start sweating after eating Indian or Mexican? Now you know. Every little bit does help, so make fresh herbs and spices a staple in your kitchen. Or get out your green thumb and grow a few different fresh herbs in little pots on your windowsill, balcony, or backyard.

Fiber: A Gal's Best Friend—Next up is all this talk about high-fiber. What's so unbelievably special about fiber? We discussed it early on in Chapter 1, but here's a quick crash course again: It's one of our best allies in the game of weight management and feeling satiated, not to mention its cholesterol-lowering benefits and ability to promote healthy, speedy digestion. Fiber-rich foods like whole grain and wheat flours, oatmeal, multigrain breads, fruits and vegetables, high-fiber cereals, and healthy grains like brown rice, whole wheat pasta, and couscous all work to stabilize blood sugar and hunger and keep our metabolism and energy levels kicking along all day at a steady clip. High-fiber foods allow us to fill up faster on fewer calories—such a classic cheating concept.

For other healthful, high-fiber items like whole grain crackers, wraps, and breads (like Wasa and Finn Crisp crackers, Ezekiel bread, and Damascus Roll-up wraps), look for 3 grams of fiber or more on nutrition labels per serving. Don't get your adorable Hanky Panky panties in a big bunch over carbohydrate grams, as they're automatically influenced (for the better) by fiber and sugar content—this isn't brain surgery, it's simply food. You might be thinking, "If it's so damn simple, what the hell's all the carb-bashing for? Carbs are evil, aren't they?" Sorry, Sherlock, you've been duped. Hard as it may be to believe, carbs are not the enemy! To reiterate the basics from Week 1, complex carbohydrates serve as our brain's optimal source of fuel and provide our body with consistent energy. On an average day, go for the good, hearty stuff (rich in fiber and whole grains) rather than refined carbs like white breads, sugar, candy, chips, etc. Think more about the ingredients of what you're eating rather than an extra few grams of carbs here or there.

The Scoop on Cereal—If you're in the market for a stand-out fiber-rich cereal, look no further than 5 grams of dietary fiber or more on the nutrition label. Aim to keep added sugars to 7 grams or less and you'll come away with a kick-ass whole grain cereal. The vast majority of cereals from brands like Kashi, All Bran, Uncle Sam's, Cascadian Farms, and Nature's Path are excellent picks. Remember to look at the serving size listed on the box so you're not pouring yourself three times the portion, which is easy to do at 7 a.m. You could also go down the path of heartier cold cereals like muesli, Grape-Nuts, and granola. Remember that a serving of these cereals is typically ½ cup—it's about the size of what you can hold in the palm of your hand.

Cheater's Secret: Keep cereal to one bowl only. If cereal tends to be an eating trigger (i.e., oops, there went half the box), think of cereal as a breakfast-only item—you're giving cereal a home and establishing boundaries without banning it completely. For whatever reason, cereal can sometimes get a little out of hand when we start munching on it outside of mealtimes. I think some of us find it a guilt-free low-calorie snack, but we end up eating bowl after bowl or handful after handful and calories skyrocket. To keep your cereal in check, keep it in a bowl, no refills! And equally important, if you find yourself starving an hour later after a bowl of cereal at breakfast (like yours truly), there's a good chance it's not the most satisfying way for you to start your day . . . so opt for something else more filling and energizing. Me personally, I rarely do cereal because I know it just doesn't do the job and leaves my stomach rumbling within sixty minutes or less. Figure out what *balanced* breakfast does the trick for you and your body, whether it's eggs; yogurt, fruit, and ¼ cup granola; or toast, peanut butter, and banana to name a few . . .

Okay, back to shopping. Regardless of what other items are on your grocery list, here's some helpful information to take note of when you're perusing those inner aisles.

Get to know ingredient lists—Please remember to check ingredient lists on food items, keeping in mind that fresh is best. If you're wondering about the nutritional value of a product, turn the box around, glance at the nutrition facts label, and then look at the ingredients list. If the list is more than twenty items long, you may want to consider leaving it on the shelf. The fewer number of items, in general the less processed the item is, and the better it is for you. And remember, if you're going to cheat, you want to make sure it counts—delicious, fresh, and the best of the best. Otherwise it's not worth it. If there are multiple ingredients you've never heard of and can't pronounce, the likelihood it's a wee bit too manhandled is high. Bye-bye, Mr. Processed Twinkie (going strong at thirty-nine ingredients, including a substance also used in rocket fuel—pass it up!). My standard rule of thumb is: If there are three or more ingredients you can't pronounce or spell, that item's staying on the shelf.

Tacky trans fats—Hydrogenated trans fats have gained major media attention over the past few years, causing many big-name food companies and restaurant chains to throw these really unhealthy fats out on the curb, thank goodness! Trans-fatty acids are ultrasaturated (or hydrogenated) fats used to preserve the shelf life of processed foods. They do heavy-duty damage and are linked to increased heart disease risk, higher levels of "bad" LDL cholesterol, and lower levels of "good" HDL cholesterol. Trans fats are most often found in processed foods, commercial baked goods and snacks (cookies, cakes, donuts, chips), fried foods, and vegetable shortening and margarines—all items you'll want to keep out of your grocery cart. Keep an eye out for red-flag words on ingredients lists that indicate trans fat, like "partially hydrogenated oil" or "shortening." Food products can advertise that they're "trans-fat-free" even if there's .5 gram on the nutrition food label. Aim to choose items that have 0 grams of trans fats as often as possible.

High-fructose corn syrup—Good old HFCS, delicious but not so nutritious. High-fructose corn syrup is the super-cheap sweetener often found on the ingredients lists of conventional brand processed, packaged foods, snack items, bottled salad dressings, ketchup, soda, and fruit drinks, to name a few. Though the verdict's still out, many studies have linked HFCS to stimulating appetite and fueling weight gain. To reiterate, the USDA recommends that the average person consume a maximum of 10 to 12 teaspoons of added sugar or caloric sweetener per day. A single 12-ounce can of soda alone contains about 13 teaspoons of high-fructose corn syrup. A conventional brand low-fat fruit yogurt, up to 10 teaspoons of HFCS. And for your fact file, the USDA reports that annual consumption of corn syrup and high-fructose corn syrup increased 400 percent from 1970 to 2003—that's 79 pounds of sweetener per person, with numbers steadily on the rise. As a society, we're eating more across the board, HFCS and beyond. Just 15 percent of American adults were obese in 1980, as opposed to more than double that a few years back. Bottom line, do a quick scan on ingredient lists for HFCS. If you spot it, the item goes back on the shelf.

100-calorie packs—They might be "perfectly portioned," but 100-

calorie packs aren't as satisfying as you might think. They're typically lacking fiber and have you downing empty calories, which can lead to munching on multiple bags. Oops, there go three bags of 100-calorie pack Oreos (which, by the way, don't even have the creamy filling, what the hell?), and now you're at 300 calories. So much for portion control. Stick to 100-calorie packs of fiber-rich popcorn or almonds, or have a more satisfying snack like fruit and low-fat cheese or whole grain crackers and almond butter—snacks that combine some healthy fat, protein, and carbs, your Cheater's triumvirate of nutrients to manage hunger and stabilize blood sugar.

Low-calorie, sugar-free brownies, cookies, and other "fake" treats—Out with the fat and the taste and in with the artificial sweeteners and chemical preservatives . . . and the calories (there are usually two servings in those sugar-free or low-calorie treats, sneaky suckers. That often equates to 400 to 500 calories in just one cookie that's marketed as "diet-friendly." Reach for the real deal and have a fresh or home-baked (not plastic-wrapped) brownie or chocolate chip cookie. Who needs an artificially sweetened ice cream bar that causes you to crave three more? You're now cheating your way to work smaller, satisfying portions of real, delectable indulgences into your diet like an MVP.

Chocolate-coated energy or protein bars—For the calories and sugar in many chocolate or yogurt-coated protein and energy bars, you could eat a Snickers bar just the same. Leave chocolate for when it's truly worth it—rather than a daily occurrence at snack time or early in the morning. Starting your day off with chocolate-coated "health food" may leave you pining for more sweets throughout the day. Instead, reach for all-natural fruit and nut bars with just three to six ingredients, like Larabar, Clif Nectar, or Kind for a boost of energy, protein, and heart-healthy fat. And if your only option at the corner deli or in an airport is a chocolate-coated energy bar, leave it for a late afternoon snack.

Organic manic—Just because something's organic doesn't mean you're home free. Organic chips, cookies, candies, and other treats often still have just as many calories, sugar, and salt as conventional brands. Keep snack portions in check and focus on organic items that really are worth the extra cost, like dairy products, meats, poultry and eggs, and certain fruits and vegetables that don't have thick skins or rinds, like berries, green beans, and apples.

Label Lingo Letdown: "Made with Whole Grains" and "High Fiber"—"Made with whole grains" has come to have a very cloudy definition. To be deemed an "excellent source" of whole grains, a product must contain at least 16 grams of whole grains per serving, according to the FDA, and a "good source" must have 8 to 15 grams. But bottom line, the best source of whole grains are those that have the fewest ingredients, like brown rice, oatmeal, basic bran cereal, quinoa, whole wheat pasta, and 100% whole wheat or whole grain breads or flour.

From yogurt to water to ice cream to sugary sweet snack bars, everything seems to have extra fiber added to it lately. Fiber in ice cream . . . gross. Why? Food marketers are working hard to take advantage of fiber's magical powers—it keeps us more full for longer, typically off fewer calories, and speeds up digestion. The catch: Added fiber powders, the type of fiber going into packaged products, are digested differently in our bodies than fiber that's found naturally in foods and doesn't provide the same health benefits. Ingredients like maltodextrin, inulin, polydextrose, and oat fiber help stake the high-fiber claim on food labels but they also increase the amount of additives and potentially the amount of fake sugars you're getting, so steer clear. Reaching for natural, whole sources of fiber from fruits, vegetables, and whole grains is always your safest, smartest decision.

Shopping Tactic #3: Never, Ever Walk into a Grocery Store Hungry!

This meaningful piece of motherly advice rings loud and clear every time I walk into a grocery store. I mean, honestly, how can you focus on getting healthy, nutritious items into your basket when your stomach sounds like a foghorn and you're having a showdown with a half gallon of ice cream in aisle 7? Even if you've got the willpower of Wonder Woman, if you enter the grocery store hungry, you'll inevitably leave with at least four or five extraneous items in your cart, healthy or not. That's precisely when mint chocolate chip ice cream for dinner starts to sound really good. Sixty minutes and six servings of ice cream later, you're lying on your couch with a massive stomachache and wishing you hadn't ever walked into that grocery store on an empty stomach! Spare your stomach, your waistline, and your wallet—stick to your list and have a snack or meal before you step out of the house.

Shopping Tactic #4: The Big Benefit of Having a Standing Online Grocery Order

Time for a quick reality check . . . if you're a self-proclaimed jet-setter and have a piece of luggage attached to your hip at all times or your proverbial plate is so darn full you literally haven't stepped foot into a grocery store in six months, should you just stop reading this book right now? Why waste time you don't have? Wait a sec, slow down there, there's still hope for you. More and more companies are popping up in cities across the nation that provide online grocery shopping and deliver directly to your home at a specific time you designate. Consumers are expected to spend more than $8.4 billion on online groceries this year—see, you can be a trendsetter even when grocery shopping!

Online grocery services allow you to have a standing order, a huge advantage when you don't have time to dillydally down the aisles. Take a bit of time on a Sunday evening, think about your typical week, and create a template. Your account information will be saved, and with the click of your mouse, you've got next day's groceries at your fingertips. Most of the services even allow you to sort by organic, all-natural, gluten-free, local, and kosher products and by health needs and nutritional value—if you're looking for low-sodium, low-calorie, high-fiber, you can often sort products accordingly and check out their nutrition labels. Thankfully, online shopping doesn't have to bust your wallet open, as many companies offer free delivery for orders of $50 or more and others frequently provide coupons. If you need a little hand-holding (and we all do sometimes), here's a sample standing online grocery list to start off with for a basic weekly or biweekly order. Of course, this Cheat

CHEAT SHEET: Bringing Home the Basics

Sample standing online grocery list

4 fruits
❑ bananas, strawberries, peaches, green grapes

5 vegetables
❑ tomatoes, bag of mixed greens or baby spinach, carrots, green beans, red bell peppers

3 whole grains
❑ I box high-fiber cereal (5 grams of fiber or more, 7 grams of sugar or less)
❑ 100% whole wheat or seven grain bread
❑ whole wheat penne pasta, brown rice, whole wheat couscous, or quinoa

3 or 4 lean proteins
❑ I package deli meat, like Applegate Farms roasted turkey, chicken, or lean ham
❑ cage-free eggs
❑ I package free-range skinless chicken breasts (or ground turkey, sirloin, pork tenderloin, etc.)
❑ I salmon fillet (or tuna, halibut, cod, etc.)

2 or 3 dairy products
❑ skim milk
❑ low-fat plain yogurt or cottage cheese
❑ I pack of string cheese or cheddar cheese

2 or 3 healthy snacks
❑ hummus (any flavor—be adventurous!)
❑ I box granola bars, like Kashi TLC, Clif Nectar, Larabar, or Health Valley

I or 2 indulgences
❑ dark chocolate bar or low-fat frozen natural or organic yogurt (something fun, satisfying, and hopefully healthy, your pick—aim for 100 to 150 calories per serving)

For Emergencies
❑ 2 to 3 frozen entrées, like Kashi or Amy's Kitchen

Sheet grocery list would serve as a phenomenal reference anytime you shop, online or when you're physically pushing the cart around the aisles.

CHEAT SHEET: Check out these online grocers in your area

Fresh Direct—www.freshdirect.com
New York City metro area
Peapod—www.peapod.com
Washington, D.C., metro area, Chicago, Midwest, New England, and San Francisco (can shop by gluten-free, low-fat, low-sodium, or other dietary guidelines)
Safeway—www.safeway.com
California, Las Vegas, Portland, Washington, D.C., metro area, Philadelphia (save big on weekly specials; use the "personal shopper" feature to make specific requests, such as green bananas, for example)
Spud!—www.spud.com
San Francisco, Los Angeles, Portland, Seattle (specializes in local and organic items; free delivery, delivery within twenty-four hours)
Netgrocer—www.netgrocer.com
(national service for groceries; carries organic and kosher brands—shipping costs apply)

But before you get ahead of yourself . . .

Okay, we're heading into reverse gear for a moment or two. In order to plan out meals and snacks for the rest of the week, we've got to start with those empty cabinets and barren refrigerator shelves. Here comes your handy cheat sheet of the top kitchen essentials and cooking tools that help make healthy cooking and eating a breeze. These are different from your ten to fifteen basic weekly staples in that many of them last longer (like your spices, herbs, and oils) and they form the foundation of a well-stocked kitchen.

CHEAT SHEET: Stock Up on Kitchen Staples

- Extra-virgin olive oil, canola oil, toasted sesame oil (note that oils can go bad quickly and should be kept for no more than a year; store in a cool area)
- Balsamic and red or white wine vinegar, rice vinegar (great for Asian-inspired dishes)
- Low-sodium chicken and/or vegetable broth (choose a free-range chicken broth if available)
- Low-sodium soy sauce, teriyaki sauce
- Spices like cumin, paprika, cinnamon, cayenne pepper, chili powder, cardamom, curry powder (spices are most flavorful when used within one year)
- Salt (regular kosher and coarse sea salt), red pepper flakes, black pepper/peppercorns
- Dijon mustard, canola oil–based mayo (use mayo sparingly!)
- Organic skim milk or unsweetened soy, rice, or almond milk
- Organic eggs (look for organic eggs that are cage-free)
- Organic or natural peanut, almond, or cashew butter
- Unsalted organic butter
- Hunk of Pecorino Romano or Parmesan cheese (get the good stuff—it's worth it!)
- A few whole grains, like brown rice, quinoa, and whole wheat couscous
- A few different pastas, like whole wheat or regular semolina penne, angel hair, or spaghetti
- Nuts—walnuts, pine nuts, almonds, pecans, pistachios, and more
- Fresh garlic, shallots, and/or onions
- Baking powder, baking soda
- Whole wheat flour, all-purpose flour
- Organic brown and cane sugar, honey or agave nectar, vanilla extract
- A few cans of beans, like chickpeas, black beans, cannellini beans, kidney beans, lentils
- Canned tuna or salmon
- Canned tomatoes, tomato paste
- Frozen veggies (preferably organic)—spinach, broccoli, stir-fry mix
- Frozen fruit (preferably organic)—berries, mango, peaches
- 2 or 3 emergency frozen meals, like Kashi frozen dinners
- 2 or 3 cans low-sodium soups, like Amy's Kitchen, Pacific, or Walnut Acres

CHEAT SHEET: Cheatin' Kitchen Essentials

- **High-quality saucepans, skillets, and baking dishes like Calphalon, All-Clad, Le Creuset**—Invest in a few good ones and it'll make a world of difference. You can go with regular or nonstick. Nonstick makes life a little easier if you're a newbie to the kitchen, as it's less prone to sticking and overheating and you're able to use a little less fat or oil to coat the pan. An 8-, 10-, or 12-inch pan, a small and large pot, an extra-large pot for soup and pasta, a casserole/baking dish or two, and maybe a cast-iron skillet, and you've got the basics down.
- **Steamer basket or rack**– So great for veggies, seafood, and fish.
- **Grater**—Allows you to shave off thin or thicker pieces of cheese, and can also be used to grate potatoes, onions, carrots, beets, and more.
- **Microplane grater**—The perfect tool for grating citrus zest, fresh ginger, onion, and garlic.
- **Chef's knife**—A 10-inch chef's knife is a must. It's like you've died and gone to heaven after finally making the switch. Test out different brands and handle weights to see what feels most comfortable.
- **Food processor and blender**—There's a world of sauces, purees, soups, smoothies, cookie and pie doughs out there.
- **Measuring spoons and cups**—Essential in any kitchen, so go get some if you don't already own them! Measuring devices actually allow you to rock out recipes and proportions with preciseness (definitely a must when you're baking desserts and sweets). And surprise, surprise, they'll also help you gain a better idea of exact portion sizes! Remember to note that dry measuring cups are different from the glass ones you use for liquids.
- **Slow cooker**—aka the seventies' infamous Crockpot. They're making a big comeback now and make healthy one-pot cooking a cinch.
- **Electric hand mixer or beater**—Makes baking desserts and mixing and whipping stuff up so much easier.
- **Indoor grill/grill pan**—If you're not lucky enough to be the proud owner of an outdoor grill, gift yourself a grill pan or indoor grill . . . serious lifesavers that make a quick meal so simple and don't require much added fat.
- **Olive oil mister**—This one's a toss-up in my opinion. I have a mister myself, but typically end up just drizzling a touch of olive oil right out of the bottle—or covering part of the spout with my finger. Misters are fantastic, however, for ensuring that you're not dousing the pan or your food with too much of a good thing. A quick misting is often all you need to grease a pan or season food.

Getting a Good Meal and Great Grains
Out of Your Groceries

"Pasta . . . I love it like a child!"

—Virginia

By this stage in the game, you should feel pretty confident in your burgeoning cooking skills and comfortable enough to tackle anything that comes across your plate—including pasta, whole grains, and other carbs. I tried to hold out as long as I possibly could (I know many of you either avoid pasta and carbs, even many of the healthy ones, at all costs), but it's time to fully embrace carbohydrates and branch out from your small safety net of whole grain bread and cereal, oatmeal, fruit, and sweet potatoes. You just conquered each aisle of the grocery store and discovered that there's a whole world of complex carbohydrates out there waiting for you, including pasta (regular semolina, whole wheat, gluten-free, and spelt), noodles (such as soba and rice), and whole grains (like quinoa, barley, bulgur, and couscous).

You've managed to cheat your way through incorporating countless other foods into your diet that you never imagined would be feasible—now do the same with pasta and grains. Because, like everything else in the land of cheating, they can be part of a perfectly balanced, healthful diet without royally screwing up the scale. You can be skeptical—I'm okay with that. But I hope you're also secretly jumping for joy right now after being given the green light to enjoy pasta and rice again. Obviously this doesn't give you the go-ahead to wolf down a massive bowl of fettuccine Alfredo or even a mountain of brown rice and turkey meatballs night after night. We know how big restaurant pasta and carbohydrate portions can be—no need to replicate that at home. The notion still stands that pasta and grains should be the plate liner addition to your meal, a carb-lover's bonus. Veggies like eggplant, peas, broccoli, and tomatoes, along with lean protein like shrimp, meatballs, grilled chicken, chicken sausage, and beans are what's really stealing the show on your plate. I often remind people, if you've traveled to Italy or many other European and Mediterranean countries, pasta is served in appetizer-size portions, about the amount you could fit onto a dainty little saucer or small plate, no more than 1 to 1 ½ cups usually. Think about it and bring it back into your own kick-ass kitchen. You're still capping portions at 1 to 1 ½ cups of pasta and ¾ cup of whole grains/rice (½ cup is a standard single serving for both, at 100 calories).

Just as you've been doing, set some standards for an average week: pasta once or twice and whole grains two or more times—having a serving of brown rice at lunch and then quinoa at dinner is perfectly acceptable. If you're a pasta freak and can't live on just twice a week, go up to three or four times, but still consider portions carefully and get some whole wheat pasta in there at least once.

Whole wheat pasta and brown rice—Here's the down-low: Whole wheat pasta and whole grains like brown rice and quinoa have more fiber and protein than your traditional semolina, white pasta, white rice, or other refined grains. Higher-fiber, complex grains keep you full longer and provide more nutritional benefit. Look for brands of whole wheat pasta that provide at least 4 or 5 grams of fiber per 1 cup serving, as opposed to the 2 grams of fiber you get in your average regular pasta. Some brands, like Barilla Plus Multigrain pasta have even added omega-3 fats and protein to their pastas. You know me and marketing claims, but the ingredients here are pretty decent, and if the multigrain pasta helps fill you up faster and you enjoy it, that's what counts.

Are white pasta and white rice off-limits?—No, nothing's restricted when you've mastered cheating. If white pasta and rice were off-limits, I'd be in a heap of trouble. There are very few whole wheat pastas that my taste buds are happy with, and I really enjoy the aromatic flavor of basmati and jasmine rice. But I also know that these more refined, lower-fiber carbs don't do much to fill me up quickly or steady my blood sugar. So I cheat and am sure to space them out over the week, about one to three times, always keeping portions in check and piling on vegetables and a protein so that I'm satisfied. And as with most foods, I do my best to scout out really great brands, the most flavorful rice, the tastiest pasta, so by the end of the meal, I'm a really happy camper and have eaten an appropriate portion.

Cheater's Secret: If you're gluten intolerant, there's still hope for pasta! There is indeed gluten-free pasta, or try out Asian rice and 100% buckwheat soba noodles, which are both gluten-free friendly. You'll find wheat-free spelt and soy noodles on the market as well. Other gluten-free grains include quinoa, amaranth, buckwheat, kasha, grits, millet, and white, wild, brown, and colored varieties of rice.

We just did a run through the grocery store and after stocking up on weekly staples and kitchen essentials, there should be at least one type of pasta or whole grain that made it home with you. You've got a lot of gorgeous fresh groceries sitting on your counter. Use them! Break out the pasta or quinoa and start cooking.

To get you started and help you reenter the wonderful world of pasta and grains, here are few of my own favorite recipes, good to the last al dente bite.

Whole Wheat Spaghetti with Rustic Marinara Sauce

Remember to add in some protein, on the side or in the sauce, to round out the meal and fill you up. A few quick ideas: grilled chicken breast or extra meat from a roasted chicken, 3 to 4 small meatballs, shrimp, or beans. My dad used to throw in leftover chunks of lean pot roast into his signature sauce . . . good stuff. Pop in a nice salad of mixed greens and you've got a well-balanced pasta meal. Note that you'll likely have sauce leftover.

Makes 8 to 10 servings

THE GOODS
    3 tablespoons extra-virgin olive oil
    3 or 4 garlic cloves, minced
    1 small onion, diced
    2 28-ounce cans crushed tomatoes
    1 6-ounce can tomato paste
    1 teaspoon sugar

¼ teaspoon red pepper flakes
Salt and freshly ground pepper
½ cup loosely packed fresh basil leaves (optional)
1 16-ounce box whole wheat spaghetti
½ cup freshly grated Parmesan cheese, for serving

THE BREAKDOWN
1. In a large heavy pot, heat the olive oil over medium-high heat. Add the garlic and onion and sauté for 2 to 3 minutes.
2. Add the tomatoes, tomato paste, sugar, red pepper flakes, salt and pepper to taste, and basil, if using. Bring the sauce to a boil, then reduce the heat to low and simmer for at least 1 to 2 hours.
3. For the pasta, bring a large pot of water to a boil. Add the spaghetti and cook for 8 to 10 minutes, until al dente. Drain and serve with the sauce and Parmesan sprinkled on top (1 cup pasta per serving).

The Facts: 300 calories; 7g fat; 2g saturated fat; 13g protein; 10g fiber

VARIATION: * If you're choosing to add meatballs to your sauce and pasta, turkey or bison meatballs serve their leaner, lower-fat purpose, but having a scrumptious real-deal meatball (made of the traditional pork/veal/beef mixture) is heaven on occasion. Have one or two fewer than you would of the turkey and you're right back in action.

Market-Fresh Tomato and Basil Summer Pasta Salad

This pasta is the ultimate summertime crowd-pleaser—it's unbelievably easy and you can make it ahead of time and chill it. I have to give credit to one of my closest college friends, Lauren, whose incredible culinary talent created this dish years ago. It's since become an all-time staple whenever our girlfriends get together and gather around the table. The key to a killer dish is getting the best quality Pecorino Romano cheese— get a good hunk of it rather than the preshredded stuff, which loses its flavor and freshness.

Makes 10 to 12 servings

THE GOODS
> 1 15-ounce box regular or whole wheat penne pasta (can substitute bow-tie pasta if desired)
> 6 to 8 ripe plum, vine-ripened, or heirloom tomatoes, diced
> 1 cup fresh basil, torn in small pieces
> ¼ cup extra-virgin olive oil
> ¼ cup balsamic vinegar
> Salt and freshly ground black pepper
> ¾ to 1 cup freshly shredded Pecorino Romano cheese

THE BREAKDOWN
1. Bring a large pot of water to a boil for the pasta. Cook the pasta for 8 to 10, until al dente. Drain the pasta and cool it.
2. In a large bowl or storage container, combine the pasta, tomatoes, basil, oil, and vinegar and mix thoroughly to evenly distribute. Season with salt and pepper, top with Pecorino Romano, and mix lightly again. Serve at room temperature or refrigerate and serve cold.

The Facts: 230 calories; 7g fat; 2.5g saturated fat; 9g protein; 2g fiber

Whole Wheat Penne Pasta with Spicy Italian Turkey Sausage, Eggplant, and Olives

This is one of my favorite cold-weather comfort meals. I love the spice of the sausage and the heartiness of the eggplant.

Makes 4 servings

THE GOODS
> 1 tablespoon extra-virgin olive oil
> 2 links spicy Italian turkey or chicken sausage, meat removed from casings
> 1 garlic clove, minced

1 small eggplant, chopped

⅔ cup pitted green and black olives, roughly chopped

1 28-ounce can whole plum tomatoes

1 teaspoon sugar

Salt and freshly ground black pepper, to taste

¼ teaspoon red pepper flakes

½ 16-ounce box whole wheat penne or rigatoni pasta

THE BREAKDOWN

1. In a large heavy pot, heat the olive oil over medium-high heat. Add the sausage meat and garlic and sauté, stirring, until the meat browns, about 4 minutes.
2. Add the eggplant, olives, tomatoes, sugar, salt and pepper, and red pepper flakes. With a wooden spoon or spatula, break the whole plum tomatoes into chunks.
3. Bring the sauce to a boil, then reduce the heat and simmer for 30 to 40 minutes, until the eggplant is softened.
4. Bring a large pot of water to a boil. Add the penne or rigatoni and cook until al dente, about 12 minutes. Drain and serve with the sauce.

The Facts: 440 calories; 12g fat; 0.5g saturated fat; 18g protein; 13g fiber

Farfalle "Butterflies" or Fresh Ravioli with Spring Peas and Fava Beans

This recipe came about by accident, and it's turned out to be one of my favorite ways to usher in warmer weather and amazing springtime produce like peas and fava beans. At the last minute, a few friends were headed to my place for a laid-back weeknight dinner. I hadn't had the chance to hit the grocery store or greenmarket, so I decided to wing it and scoured my fridge and pantry, finding some remaining farfalle pasta and a few leftover freshly made ravioli I'd picked up at the farmers' market the weekend prior. Normally I wouldn't think to toss two kinds of pasta together, but it totally worked (just be sure to use two different pots to cook them in, as they'll have different cooking times). The farfalle and ravioli provided some nice variety, a little something for everyone. Obviously, you can stick to a single pasta—either will work just perfectly.

Makes 4 servings

THE GOODS
⅓ 16-ounce box farfalle (bow-tie) pasta
12 fresh ravoli with ricotta and herbs
1 tablespoon extra-virgin olive oil
2 garlic cloves, minced
¾ cup shelled English peas
½ cup shelled fava beans
1 tablespoon grated lemon rind
½ to ⅔ cup grated Pecorino Romano cheese, plus more for serving

THE BREAKDOWN
1. Bring two large pots of water to a boil for pasta. Meanwhile, add the peas and fava beans to a medium pot of salted boiling water and blanch for 2 to 3 minutes, then drain.
2. Add the farfalle to one pot and cook for about 12 minutes, until al dente. Add the fresh ravioli to the other pot and cook for about 4 minutes, until al dente. Drain and run cool water over the pasta to stop cooking process. Place the pasta back in one of the pots.
3. In a large sauté pan, heat the olive oil over medium-high heat. Add the garlic and cook for 30 seconds, until softened but not browned. Add the peas and fava beans and cook for 1 to 2 minutes. Add the pasta and stir to coat with the oil. Add the lemon rind and Pecorino and cook an additional 1 minute. Serve on its own or with a mixed greens salad and grilled chicken.

The Facts: 240 calories; 8g fat; 3.5g saturated fat; 10g protein; 2g fiber

VARIATION: *For a quick slant on this recipe, boil up enough bow-tie pasta for just 2 servings. Thinly slice 1 zucchini and sauté in 2 teaspoons olive oil with 1 minced garlic clove. Season with salt and freshly ground black pepper and cook for another 4 to 5 minutes. Mix together ½ cup fresh part-skim ricotta cheese with 1 teaspoon each of minced fresh parsley, chives, and basil. Once the pasta is done, drain and toss in the pan with the zucchini. Divide the pasta into 2 bowls and top each with ¼ cup fresh ricotta.

Linguine with Lemon-Garlic Shrimp and Asparagus

Makes 4 servings

THE GOODS
- ½ 16-ounce box linguine
- 1 bunch fresh asparagus (about 12 spears), ends trimmed and chopped into 1- to 2-inch pieces
- 1 pound peeled and deveined shrimp
- 3 teaspoons extra-virgin olive oil
- 2 minced garlic cloves
- ¼ cup dry white wine
- Zest of 1 lemon plus juice of ½ lemon
- 2 tablespoons finely chopped chives
- 2 tablespoons finely chopped fresh Italian parsley
- Salt and freshly ground black pepper to taste
- ¼ teaspoons red pepper flakes
- 1 teaspoon unsalted butter
- ½ cup fresh grated Parmesan reggiano cheese

THE BREAKDOWN
1. Bring a large pot of water to boil for the pasta. Add the linguine and cook until done, about 8 to 10 minutes or according to the package.
2. Steam the asparagus for 3 to 4 minutes, plunge in an ice bath to stay crisp, drain, and set aside.
3. Heat the olive oil and garlic in a large sauté pan over medium-high heat. Sauté the shrimp about 2 minutes. Add the wine, herbs, lemon zest and juice, salt, pepper, and red pepper flakes to pan. Add the asparagus back in and cook for another 3 to 4 minutes.
4. Toss the pasta into the pan with the shrimp and asparagus. Add in the Parmesan cheese and butter, mix well, and serve.

The Facts: 460 calories; 12g fat; 4.5g saturated fat; 38g protein; 3g fiber

Basic Pesto

One of the things I adore the most about my local greenmarket is the incredible array of fresh herbs I'm able to find throughout the year, and the prices are generally way cheaper than at the grocery store. Basil's at its best in the height of summer—the perfect time to whip up a batch of fresh pesto. You'll never think to get the store-bought stuff again. The pesto keeps in the refrigerator for up to 1 week.

Makes about 1 ⅓ cups (Aim for a serving size of about 1 tablespoon or less—a little goes a long way!)

THE GOODS
   3 large garlic cloves
   ½ cup pine nuts
   2 ounces Parmesan cheese, coarsely grated (about ⅔ cup) (or half Parmesan and half Pecorino Romano)
   1 teaspoon salt
   ½ teaspoon black pepper
   3 cups loosely packed fresh basil
   ⅔ cup extra-virgin olive oil (you may want to decrease the amount of olive oil to ½ cup, depending on desired consistency)

THE BREAKDOWN
   With food processor running, drop in the garlic through the hole in the top and finely chop. Stop the motor and add the nuts, cheese, salt, pepper, and basil, then process until finely chopped. With motor running, add the oil through the hole in the top, blending until incorporated.

The Facts: 110 calories; 11g fat; 2g saturated fat; 2g protein; 0g fiber

VARIATION: *You've just made an entire batch of pesto and don't know what to do with it. Aside from a pasta mix-in, top grilled chicken or fish with a dollop of pesto, mix into a big bowl of steamed, sautéed, or grilled vegetables, use it as a spread for sandwiches, panini, or brushcetta, place a teaspoon or two atop an omelet, sunny-side up, or poached eggs. Try out other pesto variations: Swap the pine nuts with walnuts for a boost of healthy omega-3 fats; do equal parts arugula and basil for a peppery kick; swap the basil completely for sun-dried tomatoes or roasted red peppers for a flavorful red pesto; or try the Sicilian version of pesto, switching the pine nuts for almonds and adding in 2 or 3 plum tomatoes.

Soba Noodles with Grilled Chicken and Peanut Dressing

Makes 4 servings

THE GOODS
- 8 ounces (½ package) soba noodles
- 4 4-ounce grilled chicken breasts, cut into thin strips
- 2 carrots, julienned
- 1 red bell pepper, julienned
- 2 scallions, chopped
- 2 tablespoons chopped roasted, unsalted peanuts

THE DRESSING
- 1 scallion, chopped
- 3 tablespoons canola oil
- 2 tablespoons rice vinegar or cider vinegar
- 1 ½ teaspoons organic sugar or agave nectar
- 2 teaspoons low-sodium soy sauce
- ¼ teaspoon minced garlic
- 1 teaspoon minced ginger
- 2 teaspoons toasted sesame oil
- 2 tablespoons all-natural peanut butter

THE BREAKDOWN
1. To make the dressing, in a medium bowl, whisk all the ingredients together until well blended.

2. For the noodles, bring a large pot of water to a boil. Cook the soba noodles for 4 to 5 minutes, or as the package directs. Drain and cool to room temperature. Place in a large bowl.
3. Toss the noodles with the chicken, carrots, bell pepper, and dressing. Garnish with the scallions and peanuts.

The Facts: 550 calories; 24g fat; 3g saturated fat; 35g protein; 5g fiber

Curried Quinoa with Cashews and Currants

Makes 4 ½-cup servings

THE GOODS
1 cup quinoa, rinsed
2 cups water
2 teaspoons curry powder (add more for stronger flavor)
1 teaspoon salt
1 tablespoon extra-virgin olive oil
½ cup diced onion
½ cup low-sodium chicken or vegetable broth
1 cup cooked chickpeas
¼ cup currants or raisins
3 tablespoons chopped toasted cashews

THE BREAKDOWN
1. In a medium saucepan, combine the quinoa, curry powder, salt, and water, bring to a boil, then reduce the heat to a simmer. Cover the pot and cook until the water is absorbed and the quinoa is light and fluffy, 10 to 15 minutes.
2. While the quinoa is simmering, heat the olive oil in a large skillet over medium heat. Add the onion and sauté for 1 minute. Add the broth, chickpeas, and raisins and simmer for 3 to 4 minutes. Add the cooked quinoa and toasted cashews and mix thoroughly.

The Facts: 220 calories; 9g fat; Ig saturated fat, 6g protein, 4g fiber

Coconut Rice with Cilantro and Ginger

Makes 4 servings

THE GOODS
  1 cup jasmine rice
  1 tablespoon canola oil
  3 tablespoons minced fresh ginger
  2 garlic cloves, minced
  ½ cup low-sodium chicken or vegetable broth
  1 cup light coconut milk
  ¼ teaspoon salt
  ¾ cup chopped cilantro
  2 scallions, chopped, for garnish

THE BREAKDOWN
  1. Rinse the rice well until the water runs clear, then drain. Heat
     the canola oil in a large saucepan over medium-high heat.
     Add the ginger and garlic and sauté for about 1 minute. Add
     the rice and stir for 2 minutes.
  2. Add the broth, coconut milk, salt, and cilantro, and stir.
  3. Bring to a boil, then reduce the heat to low and simmer for
     about 15 to 18 minutes, until the rice is done. Remove from
     heat, fluff the rice with a fork, and garnish with the scallions.

The Facts: 150 calories; 7g fat; 3.5g saturated fat; 3g protein; 0g fiber

Wild Rice with Dried Cranberries, Scallions, and Toasted Almonds

This dish uses a blend of wild rice which is high in fiber, but slightly heavier in calories than regular rice.

Makes 4 servings

THE GOODS

1 tablespoon extra-virgin olive oil

1 tablespoon minced shallot

¼ cup chopped onion

1 cup wild rice blend (mix of wild, brown, and sometimes red rices)

2 cups low-sodium chicken or vegetable broth

1 cup water

¼ teaspoon salt

¼ cup dried cranberries

¼ cup toasted slivered almonds (or substitute chopped walnuts or pecans)

¼ cup chopped scallions

THE BREAKDOWN

1. Rinse the rice well until the water runs clear and drain. Heat the olive oil in a large saucepan over medium-high heat. Add the shallot and onion and sauté for about 1 minute. Add the rice and stir for 2 to 3 minutes.

2. Add the broth, water, and salt and stir.

3. Bring to a boil, then reduce the heat to low and simmer for about 35 minutes, until the rice is done. Remove from heat, add in the dried cranberries, almonds, and scallions and fluff with a fork. Let stand 10 minutes.

The Facts: 250 calories; 8g fat; 1g saturated fat; 5g protein; 4g fiber

Refresher Course—Key Goals from Weeks 1 to 6

❑ Resize portions—3 to 5 ounces protein, ½ to 1 cup rice/pasta/grain, 1 cup/piece fruit, 1 to 3 cups veggies/salad (aim to cut total portions by 15 to 25 percent and set your plate up as: ½ fruits/vegetables, ¼ lean protein, ¼ healthy, complex carbs).

❑ Eat 2 servings of fruit per day; aim to have vegetables with lunch AND dinner.

❑ Drink 1 ½ to 2 liters of water per day.

❑ Don't skip meals—you'll lower your calorie-burn capability!

❑ Cheat it up each week with one or two indulgent meals (order what you wish, but still consider portions) and one to two treats (between 200 and 300 calories each).

❑ Exercise at least three or four days this week—kick it up a notch if you have a heavy week of drinking and/or eating ahead.

❑ Cut your alcohol intake per week by at least 25 percent.

❑ Food journaling . . . DO IT!

❑ Bring three to five basic office staples to work for snacks and emergencies.

❑ Re-plate and re-portion takeout and delivery food. Aim for half to three quarters of the to-go container.

❑ Watch portions like a hawk at restaurants, and leave at least 5 bites on the plate, if not a quarter to half. If the bread isn't awesome, lose it.

❑ Put all snacks and meals on a plate to halt mindless eating.

❑ Artificial sweeteners should be completely kicked to the curb by now.

❑ Get back on board with the basics after a long night out and a hangover.

❑ Stock up on your staple groceries each week.

CHAPTER 7—WEEK 7

Fresh for the Taking: Loving Local and Seasonal Food

"Going to the farmers' market makes me want to go on a fruit and vegetable shopping spree."

—Amy

WEEK 7 GOALS

- Learn to love the best by tasting the best.
- Go to your local greenmarket and explore.
- Purchase a new seasonal fruit or vegetable to test out.
- Keep driving home goals from Weeks 1 through 6: revised portions, increased exercise and water intake, at least 2 fruits and 2 veggies per day, no skipping meals, adjusted alcohol down by 25 percent, plate out your food, kick stress and emotional eating and artificial sweeteners to the curb.
- Congrats, you've successfully built a solid foundation of healthy eating goals that have now turned into daily habits—keep going strong!

We're now into Week 7, and if you never imagined you'd be grocery shopping, cooking, exercising, losing weight, enjoying dessert, and feeling pretty darn amazing all within a few short weeks, well . . . surprise! By now, you're likely down a good ten to fifteen pounds and still going—not too shabby. Your last big challenge is to hit your nearest farmers' market and get to know the goodness of seasonal produce and local meats, cheeses, and breads. Personally, I've been a fan of going local for as long as I can remember—I have vivid childhood memories of stopping by roadside farm stands during painfully long rides to the Delaware shore. Even at the age of five or six, the taste, smell, and vibrant colors of heavenly ripe cantaloupe, juicy white peaches that nearly melt in your mouth, and sweet, crisp golden corn were enough to win me over. A big thank-you to Mom and Dad for dragging my brother and me, despite woeful whining from the backseat.

If you've never thought to venture to your local farmers' market on a sunny Saturday morning, you're missing out big-time. And yes, your town or a town nearby most likely has at least one market— check out www.localharvest.org to find one. Don't worry, you will not be accosted by a crunchy crowd of farmers and health nuts. You will find there instead chefs, gourmets, and regular folk who have also discovered that farm foods close to home are fresher and cheaper, are more sustainable (better for the environment and local agriculture), and simply taste better. And as you know by now, finding the best-tasting foods is one of the keys to cheating. Why eat something if it's mediocre?

The Plan

This is the week to get a little closer to fresh food in order to keep losing those pounds. Greenmarkets and farm stands embody the Cheater's philosophy at its very core—the best of the best in its prime. By exploring your nearest farmers' market you'll gain a better appreciation for really fresh, high-quality, great-tasting food. In seeing a rainbow-colored bastion of seasonal produce, I'm hoping you'll be inspired to try a new fruit or vegetable, or create an entire recipe on your own. I'm anticipating that you'll be excited about a loaf of fresh-baked whole wheat bread with sunflower seeds and will jump at the thought of bringing home a log of herbed goat cheese that's unbelievably creamy. Your primary goal this week, and for weeks to come, is to take more ownership of your food, build discriminating taste buds, and gain a sense of how to form a good meal from simple, fresh ingredients. And in the process, be better equipped to keep cheating—to keep losing weight or maintaining your loss because you've uncovered the hidden gem of quality rather than quantity. Here's a snapshot of your week ahead incorporating farm-fresh food:

Week 7: Sample—Farmers Market Fresh
based on 1400-1600 calories

Week 7:	Monday	Tuesday	Wednesday
BREAKFAST 300-400 calories 7-9:30 a.m.	A.M. Run Outdoors (45 mins) Banana pre-workout ½ cup 2% cottage cheese with fresh berries and 1 tablespoon flaxseed	6 ounces low-fat plain yogurt with ¼ cup homemade granola (pg 362) and berries	HIT THE GYM 1 cup high-fiber cereal (more than 5 grams fiber) with 1 cup strawberries (or a serving of fruit) with skim or low-fat soy milk
SNACK ~100 calories 10-11 a.m.	Skip it	Iced coffee	Skip it
LUNCH 400-550 calories 12-2 p.m.	Make-Your-Own Salad You know the drill . . . 1. mixed greens, spinach, or arugula 2. some type of protein 3. whatever veggies or fruits you wish to add 4. a sprinkle of 1-2 of the following: cheese, dried fruit, nuts, olives, and/or avocado 5. 1-2 tablespoons vinaigrette dressing or olive oil/lemon	"Farmers' market" salad from home ½ cup cooked barley, ½ cup cannellini beans, ¼ cup cooked peas, ¼ cup chopped tomato, 1 tablespoon fresh mint, 1 ounce feta cheese, 2 teaspoons olive oil and lemon juice	½ fresh roasted turkey sandwich on whole grain with apple slices and 1 slice cheddar cheese, or a small amount of brie *make it fancy and mix ½ teaspoon raspberry preserves with ½ tablespoon Dijon mustard as a spread Remaining ½ of apple
SNACK 100-200 calories 3-5 p.m.	CHEAT TREAT #1 Crap day and it's only Monday, coffee break with your girlfriend Iced tea and split ½ gigantic peanut butter cookie	1 cup red and yellow pepper strips with 3 tablespoons store-bought light onion dip or hummus	2 dried apricots and 5 yogurt-covered almonds sitting out on your coworker's desk

Thursday	Friday	Saturday	Sunday
1 egg on a whole wheat English muffin with tomato slices Iced coffee	Quick breakfast smoothie with 6 ounces low-fat plain yogurt or skim/soy milk + ½ cup frozen mango + ½ banana + 1 tablespoon ground flaxseed + 1 teaspoon agave nectar	Hit the farmers' market and stock up for the dinner party you're hosting tonight! 6 ounces low-fat plain yogurt with ¼ cup home-made granola (pg 362) and berries	SLEEP LATE Tennis with friends (or your choice of exercise, 60 minutes) Small bowl (¾ cup) of high-fiber cereal and skim milk with ½ fresh peach to get you out the door
Peach or plum	1 hard-boiled egg	Raspberry iced tea while strolling the greenmarket	
Make-Your-Own Salad You know the drill . . . 1. mixed greens, spinach, or arugula 2. some type of protein 3. whatever veggies or fruits you wish to add 4. a sprinkle of 1-2 of the following: cheese, dried fruit, nuts, olives, and/or avocado 5. 1-2 tablespoons vinaigrette dressing or olive oil/lemon	Work lunch Grilled steak salad 1 small raisin-nut roll (you love raisin-nut bread, go ahead and have the small roll!)	Light lunch at home Open-faced sandwich (1 slice whole grain bread with 1 ounce feta cheese, 2 tomato slices, 2-3 basil leaves, 1 teaspoon olive oil and fresh pepper . . . pop into the toaster oven to lightly warm)	Poached Eggs with Asparagus, Parmesan, and Pepper (pg 167) 1 slice whole wheat sunflower bread from the farmers' market!
2 whole grain crackers with 1 ounce goat cheese or Laughing Cow Yoga or Pilates class after work	1 apple with 1 tablespoon almond or cashew butter (try something new!) Body conditioning class after work	1 cup fresh watermelon chunks or fruit salad	4 fresh figs from the farmers' market with 2 tablespoons goat cheese

Continued

Week 7:	Monday	Tuesday	Wednesday
DINNER 400-600 calories 7-8:30 p.m.	Have a light meal, that cookie did you in. Poached Halibut with White Wine, Lemon, and Thyme (pg 164) with veggies and small sweet potato or 1 cup butternut squash *make lunch for tomorrow ahead of time	Grilled chicken or tofu salad with Cheater's Caesar Dressing (pg 129)	Office happy hour 2 beers Grab takeout on the way home Greek salad with feta cheese 1 cup lentil soup OR Fresh herb, cucumber, and tomato salad and grilled chicken kebab with roasted tomatoes and mint
SNACK 100-150 calories 8:30-9:30 p.m. (If you're not hungry SKIP IT! Work in desserts and treats when you really want them and they're damn worth it!)	Skip it	Still a tad hungry after a run and a light dinner . . . Banana-date smoothie (⅔ cup unsweetened almond milk + ½ banana + 3 dates, chopped + ½ teaspoon vanilla extract + ½ cup ice. Throw it all in the blender!)	2 pieces dark chocolate
WATER	1.5 liters	2 liters	2 liters
ALCOHOL/ OOPS!			2 beers
EXERCISE	Run/jog outdoors		Gym

Thursday	Friday	Saturday	Sunday
CHEAT MEAL #1 Fancy date night 4 ounces duck breast with blackberry glaze Sautéed spinach and parsnip puree	Fish soft tacos with mango or peach salsa 2 small corn tortillas with 4 ounces grilled snapper or shrimp Salsa: ½ cup diced mango + 2 teaspoons minced red onion + juice from ½ lime + 1 teaspoon cilantro + pinch of salt Serve with 2 cups mixed greens	2 cups Arugula Salad with Grilled Peaches and Mozzarella (pg 335) 3 ounces Seared Scallops with Fresh Corn and Tomato Relish (pg 336) ¾ cup Fingerling Potatoes with Pesto (pg 337)	Bison burger (pg 113) with 1 ear fresh corn (leftover from yesterday) and 2 cups heirloom tomato and basil salad dressed with 2 teaspoons olive oil, 1 teaspoon balsamic vinegar
CHEAT TREAT #2 Share dessert Berry or apple crisp with vanilla ice cream	Skip it	1 cup balsamic strawberries with 2 tablespoons home-made whipped cream (pp 337–338)	Leftover strawberries!
1.5 liters and seltzer	2 liters	2 liters and 1 glass seltzer with lime	2 liters
2 glasses wine		3 Lemonade Vodka Spritzers—they're a little too good! (pg 266)	
Yoga or Pilates	Body conditioning class		Tennis or exercise

Week 7—Cheater's Shopping List:

- ❑ Vegetables: 3 to 5 (or more) for the week: 3 tomatoes, red and yellow bell pepper, asparagus, peas, arugula, 3 ears fresh corn, red onion
- ❑ Fruit: 2 to 4 types (or more), your pick (enough to get you through 5 to 7 days, 2 servings a day): peaches, apples, watermelon, strawberries, figs
- ❑ Protein: 4 ounces halibut, 4 ounces snapper, 1 pound scallops, ¼ pound fresh roasted sliced turkey, 4 ounces ground bison, eggs
- ❑ Healthy carbs: whole grain cereal (more than 5 grams fiber, less than 7 grams sugar), whole grain bread, soft corn tortillas, sweet potato, barley
- ❑ Dairy/calcium: feta cheese, cheddar, 3 to 4 low-fat plain yogurts or cottage cheese, skim/soy/almond milk
- ❑ Other: 1 can cannellini beans
- ❑ Seasonings and spices: basil, garlic, mint, 1 lemon, 1 lime
- ❑ Snack stuff and staples: jar of almond or cashew butter (or finish your peanut butter), hummus
- ❑ Dessert/treat: heavy cream for the whipped cream! dark chocolate

But Seriously, Why Go Local?

Greenmarkets are sprouting up across the nation, 4800 of them offering bushels and baskets loaded sky-high with produce, baked goods, cheeses, dairy products, and more from local farmers and purveyors (local being defined as within about 100 miles of your home or less). Something's obviously catching on. That *something* is tied directly to the recent rise of the sustainable food and agriculture movement, environmentally conscious, go-green efforts around our food system that are catching the eyes and ears of celebrities, high-profile political figures, the media, and the common consumer. Foodie First Lady Michelle Obama, *Omnivore's Dilemma* author and food activist Michael Pollan, and celebrity hottie Leonardo DiCaprio would certainly applaud you for lowering your carbon footprint by sauntering over to your local market. Emphasis on locally and organically grown food and a more nutritious and sustainable food supply is building momentum, and with any luck, political power.

But aside from gaining some praise from a political figurehead and a scrumptious Hollywood heartthrob, why bother going to the farmers' market? Why does buying local or supporting sustainability honestly matter? Is being "green" or "going local" just the latest yuppie or hipster fad? Concerns about our food supply, food safety, and environmental consciousness continue to garner some serious attention—it's not just a California or an NYC or a Portland thing. It affects all of us and it affects the quality, taste, and cost of our food and can really impact our overall relationship with food. I've found that the closer you are to your food source, the more you appreciate what you're eating, the more you savor it, and the more whole, fresh, nutritious food you end up eating—which generally translates to fewer calories, greater satisfaction, and smaller quantities . . . and, of course, better health overall.

When talking about proximity and how your food is getting onto your plate, the average piece of conventional produce, from apples to asparagus, travels an estimated 1500 miles and sometimes across several continents before it lands on your dinner plate. "Food miles" refer to the number of miles your food travels from the farm to your table and they can rack up quite quickly. The estimated food miles of many conventional items sold in grocery stores are twenty-seven times greater than those purchased from a local farmer or vendor. Those apples sitting in your fridge may have taken 1726 miles to get there, not to mention a whole lot of fossil fuel that spews carbon dioxide and other pollutants into the atmosphere.

Doesn't sound too good, does it? Obviously, buying *all* your food local is a pretty serious undertaking, particularly if you lead a busy life. If you don't always have access to a farmers' market or can't make it there each and every week, is it an absolute sin to purchase apples from the grocery store? No, of course not, but given the opportunity, the more you can buy local the better.

Week 7:	Monday	Tuesday	Wednesday
Week 7: Your Weekly Food Journal			
BREAKFAST 300-400 calories *(Note your hunger level on a scale of 1 to 10 after each meal!)*			
SNACK *~100 calories (If you're not hungry, skip it!)*			
LUNCH 400-550 calories			
SNACK 100-200 calories			
DINNER 400-600 calories			
SNACK 100-150 calories *(Aim for at least 2 hours before bed!)*			
WATER			
ALCOHOL/ OOPS!			
EXERCISE			

Thursday	Friday	Saturday	Sunday

Cut to the Chase—What Local Food Can Do for You

1. *Local food tastes better*—Ever had an underripe, mealy, tasteless tomato from the grocery store? It's likely because the poor little guy spent a week traveling cross-country stuck in a truck, train, or plane and then chilled out in a warehouse for another full week before landing directly on your plate or because he was genetically engineered in a greenhouse somewhere in the middle of South Dakota. If you go local and get food that's straight from the source, the farmer's own two hands, the flavor is often incomparable and you get to know where your food is coming from. Make friends with your farmers!

2. *Local food is better for you*—The shorter the time between the farm and table, the fewer vitamins and minerals that are lost. Produce is most healthful at peak freshness, so eat up. You have access to the people providing you food and you can easily ask about what farming methods they employ, if the produce or food item is organic, and if pesticides are used in any way.

3. *Local food strengthens a sense of community*—So it may sound like I've been sitting around the Girl Scout campfire a little too long, but farmers' markets build a sense of community; you're connecting with your food and who brought it to you. By purchasing food from local purveyors, you're also supporting your local environment, agriculture, and the farmers.

4. *Local food often costs less*—Save a buck or ten by buying local rather than the jaw-dropping prices you'll often find at grocery stores. Save some cash and that to-die-for new handbag is that much closer to having a home in your closet.

5. *Local food helps you cheat and maintain a slim, trim figure*—As your scale can confirm, fresh food is definitely best for losing weight and keeping it off, feeling more perky and energized, filling up faster on less, and finding real delight in what you're eating. This is really what cheating's all about and is precisely why it's so successful. The better quality the food is, the more flavor

and healthful indulgence, and the less processed and packaged something is, you wind up with the perfect recipe for cheating the system: slimming down without giving up the good stuff. If that's not a reason to go local, I don't know what is.

* Check out www.sustainabletable.org for more information on local and sustainable food.

CSA Chic

If you find yourself smitten by the greenmarket and really want to take the next step toward connecting with your local farming community, you might consider purchasing a share in a CSA, Community Supported Agriculture. In joining a CSA, you support a local farm by purchasing produce and goods in advance. This system helps finance the farmer's crop each season. You, the consumer, in turn receive a portion of what's been harvested each week. CSAs generally have accessible pick-up points for their members living in both urban and suburban areas. A mere disclaimer rather than a deterrent—CSAs can be a bit of gamble. If it's been a bountiful harvest, you can hit the jackpot, but if the harvest isn't so plentiful, your bags may be on the skimpy side. That said, the CSA is an excellent endeavor for the adventurer who likes living on the edge and cooking off the cuff, as you never know what you'll receive each week. You might find yourself knee deep in five pounds of beets and peaches one week, squash and fresh peas the next. Never knew you could prepare beets fifteen different ways, did you? To learn more about CSAs near you, check out www.sustainabletable .org/shop/csa, www.localharvest.org/csa, or www.myfarmshare.com (New York metro area only).

When to Buy Organic

After all this local food and greenmarket chatter, you're likely wondering where "organic" falls into the picture. By definition, organic denotes that a food has been produced or grown without any form of pesticides, hormones, additives, colorings, antiobiotics . . .

need I continue? Look for the big green USDA organic stamp on food labels to ensure it contains at least 95 percent organic ingredients. Many farmers and vendors you'll come in contact with at the greenmarket employ organic farming or food preparation methods.

Unfortunately, organic items often come at a hefty price. Thankfully, you don't have to buy everything organic. Buy smart and soundly to keep your hard-earned dollars where they belong—saving up for that gorgeous handbag you've been drooling over for months. You'll likely find both organic and nonorganic local vendors at your greenmarket. You can shop with both and can always inquire whether or not a particular farmer uses organic methods. Oftentimes, red tape can snag the certification process. Many local nonorganic farmers still don't use harmful pesticides or hormones. They just haven't been given their certification yet.

CHEAT SHEET: The Dirty Dozen—Top Foods to Buy Organic

- Apples
- Cherries
- Grapes
- Berries
- Potatoes
- Milk
- Beef and poultry
- Celery
- Bell peppers
- Spinach
- Peaches
- Pears

Cheater's Secret: The Environmental Working Group, a nonprofit organization that informs the public on health and environmental issues, has identified the "dirty dozen," items with the greatest exposure to pesticides and hormones because of thin skins and permeability (produce) or added hormones and antibiotics (dairy, meat, and poultry). These items *should* be on your organic/locally grown list as often as possible: **apples, cherries, grapes, berries, potatoes, milk, beef and poultry, celery, bell peppers, spinach, peaches, and pears.** Produce with protective skins, coverings, or rinds like melon, avocado, and pineapple can be bought conventionally without too much worry.

High Season

The notion of seasonality might seem a bit foreign in our country of plenty, where virtually anything and everything is accessible at all times of the year thanks to importing. Many of us have come to expect to be able to find deliciously sweet mangos on any given day even though mangos aren't native to the United States, nor are they in season in the dead of winter. Deliciously juicy strawberries in January? You've got to be joking. They're in season in North America June through August. By simply walking around the farmers' market, you can get a pretty clear picture of what is actually in season in your geographic area and therefore what will taste the best in your mouth and do your body good. This is what we call seasonality, working with what the earth provides us throughout the year. Your taste buds will thank you. You can check what's harvested and when it's harvested in your neck of the woods on the Seasonal Ingredient Map at www.epicurious.com.

Taking the Farmers' Market by Storm and Cooking for Others

It's the weekend and you're faced with the task of cooking dinner for three of your closest friends. The key to any successful soiree is making it appear effortlessly chic and healthfully gourmet. Even your most "healthy food–fearing" friend will be blown away by your masterful skills! Thankfully, I've convinced you

CHEAT SHEET: Seasonal Produce Guide

FALL		WINTER	
apples	potatoes	blood oranges	kiwi
Asian pears	quince	Brussels sprouts	leeks
beets	radicchio	cabbage	parsnips
broccoli	squash (acorn,	citrus fruits	potatoes
broccoli rabe	butternut,	collard greens	rainbow chard
Brussels sprouts	pumpkin,	cranberries	sweet potatoes
pears	kabocha)	grapefruit	Swiss chard
persimmons	sweet potatoes	kale	turnips
pomegranates			

SPRING		SUMMER	
apricots	okra	arugula	green beans
asparagus	raspberries	avocado	honeydew
blueberries	rhubarb	beets	nectarines
cantaloupe	spinach	bell peppers	peaches
cherries	strawberries	blueberries	plums
figs	sugar snap peas	cantaloupe	strawberries
fennel	Swiss chard	corn	summer squash
		cucumber	tomatoes
		eggplant	watermelon
		grapefruit	zucchini

to head to your farmers' market (when it's up and running during the season) for some culinary inspiration and to pick up the best produce in town for dinner and for the rest of the week. Let's take a simulated tour of your neighborhood greenmarket during the summertime, at the height of fresh produce's glory. Before you arrive, sketch out your proposed meal from appetizer to dessert in your head or on paper. Most important, make it easy on yourself. Prepare things you're comfortable with and you're guaranteed to be a hostess with the mostess. Aside from the fantastic recipes scattered throughout these pages, if you find it helpful to flip through a cookbook, a cooking magazine such as *Cooking Light* or *Bon Appétit*, or a Web site like Epicurious.com, Culinate.com, or Foodnetwork.com, do so. You've got a hankering for some sort of seafood, shrimp, or scallops, and maybe a bright big salad and a simple side dish like couscous or roasted potatoes? You're a cook on a mission!

Come prepared with three things: 1) cash, as most outdoor vendors aren't equipped with credit card machines and don't accept personal checks; 2) a large canvas tote bag or small cart to carry your purchases in so you're not loaded down with a zillion different plastic bags; and 3) a shopping list and/or your dinner menu so you don't space out and forget what the hell you wanted to make. Leave room, however, for additions or edits to your list. Get inspired by what produce looks best and tailor your list accordingly. I call this renegade shopping and cooking—allowing yourself to experiment without a specific recipe and get creative with flavors and ingredients. If you plan to purchase perishable items like eggs, meats, seafood, or dairy products, you may also want to bring an ice pack or small cooler if it's really hot out.

- **Decoding the Greenmarket**—Game time. Canvas bag in hand, let's head into the market and see what we discover. The first vendor you stumble upon is a farmer selling brown and white "free-range" eggs and "pasture-raised" chicken breasts. What does that mean? First off, different colored eggs simply come from different varieties of hens, but taste and nutrition are exactly the same. Conventional "factory farmed" chickens are often raised in cramped quarters, fed genetically modified grains grown with pesticides, and given doses of antibiotics or hormones to prevent disease and promote a bigger, meatier bird. Free-range birds are free of hormones and antibiotics and have a higher amount of healthy omega-3 fats, which translate directly to the eggs they lay, which benefits you when the eggs are on your plate. "Free-range" indicates that the hens were raised in an unconfined environment where they were able to roam freely outdoors for at least five minutes daily, and they're pasture-fed. "Pasture-raised" hens and other animals roam freely in their natural environment and eat nutrient-rich grasses and plants that their bodies are adapted to digest. Pasturing is best for the animal and the environment and translates to leaner, more flavorful meat, eggs, and dairy products for you. Free-range chickens have 21 percent less fat and 28 percent fewer calories than factory-farmed chickens and eggs from pasture-raised hens contain 400 percent more omega-3 fats. In turn, your cardiovascular system and your figure will reap the benefits. Your taste buds will also thank you, as organic and locally pasture-raised poultry (beef/meat and dairy, along with wild seafood) tends to taste noticeably better. You don't need eggs for your girls' dinner, but pick some up for the week ahead and make a few great-tasting omelets for breakfast or speedy dinners.

- **Grass Versus Grain: The Verdict on Meat**—Next to the eggs, you notice a vendor selling grass-fed beef. Take note. Most cattle in this country are fed grain-heavy diets (a diet higher in refined carbs, like corn), which fattens them up quickly and cheaply. Grain-fed cows are often raised in cramped quarters and given a lot of antibiotics to ward off disease. Corn, protein supplements, and growth hormones beef them up, literally, so they can be slaughtered more quickly. However, grass-fed beef contains a third less fat than grain-fed beef and generally tastes phenomenally better. Grass-fed cows produce milk and meat that is almost twice as high in heart-healthy omega-3 fats and CLA (conjugated linoleic acid), an unsaturated fat that may decrease heart disease and has been linked to the reduction of body fat.

- **Plentiful Produce**—After buying your meat you visit a stand with richly colored summer fruits and veggies. A resplendent mountain of red and yellow tomatoes, midnight purple eggplant, and emerald green arugula lies before you. You ask the farmer about the tomatoes and he tells you they're heirloom. Another word to add to your culinary crib sheet. "Heirloom" means the fruit or vegetable stems from its original varietal. These puppies are purebred, by nature and nature alone. The taste difference speaks for itself. Grab a few and test out the arugula while you're at it. You also spot, or rather smell, some incredible summer basil and fresh cilantro. You're not sure what you'll end up doing with them, but you decide these herbs are a must-have and toss them in your bag as well.

◆ Tomatoes are packed with disease-fighting antioxidants and are particularly rich in lycopene, an antioxidant and phytochemical that may help in preventing cancer.

◆ Arugula, also known as rocket and rucola in other countries, has roots stemming from the Mediterranean and is a dark leafy green with a particularly peppery flavor. It's got a bite and it's one of my absolute favorites for salads and side dishes! Rich in vitamins A and C and folate, arugula is one leafy green not to be missed.

When purchasing fruits and vegetables, here's a basic rule of thumb: Actually feel the fruit and vegetables. Melons, peaches, pears, plums, tomatoes, and the like should be firm but slightly soft and supple to the touch. You should also smell produce to determine the degree of ripeness. Sniff your heart out. If you don't plan on using the produce for three or four days, choose items that are firmer and allow them to ripen at home. Tomatoes, peaches, nectarines, bananas, pears, avocados, and other fruits can all be stored in a brown paper bag on your kitchen counter to speed up the ripening process.

• **Better Bread, Freshly Baked**—Last, you find a local baker whose artisan bread looks irresistible. Grab a loaf of crusty Italian ciabatta for your dinner party. Ciabatta's a white bread, but this is a great example of when to incorporate a small piece of really good refined carb into your week. Skip the mediocre bread at restaurants and reach for the best breads once or twice a week. Also pick up a hearty, fiber-rich loaf of seven grain bread for sandwiches this coming week.

So there's your whirlwind tour of your local greenmarket— thanks for coming out. In one short trip you purchased the majority of ingredients for a suppertime soiree and a few fresh staples for the coming week.

From Farm to Table—Cooking with Seasonal Ingredients

Now that you've successfully toured the greenmarket and hopefully come away with some gorgeous produce, let's head back into your kitchen for a little something I like to call "renegade cooking." Whatever it was that excited you at the farmers' market, maybe some fresh ears of corn, summer peaches, ruby red tomatoes, purple potatoes, or crisp green beans, start allowing your imagination and creativity to flow (and yes, I realize how difficult this might be for some of you type-A'ers, but free-forming it can be incredibly rewarding). How could you incorporate those peaches or that corn into a meal? What else would pair well with it? Let your taste buds and what looks incredibly delicious to you guide your cooking decisions and menu planning. You'll be cooking "off the cuff" in no time, no recipe required.

One of the primary goals throughout this book is to build your confidence in the kitchen. Cooking like the renegade you are is the pinnacle; you're coming into your culinary own. When we're talking about "off the cuff" cooking, seasonality definitely plays a major role. People often ask how I cook without exact recipes, how do I know what tastes good together, or how much of an ingredient to use. My answer: a) getting inspired by what seasonal items I see at the grocery or the greenmarket, and b) a lot of trial and error in the kitchen. It's okay to screw up; you always learn something from it. Cooking by season allows you to use the most nutrient-rich ingredients available at a given time of the year, it ensures you've got variety going on in your diet, and it inspires you to experiment with new dishes with new ingredients . . . or bring back some great seasonal standbys you forgot about. And to bring the message of cheating home once again, fresh ingredients, superb quality, and great flavor means greater satisfaction for you and fewer pounds showing on the scale.

In the spirit of the summer and of the greenmarket, I've devoted the remainder of this chapter to some of the freshest and most flavorful dishes that came out of my own trips to the greenmarket when

I free-formed it and let my creativity run a little more wild than normal. Below, I've provided just a sampling of irresistible spring-summery dishes, when the farmers' market is at its peak. I've structured the recipes so they're the perfect setup for an impromptu (or well-planned) dinner party for four that's deliciously, nutritiously, and exquisitely executed.

Arugula Salad with Grilled Peaches and Fresh Mozzarella

Makes 4 servings

THE GOODS
　　2 large peaches, halved and pitted
　　Extra-virgin olive oil for brushing
　　1 large bunch arugula or 8 cups prewashed baby arugula
　　1 large ball fresh mozzarella, sliced in 8 thin rounds (if there's a
　　　　cheese vendor selling it at the farmers' market, try it out!)

THE DRESSING
　　3 tablespoons extra-virgin olive oil
　　2 tablespoons balsamic vinegar
　　1 teaspoon Dijon mustard
　　Salt and freshly ground pepper

THE BREAKDOWN
1. Heat a grill pan or outdoor grill. Brush the peach halves with olive oil and grill cut-side-down for 3 to 4 minutes, until light grill marks are made. Remove from the grill, cool, then slice the peaches about 1 inch thick.
2. In a small bowl, whisk together the ingredients for the dressing.
3. Arrange the arugula, mozzarella, and peaches on plates, and drizzle each with 1 tablespoon of the dressing.

The Facts: 220 calories; 18g fat; 5g saturated fat; 6g protein; 2g fiber

Seared Scallops with Fresh Corn and Tomato Relish

Makes 4 servings

THE GOODS
2 ears of fresh corn
3 medium vine-ripened tomatoes, diced
3 tablespoons extra-virgin olive oil
Juice of 1 ½ lemons
1 small garlic clove, minced
½ cup fresh basil leaves, plus more for garnish
Salt and freshly ground black pepper
1 pound fresh-caught large scallops
2 teaspoons unsalted butter

THE BREAKDOWN
1. Cook the corn in boiling water for 8 to 10 minutes. Drain, cool, and cut the kernels off the cobs. Place in a large bowl and add the diced tomatoes.
2. In a food processor, combine the olive oil, lemon juice, garlic, and basil and blend until smooth. Pour three quarters of the mixture into the corn and tomato mixture and season with salt and pepper.
3. Season the scallops with salt and pepper. In a large skillet, melt the butter over medium heat. Add the scallops and cook for 3 to 4 minutes on each side, until golden brown.
4. Divide the corn-tomato salad among 4 plates and place the scallops atop the salad. Drizzle the plates with the remaining basil oil and sprinkle extra basil (torn into small pieces or cut into a chiffonade) on top of the scallops.

The Facts: 280 calories; 14g fat; 3g saturated fat; 22g protein; 2g fiber

Fingerling Potatoes, Cherry Tomatoes, and Sugar Snap Peas with Pesto

One of my favorite restaurants, `inoteca, in New York's Lower East Side, inspired this recipe. The vibrant colors, fresh produce, and flavorful herbs just scream farmers' market and seasonal eating.

Makes 6 to 8 servings

THE GOODS
1 pound fingerling potatoes
1 teaspoon salt
1 pint cherry tomatoes, halved
3 cups sugar snap peas
¼ cup Basic Pesto (page 310)

THE BREAKDOWN
1. Add the potatoes and salt to a large pot filled with 1 quart water and bring to a boil. Cook for about 25 minutes, until the potatoes are tender. Drain and allow cool to room temperature.
2. In a separate pot, steam the peas for 3 to 4 minutes. Cool to room temperature.
3. In a large bowl, mix the potatoes with the tomatoes, peas, and pesto, and toss to coat evenly.

The Facts: 120 calories; 6g fat; 1g saturated fat; 4g protein; 2g fiber

Balsamic Berries with Homemade Whipped Cream

Makes 8 servings

THE GOODS
⅓ cup balsamic vinegar
2 teaspoons plus 1 ½ tablespoons sugar

Juice from ¼ lemon

3 pints fresh berries (mix it up with raspberries, blackberries, and strawberries; stem strawberries and cut in half or quarters)

Homemade Whipped Cream (recipe follows)

THE BREAKDOWN

1. Combine the vinegar, 2 teaspoons sugar, and lemon juice in a small saucepan. Stir over medium heat until the sugar dissolves.
2. Simmer until the vinegar becomes syrupy and reduces, 3 to 4 minutes. Set aside and allow to cool. You can make this ahead of time and refrigerate.
3. Place the berries in a large bowl and sprinkle with the remaining 1 ½ tablespoons sugar and drizzle with balsamic syrup. Toss to coat evenly. Divide the berries among small dessert bowls, cups, or martini glasses. Top each with a dollop (about 2 tablespoons) of whipped cream.

The Facts: 130 calories; 6g fat; 3.5g saturated fat; 1g protein; 2g fiber

Whipped Cream

Homemade whipped cream is one of the easiest, deliciously indulgent things ever. A little of this stuff won't make a huge dent on a light dessert like berries, but it'll bust your cheat factor through the roof when you're looking for dessert. Just be careful, this stuff can be addictive; aim for about 2 to 3 tablespoons per serving.

THE GOODS

2 cups heavy cream

¼ cup sugar

1 to 1 ½ teaspoons vanilla extract (I like my whipped cream with a strong vanilla flavor, so I always opt for a little more)

THE BREAKDOWN

Place all the ingredients in a large bowl, get out your electric beater or electric whisk if you have one, and beat on a low setting until soft peaks form—don't overbeat or the cream can get stiff and curdle. If you don't own an electric beater, you can always use a regular whisk and get a killer arm and wrist workout! The whipped cream can be refrigerated for up to 4 hours before serving.

The Facts: 60 calories; 6g fat; 3.5g saturated fat; 0g protein; 0g fiber

VARIATION: *For a flavorful twist on whipped cream for any occasion, cut the vanilla in half and add 2 teaspoons rum, brandy, or a liqueur like Irish cream or Kahlùa. Or for a lemony whipped cream, add 1 teaspoon lemon zest or 2 teaspoons store-bought lemon curd.

Refresher Course—Key Goals from Weeks 1 to 7

- ❑ Resize portions—3 to 5 ounces protein, ½ to 1 cup rice/pasta/grain, 1 cup/piece fruit, 1 to 3 cups veggies/salad (aim to cut total portions by 15 to 25 percent and set your plate up as: ½ fruits/vegetables, ¼ lean protein, ¼ healthy, complex carbs).
- ❑ Eat 2 servings of fruit per day; aim to have vegetables with lunch AND dinner.
- ❑ Drink 1 ½ to 2 liters of water per day.
- ❑ Don't skip meals—you'll lower your calorie-burn capability!
- ❑ Cheat it up each week with one or two indulgent meals (order what you wish, but still consider portions) and one or two treats (between 200 and 300 calories each).
- ❑ Exercise at least 3 or 4 days this week—kick it up a notch if you have a heavy week of drinking and/or eating ahead.
- ❑ Cut your alcohol intake per week by at least 25 percent.
- ❑ Food journaling . . . DO IT!
- ❑ Bring three to five basic office staples to work for snacks and emergencies.

❏ Re-plate and re-portion takeout and delivery food. Aim for half to three quarters of the to-go container.

❏ Watch portions like a hawk at restaurants, and leave at least 5 bites on the plate, if not a quarter to half. If the bread isn't awesome, lose it.

❏ Put all snacks and meals on a plate to halt mindless eating.

❏ Artificial sweeteners should be completely kicked to the curb by now.

❏ Get back on board with the basics after a long night out and a hangover.

❏ Stock up on your staple groceries each week.

❏ Shop at your local farmers' market, the best of the best.

Cheating All Year Long: Special Occasions, Holidays, Travel, Aunt Flow, and More

"Just because it tastes good doesn't mean you need to have a ton of it."

—Johanna's mom

WEEK 8 GOALS

- Plan ahead and mentally prepare for special occasions, holidays, and travel, and have a plan of attack for PMS cravings and food-heavy situations.
- Pick up food journaling when needed in the months ahead. Hit the wall for a few days or screw the pooch on vacation? Grab your food diary and get writing for at least three to five days to get back to healthy eating and cheating habits ASAP. Accountability and structure can work wonders.
- Keep driving home goals from Weeks 1 through 7: revised portions, increased exercise and water intake, at least 2 fruits and 2 veggies per day, no skipping meals, adjusted alcohol down by 25 percent, plate out your food, kick stress and emotional eating and artificial sweeteners to the curb, weekly grocery and greenmarket shopping.

We're coming up to the finish line and preparing to send you off all on your own. Deep breaths, you'll be just fine. You're armed and dangerous, having built up an arsenal of useful tools, tricks, and tactics over the past seven weeks and seven chapters. I hope they've built upon one another and you're now feeling confident, collected, and quite coquettish in your well-fitting skinny jeans and little black dress. The game plan for this chapter is to cement and solidify all the healthy eating and cooking habits that you've taken in thus far, address a smattering of miscellaneous but ever-important topics—like stomach issues, family holidays, frozen yogurt, and PMS—and send you on your merry martini-making way. So here we go . . .

- **Handling the Holidays**—As joyous and exciting as the holiday season is, it can often end up being a month-long free-for-all of cocktails, heavier meals, and your favorite childhood sweets. Inevitably you're faced with a boozy holiday season each and every year, so prep yourself for a slightly bumpy ride in hopes of avoiding chaining yourself to the treadmill for the entire winter. By early to mid-December, you've likely already logged a handful of holiday parties and have four more to go, are still reeling from last Saturday's Santa pub crawl (doesn't wearing a blazing hot Santa suit burn off extra beer calories?), are gearing up for your office party, and are prepping yourself for the onslaught of overbearing, eggnog-pushing relatives come the actual holidays themselves. So if you're counting down, by the time all is said and done, the tally comes to: 12 pigs in a blanket, 11 mini egg rolls, 10 bacon-wrapped dates, 9 pieces of fudge, 8 pieces of Brie, 7 shots of spiced rum, 6 handfuls of cocktail nuts, 5 stuffed mushrooms, 4 glasses of that damn eggnog, 3 candy canes, 2 pieces of chocolate cheesecake, and enough cocktails and Christmas cookies to make your head spin and send your weight off the Richter scale. Thank goodness for New Year's resolutions right?

If the sirens are sounding in your head, put the brakes on . . . the scale isn't totally tipped just yet. Most of us typically gain just one single, teeny-weeny pound per holiday season. Not terrible, but the downfall is that single pound that adds up to five, ten, or more over the years. Damn all those unsuspecting handfuls of red and green M&M'S.

I love to indulge during the holidays as much as anyone else. Here are ten no-fail tips to get you through the holidays unscathed and with cheer, enjoyment, and delight without busting your bathroom scale. If you still find yourself chained to the treadmill come January 2, that's your own call.

10. The holidays occur on simply a few DAYS—that doesn't give you a free hall pass for the entire month of December! Use your two weekly *cheat and eat* meals and treats wisely and apply them to holiday-specific meals and events, such as your office holiday party or cocktail hour. Remember you can swap a single treat for two or three extra cocktails if it's a particularly booze-heavy week of holiday parties. On the actual holiday itself, enjoy the day to the fullest, indulge—smartly—without having a daylong smorgasbord.

9. Continue with your typical workout and eating routine (refer back to page 339 for a summary of Weeks 1 to 7's key goals) throughout the month so that you can add in extra cocktails and treats and a holiday meal here and there without getting derailed. Start your day off with your head in the game. Just as you normally would, set the tone of your day with a healthy, balanced breakfast—like a poached egg, slice of whole grain English muffin and fruit, or a warm cup of steel-cut oatmeal with banana slices rather than a cinnamon roll and a piece of fudge so you can ward off a snowball of mindless nibbling, sweet cravings, and heavy eating. Starting off right keeps your mood and energy levels running at full speed.

8. If you have multiple social engagements in a given week, refer back to Chapters 3 and 5 and keep tabs on the booze intake (ideally eight drinks or under), plug in one or two special (i.e., calorie-heavy) meals, and balance things out with a little more exercise (four to six times a week, even if all you can get in is a brisk wintry walk for thirty minutes), at least 2 liters of water, and lighter fare (read: pack in extra fruits and vegetables, focus on smaller portions at mealtimes).

7. Take a second look. Scaling back just 15 to 20 percent on portion sizes at meals and snacks will allow you to account for the extra 100 to 300 calories, or more, you're downing on a party-hardy day. Leaving behind one fifth of your sandwich at lunch or fruit-nut bar at snack isn't really that much to ask. Don't feel bad about wasting food—you'll make up for it with an extra glass of champagne soon enough and can help the homeless or malnourished children in other ways.

6. Cocktail party situation: Before you lay a finger on a coconut shrimp, scan the room, assess your options, and build your plate with strategic confidence. Fill up on fruit and vegetables and light appetizers if they're available and then choose two or three naughty (but oh so nice) hors d'oeuvres, such as fried goat cheese and crab dip, and you're good to go. *Don't* stand directly next to the table with the bowl of cocktail nuts, chocolate truffles, or tortilla chips (willpower doesn't come easy, why punish yourself?). Engage in conversation—whether it's with a friend, colleague, or if you're unattached, a romantic prospect. Hey, they hung mistletoe for a reason!

5. The best cocktail for all you boozehounds (and you know who you are): If you're going for the bottle and it's going to be a long night, skip the calorie-rich eggnog, rum punch, and chocolate martinis. Champagne's a "boozy best" at 85 calories a glass. There isn't anything wrong with a little bubbly. Otherwise, stick to the basics . . . red or white wine, vodka and club soda, Johnny W. on the rocks or with a splash of ginger ale. Stick with what you know . . . and an amount your body can tolerate. Nothing's more humiliating than getting smashed at your office party and telling your boss something you probably shouldn't.

4. Save dessert for when it's really worth having. Store-bought cookies that have been sitting on the shelf for weeks don't generally taste that good. Again, seek options that are either fruit-heavy, bite-size, or incredibly rich that four or five forkfuls

will satisfy your sweet tooth. Decide between a chocolate-covered strawberry and a mini cupcake, a baby cannoli and a walnut-rum ball, or four or five bites of chocolate mousse or raspberry cheesecake and conquer the dessert table.

3. The office issue. Every year your office gets inundated with gift baskets, boxes of chocolates, random brownies, cupcakes, and sugar cookies and the endless bowls of candy wherever you turn. Turn autopilot off and step away from the candy bowl. Think about what you're reaching for and save those calories for when you really want them . . . just two palmfuls of M&M'S or four teensy Hershey's kisses can rack up an easy 100 calories in no time flat.

2. Get sufficient sleep and drink enough water, at least 1 ½ to 2 liters a day . . . it'll help with those morning-after hangovers.

1. After a night of holiday cheer, bring back your cheating basics: balanced meals (refer back to the Cheater's Triangle on page 33 in Chapter 1), smaller portions, and lots of fruits and veggies. Get right back on the horse and you'll prevent the slippage and skidding that can lead us into a very sticky New Year.

- **Birthday Girl**—I am firm believer that on your birthday, you have full reign to cheat it up and indulge to your heart's content. Have a full-out freebie day—that's my birthday gift to you. Just remember that your birthday is one single day only . . . not the entire week. A one-day freebie and you're back to the basic plan as usual the very next morning.

- **Weddings Without the Crash and Burn**—Weddings are a piece of cake. If there's an open bar, you might be in a bit of trouble (stick to the basics like vodka-sodas and champagne), but aside from that, meal portions tend to be tiny and the food is generally nowhere near stellar, so you're not inclined to eat all that much. During the cocktail hour, snap up a few appetizers, one small plate, or three or four passed hors d'oeuvres, and try to make at least half of them relatively healthful. Have a small slice of the wedding cake, watch the alcohol consumption over the course of the evening, and wear something that makes you feel drop-dead gorgeous, and you'll be good to go. And, if you're like me, you'll be on the dance floor burning it up most of the evening—there's a few extra calories burned. Enjoy yourself and go back to your standard eating routine the following day. As for all the festivities preceding the big day—the engagement party, bachelorette party, and bridal shower—the same principles apply here as they would at any other event. Do a lap around the buffet table first, assess your options, and build a balanced plate accordingly—fruits and veggies first if you can, to fill up on healthy treats so that you'll have the perfect amount of room for the really sinful ones. If you're anticipating sweets, dessert, and/or alcohol being served (and consumed) at these events, adjust your week to keep treats and calories on track. You've got two *cheat and eat* treats to work with, so use them wisely.

- **Traveling Without Excess Baggage**—We touched a good bit on travel in Chapter 2 with respect to work trips and en route travel tactics, but let's not forget to establish a good game plan for weekend getaways and vacations. Follow these cheating rules of thumb and you'll survive any five-day trip to wine country or two-week escape to Thailand.

  ◆ **1. Pack snacks for the plane ride or car trip AND for your stay.** You're already doing this for work trips, but pack extra not only for the trip over, but your full stay as well—just as a precautionary measure. Who knows where you might find yourself at a meal- or snack time and what options are or aren't around. Come prepared and pack travel-friendly snacks like nuts, granola, and fruit-nut bars. Crazy as it sounds, you might even consider packing an unopened jar of peanut or almond butter (plastic so it won't break). Nut butter can be a filling protein- and healthy-fat-packed life-saver in many situations.

◆ **2. Eat like a local.** When traveling, you know you've stumbled on a great restaurant when you don't see another tourist in sight and, if you're in a foreign country, hear very little English being spoken. Certainly two signs that often indicate fresh, home-cooked, quality fare. Absolutely taste local signature dishes and try specialties you might otherwise steer clear of normally at home (like sweets and fried or olive-oil drenched items). "Taste" and "try" are vital words here, though. Keep your overall meals and snacks each day as even-keeled as possible by focusing on fruits and vegetables at each sitting (when they're available) and lean protein sources like the incredible grass-fed beef in Argentina or the fresh-caught fish in Greece. Your well-sized Cheater's portions remain intact of course. This way, even if your only option is bread, cheese, and jam for every breakfast in France, you'll still be able mitigate the potential extra pound or two gained. And if you do happen to go overboard at a meal or two, thankfully the large amount of walking and sightseeing you're doing will keep things in check.

◆ **3. Beach vacations and buffets.** Sometimes a lazy, lay-by-the-pool or on-the-beach type of vacation is exactly what you need. Just because you're not trekking all over Rome for eight hours straight doesn't mean you can't stay physically active in the Caribbean. Do something different and aim to exercise at least 50 percent of the time you're away (you do need a little break after all). Surfing, tennis, a run or sixty-minute walk on the beach, biking, hiking, swimming . . . just to give you a few ideas. If you're staying at an all-inclusive resort where meals are buffet-style bountiful twenty-four hours a day, approach each meal just like you would at a party or holiday. Scope all your options first, build a balanced plate in your head (½ fruit/veggies, ¼ protein, ¼ carbs) and then make your move. One plate, one round, same portions as you'd do at home. If something looks unbelievably mouthwatering, most definitely cheat—you're on vacation! Bring back the three to five bite rule when adding extra indulgent tastes to your plate.

◆ **4. The alcohol situation.** It's vacation, and if you're a drinker, you're bound to up the ante on alcohol consumption. If you're away just for three or four days and want to have a drink or two each night, do it. Just try to keep your total intake in the realm of reason, we'll say four to eight drinks to be nice (your body should be asking for a weeklong respite from the bottle when you return home to get you back up to speed weight-wise). If you're taking an extended trip, five days or more, attempt to simulate drinking as you would over an average week at home, eight drinks or so. Being that it's vacation, if three or four extra happen to sneak in, don't stress, but consider skipping alcohol altogether over the next day or two after.

◆ **5. Back to business at home.** Your Cheater's foundation is back in action the second you step off the plane and head home. Enough said. Try to break the excuse of "transitioning" back into your normal routine that somehow takes two weeks. Consistent meals and snacks, on-target portion sizes, veggies and fruit at every meal, 1 ½ to 2 liters of water daily, and three or more bouts of exercise a week. Your body's probably ready for its feel-good routine again. Welcome home.

• **Aunt Flow's Monthly Visit**—Oh yeah, we all can relate to this one. Who doesn't love feeling beyond bloated, emotionally whacked out, and lethargic as hell for a good week out of every month? You love the female gift of menstruation, not to mention the boatload of food cravings (chocolate, carbs, and red meat) that often accompany PMS. Whether you've employed certain combative tactics in the past or simply surrender the white flag each month, there are a few cheating tips to lessen the blow. Fact: It is quite common to gain three or four pounds in water around the time of your period, so don't freak out if you step on the scale and see a significant shift. Better yet, if you know it's going to bother you, don't step on the scale at all! Cleaning up your diet by following the

Cheater's Diet will certainly help minimize cravings, cramps, and any associated headaches or migraines . . . at least a little. Hormones are hormones, though, and your body may just be prone to craving salt or a boost in pleasure-inducing serotonin from chocolate. If you're a red meat, burger craver, your body's likely in need of some iron. No big surprise, you lose a decent amount each month during your period. Bottom line, listen to your body, have the burger (maybe cut it in half, leave half the bun, and/or skip the fries) and try to recognize and anticipate typical cravings. Plan a day or two during the week where you work in a chocolate chip cookie or a few extra pieces of dark chocolate, but do your best to keep the foundation of your day as rock-solid consistent as possible.

- **Ditch Digestive Distress**—It's incredible what people will tell you about their bathroom habits when they get comfortable with you. Actually, the state of your digestive system is often directly linked to what's going on with your diet. Countless individuals I work with complain of IBS symptoms (short and discreet for irritable bowel syndrome)—from bloating and gassiness to constipation and/or diarrhea and sharp stabbing abdominal pains. Not so fun or dainty, but unbelievably common. Unfortunately, IBS tends to be an umbrella (read: BS) diagnosis—there's no set of textbook symptoms, causes, or remedies. You can, however, try to pinpoint certain things that exacerbate it. The biggest culprit by far is stress, as it can wreak havoc on your sensitive stomach. Add a bunch of artificial sweeteners, alcohol, greasy or heavy food, and excess coffee to the situation and you've got a recipe for digestive disaster.

If you're simply backed-up and constipated, you should be much less so by Week 8, after making some significant shifts in your eating and drinking habits. A few other quick suggestions: Work in daily a tablespoon or two of ground flaxseed meal and an omega-3 fish oil supplement (1 to 2 pills depending

CHEAT SHEET: Helpful Tips to Alleviate IBS

- **What to steer clear of**—Things that bloat you and throw your digestion into overdrive (or underdrive) and contract your intestinal muscles, such as: caffeine, chocolate, alcohol, gum, carbonated drinks, fat-free anything (too many preservatives and additives), super-sugary foods and sweets, artificial sweeteners, cigarettes, bean-heavy dishes and soups. Also beware of fried, greasy foods and creamy dairy products. You might find that you're more lactose sensitive or intolerant with creamier dairy like Brie and Camembert cheese, milk, and ice cream. We want to bring down the gas quotient as much as possible, so skip the cheese and beans unless you're chilling at home by yourself.

- **What helps**—Eating a healthful diet full of fresh, real foods in smaller portions will definitely help calm your digestive system. Pacing yourself at meals and eating slowly can also make a big difference. The last thing you want to do is "dump-truck" your food down the hatch and overload your stomach. Not only will you end up consuming too many calories because you're inhaling your food, you're essentially backing up the roads and causing a traffic jam that your stomach has to work hard to clear. Not smart to tax a sensitive stomach. If you're prone to constipation, try boosting your water intake and fiber intake with fresh fruits and vegetables and whole grains. You may also want to consider taking a tablespoon of flaxseed oil or ground flaxseed meal on a daily basis to boost healthy fats and fiber. The healthy fats will help lube up your intestinal system and the fiber will get things moving along more readily. Sprinkle ground flaxseed meal into cereal, oatmeal, yogurt, or smoothies. If you're prone to diarrhea or are typically regular, you likely don't need much help in the fiber department, but calming those intestines can't really hurt. Try an omega-3 fish oil supplement to decrease inflammation and bloating, and you might see some positive results.

- **When in doubt**—Drink some peppermint or chamomile tea when you're doubled over in pain, likely from gas trying to move through your GI system. Not the prettiest picture, but the peppermint tea acts as an effective muscle relaxant and the chamomile tends to be fairly soothing and calming.

- **If you're a stress case**—Do something to ease up a little, like yoga, reading, or knitting if you're into it. Frequent exercise, four or five times a week, can be extremely helpful as well in managing symptoms.

on the bottle's serving amount), increase exercise if you're not doing much now, from two or three to five times a week, and try starting your morning off with a cup of hot water and half a lemon—I swear it's helpful. You're basically jump-starting your digestive system. Citrus is astringent—you could clean your sink with a lemon . . . we're just trying to send a cleanup crew to your digestive system.

If your lower half is running smoothly but you're frequently hit with heartburn, or GERD (gastroesophageal reflux— i.e., acid reflux), we've got other issues to tackle. Acid reflux is harder to relieve, and sometimes medication can be helpful. The big triggers to be watchful over are citrus, tomatoes and other nightshade vegetables like eggplant and peppers, all things acidic, caffeine, chocolate, cigarettes, fried foods, carbonation, alcohol, garlic, and onions. Some of these may affect you more, some less. Test the waters and play detective.

- **Wheat, for Better or Worse?**—There seems to be a rise in wheat-bashing in recent years, or possibly just greater awareness of those who can't eat it. For those who suffer from full-blown wheat and gluten intolerance, or Celiac disease, wheat and wheat protein (gluten) in any form is totally off the menu. The good news is that those with Celiac disease have a growing number of gluten-free food options to work with. The not-so-good news is that Celiac disease can be tricky to diagnose. Wheat issues can cause bloating, gas, diarrhea, abdominal pains, anemia, GERD (heartburn, reflux), and weight loss or gain. You might wonder if you have a slight wheat allergy, which can become more pronounced when wheat flour and wheat products are eaten in larger quantities. If you're concerned, definitely consult your doctor or a gastrointestinal specialist. Bottom line, if you feel you might be a bit wheat sensitive, watch your intake and try to pinpoint what items (breads, pasta, pizza, cookies, etc.) significantly bother you or if you're able to have them in small amounts without any trouble. Check out www.celiac.org for more info.

Cheater's Secret: On a less formal, less medical note, bready products are known to bloat us, particularly around our midsection, if we overindulge . . . too much of good thing. We've all stressed at least once or twice about an upcoming event where we'd like our waistlines to feel a little more svelte for the evening or for a certain outfit. Kick the bready bread and refined white stuff (flour and sugar) a few days before the event. And if you're lactose sensitive, kick milk products, too. I don't mean to parrot the no-carb diet fads, but reducing refined carbs will help minimize bloating. Clearly we love and *need* our complex carbs, but cut out the refined stuff and keep your servings of bread and pasta to zilch per day for a day or three and I think you and your stomach will be pleasantly surprised.

- **Facedown in Froyo**—Let's take a moment to discuss the issue of frozen yogurt. If you view fat-free, virtually calorie-free froyo as a godsend that's turned into a nightly treat (or ritual), you might want to think again. Think about how your stomach looks and feels after spooning down a small or medium cup. Is the gas and looking three months pregnant worth it? Ever consider why you can't recognize half the words on the ingredients list? It's only 160 calories for 4 ounces, but after they top you off, it's more like 6 or 8 ounces. Add a few toppings and we're talking well over 300 calories. Wouldn't you rather have a scoop of real, full-flavored ice cream and skip the urgent rush to the restroom? I don't mean to bash frozen yogurt, and please note that I'm not speaking about the good stuff you're able to get in the grocery store, like Stonyfield Farms and Häagen-Dazs, I'm talking about soft-serve frozen yogurt shops that boast the bizarrely low-calorie stuff—that generally has zero flavor and often serves to trigger your sweet tooth rather than satisfy it because of added artificial sweeteners. Most of this froyo is laden with artificial sweeteners, additives, and lord only knows what else. There are a few chains that have a leg up, boasting more "natural" plain yogurt, but they're still packed with too much sugar and too many additives.

Cheater's Secret: Skip the fake stuff when it comes to frozen treats, and when you're dying for something cool and creamy, use one of your *cheat and eat* treats and have a single small scoop, about the size of a tennis ball, of REAL ice cream on occasion. Your sweet tooth will be satisfied in no time, and big bonus, your stomach won't rumble for the next four hours. Balance out the indulgence with lighter meals during the day and make those extra calories work for you.

- **Quick Fixes for a Flat Belly**— You've got forty-eight or seventy-two hours before your best friend's wedding or a weekend away at the beach and you would prefer it if your stomach was a wee bit more toned and svelte. Clearly the Cheater's Diet does not promote cheap, far-out fad "fixes"— like starving yourself for the next two days, popping a few "metabolism-upping" pills, or knocking back a couple of meal-replacement shakes. That said, there are a few smart, natural quick tips you can utilize to de-bloat and trim your tummy just slightly in a matter of a few days.

  - ◆ **What to skip**: Things that add air to your stomach, like carbonated beverages (diet sodas, seltzer, etc.); gum chewing; drinking through a straw; artificial sweeteners that can cause bloating, including the pink, blue, and yellow packets, as well as sugar-free gum, diet drinks, and no-sugar-added foods; salty and sodium-rich foods that cause water retention, like canned soups, soy sauce, french fries, and cold cuts; refined white carbohydrates that can make you feel puffy, like fluffy breads, pizza, and pasta; refined, processed white sugars, like sweets, candy, cookies, cake, and ice cream; heavy, greasy meals out.
  - ◆ **What to reach for**: More water (at least 2 liters a day), lots of fresh fruits and veggies at every meal (if for some reason you're lagging, increase), citrus fruits to help release any excess water weight.

- **The Big 3-0, the Big 4-0: Metabolism Meltdown**—Metabolisms are tricky. To our dismay, they start slowing down around our thirtieth birthdays. The aging process sends us into uncharted territory, and at times it isn't so fun. Thankfully, metabolism only drops 1 to 2 percent each decade, but this downshift can lead to a drop in lean muscle mass and an increase in body fat, which is where we get the lovely phrase "middle-aged spread." I mean, it sounds like a death sentence. No fear, and certainly no frantic thoughts about lipo, please. Everything you've read in this book, and all the habits you're currently incorporating into your life, are arming you against the throws of aging and a slowdown in metabolism. Smaller portions, eating more frequently, and lots of healthy fats and antioxidant and calcium-rich foods . . . all of these things will help keep you feeling and looking *fine* far into the future. And to give another nod to the importance of physical activity, research finds that weight training helps females in their twenties to forties drop 7 percent abdominal fat and 4 percent total body fat. Get active at least three or four times a week, if not five, to fight the spread. Maybe that body conditioning class you take twice a week (along with two days of running and a yoga class) isn't so unbearable after all?

- **Don't Get Cocky!**—I will leave you with this final piece of advice, harsh as it might be. You've come this far and are doing great, so *don't get cocky*. Don't scoff or shake your head at me, I'm dead serious and I've seen this happen one too many times. You hit a good stride for a number of weeks, energy is high, weight is down, and then bam—somehow you feel like those extra desserts or those three extra cocktails can weasel their way back into the picture, no big deal. Of course, once in a while this can and will occur, but if you allow "extras" and old dirty habits to sneak back into the picture on a constant basis, you're risking a snowball back-spiral, which is clearly not what we want. Keep your head above water and try to take things day by day. If you find that you've hit a snag or are experiencing a period of continued slippage, consider going back to food journaling—even if just for a few days to get you back on track again thanks to a little accountability and structure. Regroup, refocus, and charge ahead on the path of cheating and eating for many well-fed years to come.

To bring it all home succinctly, we're pulling out this chapter's refresher course a little early. The goals you've been implementing over the past number of weeks have helped you drop extra weight (and will continue to do so). And when your body achieves its own personal healthy weight and size, whether it's 120 or 160, a size 2 or 10, the fundamental tenets of the Cheater's Diet will allow you to easily and indulgently maintain that loss for the foreseeable future. Here is a final glance at the core criteria that will help you continue to achieve and sustain a gorgeous, healthy, fit, and confident body (inside and out) . . . eating AND drinking everything you love!

The Cheater's Diet Take-Home Tips to Live, Eat, and Drink By:

- ❑ Resize portions—3 to 5 ounces protein, ½ to 1 cup rice/pasta/grain, 1 cup/piece fruit, 1 to 3 cups veggies/salad (aim to cut total portions by 15 to 25 percent and set your plate up as: ½ fruits/vegetables, ¼ lean protein, ¼ healthy, complex carbs).
- ❑ Eat 2 servings of fruit per day; aim to have vegetables with lunch AND dinner.
- ❑ Drink 1 ½ to 2 liters of water per day.
- ❑ Don't skip meals—you'll lower your calorie-burn capability!
- ❑ Cheat it up each week with one or two indulgent meals (order what you wish, but still consider portions) and one or two treats (between 200 and 300 calories each).
- ❑ Exercise at least three or four days this week—kick it up a notch if you have a heavy week of drinking and/or eating ahead.
- ❑ Cut your alcohol intake per week by at least 25 percent.
- ❑ Food journaling . . . DO IT!
- ❑ Bring three to five basic office staples to work for snacks and emergencies.

❏ Be prepared when traveling and pack a meal and/or snack(s).

❏ Be sure to have an energizing snack before a workout, and a balanced meal or satisfying snack afterward.

❏ Take a chance with a new recipe and experiment in the kitchen. Cook at home at least two to three times a week.

❏ Re-plate and re-portion takeout and delivery food. Aim for half to three quarters of the to-go container.

❏ Watch portions like a hawk at restaurants, and leave at least 5 bites on the plate, if not a quarter to half. If the bread isn't awesome, lose it.

❏ Put all snacks and meals on a plate to halt mindless eating.

❏ If you hit a plateau, jump-start your metabolism again: For three to five days, boost fruit and veggie intake by 25 percent (make them the focus of every meal), and skip alcohol, coffee, dairy (except yogurt), and wheat products.

❏ Artificial sweeteners are no longer in your vocabulary.

❏ Get back on board with the basics after a long night out and a hangover.

❏ Stock up on your staple groceries each week.

❏ Shop at your local farmers' market, the best of the best.

❏ Keep eating and keep cheating! Sometimes coming back to the basics is our best, most satisfying secret weapon.

Parting Gifts: Cheating Sweets and Treats

"Wait . . . sugar isn't one of the five basic food groups?"

—Lisa

I thought it'd be nice to finish off this book in true Cheater's fashion . . . on an indulgent, sweet note. I tend to enjoy cooking much more than baking—that whole requirement to follow a recipe like it's a chemistry experiment kind of kills it for me every time. Like every good Cheater, I just don't like following directions. But baking confections, treats, and desserts can most certainly be exciting, fun, creative, and even relaxing. It can also cause some pretty intense anxiety for a lot of us. The primary concern on the minds of many women I speak with is that if they bake something and it's sitting pretty in their kitchen, it's not going to last very long—a day, three days, a week at most before we devour it all by ourselves. Remember the *Sex and the City* episode when Miranda threw her just-baked chocolate cake into the garbage to keep herself from polishing it off in ten minutes? And remember when she dug it out of the bin five minutes later? Not exactly one of Miranda's finer moments, but it definitely makes a point about the whole screwed-up, "all or nothing," restrictive and emotional relationship many women (and men) have with sweets and chocolate. You can make the argument about self-control, or lack thereof, but oftentimes it's simply the need to achieve a better mood or shove back feelings or anxieties we just don't want to deal with at the moment. Sugary sweets and chocolate release serotonin and endorphins, neurotransmitters or brain chemicals, and we're momentarily happy and flying high . . . until, of course, your sugar crash sets in and that horrendous feeling of guilt returns.

But, and this is a big BUT, now that you've read the book, I hope we've effectively shot the idea of all-or-nothing, guilt-ridden restriction of certain foods (including scrumptious sweets) straight to hell. So let's bust out some baked goods. If you're still a bit uncertain about keeping stuff around the house, bake for a specific occasion or bring your creations into the office—your coworkers will love you. As with most things, if I'm going to indulge in sweets, a piece of cake, a cookie or a muffin, or some chocolate, I want it to be mind-blowing. This philosophy directly impacts how I bake—you won't find any low-fat, sugar-free, zero-flavor, apple juice–sweetened brownies or blondies or chocolate chip cookies in the pages that follow. Sure, I might substitute in some whole wheat flour on occasion, or a little applesauce or an extra egg white to lighten up a batch of banana bread or oatmeal butterscotch cookies, but generally speaking, I stick to the basics. Real-deal, full-fledged fat- and carbohydrate-laden ingredients like eggs, sugar, butter, good-quality chocolate chunks, nuts, and heaven forbid a nutritionist endorse this, but even a bit of heavy cream sometimes, shhh. . . . Some things just aren't worth eating if they're not sinfully good or super-light, moist, airy, crisp, buttery, chocolaty, or gooey.

CHEAT SHEET: Quick and Dirty Sweets and Snacks (averaging 100 to 200 calories)

- 0% or 2% plain Greek yogurt with cherries peaches, or honey on the side
- 0% or 2% plain Greek yogurt topped with 1 tablespoon dark chocolate or butterscotch chips, or 1 teaspoon honey and 2 teaspoons chopped pistachios or rum-soaked raisins (yum!)
- 2 to 3 squares of GOOD chocolate (ideally dark!) and 10 to 15 unsalted nuts of your choice—look for chocolate brands like Green & Blacks, Ghirardelli, Dagoba, Divine, Endangered Species, and Lake Champlain (keep your blood sugar balanced with the protein and healthy fat in the nuts for a more satisfying, filling snack)
- sweetriot chocolate-covered cocoa nibs (the entire container is just 140 calories!)
- 2 graham crackers with 2 teaspoons Nutella (chocolate-hazelnut spread) topped with banana or strawberry slices
- Makeshift S'mores—make a sandwich out of 2 graham crackers with 1 or 2 small squares of dark chocolate and a marshmallow in between. Pop it in the toaster oven or under the broiler fo 30 to 60 seconds until the marshmallow browns and the chocolate melts.
- Frozen banana slices dipped in melted dark chocolate and rolled in chopped walnuts, peanuts, pecans, or shredded coconut
- ½ cup organic chocolate, vanilla, or rice pudding
- ½ cup frozen yogurt or regular ice cream—look for organic, all-natural or local brands with all-natural ingredients, like Stonyfield Farms, Häagen-Dazs Five (just five ingredients), Ben & Jerry's Organic, and Breyers Smooth & Dreamy
- Stonyfield Squeezers (yogurt tubes—pop them in the freezer!)
- 100% frozen fruit bars
- Laura's Wholesome Junk Food (2 bite-lettes)—flavors like X-Treme Chocolate Fudge and Oatmeal Chocolate Chip
- Kashi TLC Cookies (1 to 2)
- Newman's Own Fig Newman's, Hermits, or Newman-O's (chocolate crème–filled cookies) (aim for 2)
- ¼ to ⅓ cup trail mix

The Cheater's mantra follows through to the last few pages— make it incredible, eat less in the long run, cheat yourself, and love it. And with that, here are a handful of delightful, delicious desserts, treats, and even a few healthful, energizing snacks thrown into the bunch!

If you're looking for a quick sweet fix without having to turn on the oven, we've got that, too—a handy list of lighter treats and simple snacks that won't break your calorie bank, averaging 100 to 200 calories. All of which you can work into your one or two *cheat and eat* treats a week.

Strawberry Rhubarb Crisp

Serves 8 to 10

THE GOODS

¾ cup sugar

1 tablespoon cornstarch

3 cups chopped rhubarb (about ¾- to 1-inch-wide pieces)

4 cups strawberries (leave small berries whole; slice larger berries in half)

½ teaspoon fresh lemon juice

⅔ cup brown sugar

½ cup unsalted butter

½ cup all-purpose flour

½ cup quick-cooking oats

2 teaspoons ground cinnamon

THE BREAKDOWN

1. Preheat the oven to 350°F.
2. In a large bowl, combine the sugar, cornstarch, rhubarb, berries, and lemon juice. Mix together well, then spoon into a lightly buttered 1 ½-quart baking dish.
3. In a separate bowl, combine the remaining ingredients to form coarse crumbs (I just mix them with my fingers). Sprinkle the crumbs over the strawberry-rhubarb mixture.

4. Place in the oven and bake for 30 to 40 minutes, until the crumb topping is lightly browned.

The Facts: 220 calories; 9g fat; 6g saturated fat; 2g protein; 2g fiber

Warm Strawberry-Rhubarb Compote with Low-Fat Yogurt or Ice Cream

---

Take any leftover strawberries and rhubarb from your crisp and stew them into a tasty compote. You'll end up with a low-calorie, delicious sauce to use over just about anything, whether ice cream or even low-fat plain yogurt as a sweet afternoon snack.

Makes 4 servings

THE GOODS AND THE BREAKDOWN

Combine 1 cup chopped strawberries and 1 cup chopped rhubarb with 2 teaspoons sugar, a dash of lemon juice, and ½ teaspoon vanilla extract in a saucepan and simmer for 5 to 8 minutes. Remove from the heat and cool. Spoon about ¼ cup of compote over ½ cup low-fat plain yogurt, frozen yogurt, or ice cream.

The Facts (compote only): 25 calories; 0g fat; 0g saturated fat; 0g protein; 0g fiber

Date-Nut Energy Bites

With the combo of dates and walnuts, these really are bite-size bursts of quick, lasting energy and will healthfully satisfy an afternoon sweet tooth in seconds. They're like your very own version of a Larabar. My mom had these in the freezer for us when I was a kid (they're great cold). And she still sends me a batch or two every year!

Makes about 24 mini bites

THE GOODS
  3 eggs
  ⅓ cup sugar
  1 cup chopped dates
  1 cup chopped walnuts

THE BREAKDOWN
  1. Preheat the oven to 375°F.
  2. In a medium bowl, mix the eggs with a fork. Add the sugar, dates, and nuts and mix. Place in mini cupcake liners in mini muffin pans. Bake for 15 to 20 minutes, then remove from the pan and cool.

The Facts: 70 calories; 3.5g fat; 0g saturated fat; 2g protein; 1g fiber

Whole Wheat Banana-Walnut Bread

Makes 12 to 16 slices

THE GOODS
  3 ripe small-medium bananas, mashed
  1 teaspoon baking soda
  2 tablespoons unsalted butter
  ¾ cup sugar
  2 eggs
  1 cup whole wheat flour
  1 cup all-purpose flour
  1 teaspoon cinnamon
  ¼ cup chopped walnuts plus 2 tablespoons for topping
  1 teaspoon vanilla extract
  2 tablespoons brown sugar

THE BREAKDOWN
  1. Preheat the oven to 350°F.
  2. Mash the bananas in a medium bowl and mix in the baking soda. Let stand while creaming the butter and sugar with an electric beater.

3. Add the eggs, flours, cinnamon, nuts, extract, and bananas to the butter-sugar mixture and mix thoroughly. Pour the mixture into a greased 9-inch loaf pan. Mix together the extra walnuts and brown sugar, and sprinkle the mixture evenly on top of the batter.

4. Place in the oven and bake for about 1 hour, or until a tester toothpick comes out clean from the center of the loaf. Cool for 10 minutes, then remove from the pan. It's best served when warm.

The Facts (per slice): 160 calories; 4.5g fat; 1.5g saturated fat; 2g fiber; 4g protein

Really Good Granola

Makes 16 servings (¼ cup per serving)

THE GOODS
  2 cups rolled oats
  ¼ cup canola oil
  1 cup chopped walnuts
  1 tablespoon vanilla extract
  ¼ cup maple syrup
  2 tablespoons agave nectar
  ¾ cup dried cherries
  ¼ cup chopped dried apricots

THE BREAKDOWN
  1. Preheat the oven to 375°F.
  2. Combine the oats, canola oil, walnuts, vanilla, maple syrup, and agave nectar in a large bowl and stir well. Transfer the mixture to a baking sheet and bake for 25 minutes, stirring halfway through. Remove from the oven and add the dried cherries and apricots. Cool and store in an airtight container.

The Facts: 160 calories; 9g fat; 1g saturated fat; 3g protein; 2g fiber

Dark Chocolate Cherry Holiday Biscotti

The holidays are great time to indulge, in moderation, and enjoy the company of family and friends. These biscotti serve as a deliciously healthy treat and are rich in disease-fighting antioxidants from dark chocolate, pecans, and dried cherries!

Makes 40 biscotti (serving size: 1 biscotti)

THE GOODS

    2 cups all-purpose flour
    ¾ teaspoon baking soda
    ¼ teaspoon salt
    1 cup sugar
    2 eggs
    2 egg whites
    1 tablespoon vegetable oil
    1 teaspoon vanilla extract
    2 teaspoons almond extract
    ⅔ cup dried tart cherries
    ½ cup chopped toasted pecans
    ½ cup good-quality dark chocolate chips or chunks (like
        Ghirardelli or Green & Blacks)

THE BREAKDOWN

1. Preheat the oven to 350°F.
2. Combine the flour, baking soda, and salt in a large bowl; stir well with a whisk.
3. Beat the sugar, eggs, and egg whites with a mixer at high speed or by hand until well blended, about 4 minutes. Add the oil and extracts, beating until well blended. Add the flour mixture, beating at low speed just until blended. Stir in the cherries, pecans, and chocolate chips.
4. Divide the dough in half and turn out onto a lightly greased baking sheet. Shape each portion into a 10-inch-long roll and flatten to 1-inch thickness.

5. Place in the oven and bake for 25 minutes, or until lightly browned. Remove the rolls from the baking sheet and reduce oven temperature to 325°F.
6. Cool for 10 minutes on a wire rack, then cut each roll diagonally into 20 ½-inch slices. Place the slices, cut-side-down, on the baking sheet and bake for 10 minutes. Turn the cookies over, and bake an additional 10 minutes (the cookies will be slightly soft in the center but will harden as they cool).
7. Remove from the baking sheet and cool completely on a wire rack.

The Facts (per biscotti): 90 calories; 3g fat; 1g saturated fat; 2g protein; 1g fiber

Bourbon Chocolate Tart with Fleur de Sel and Raspberry Coulis

I had to sneak in at least one unbelievably decadent dessert into this book—that's what cheating's all about after all. This tart isn't exactly light, but it's so wonderfully rich, you'll be more than satisfied with a very thin slice. If you're looking to make a good impression on just about anyone, look no further, and don't be put off by the lengthy instructions. It's much easier than it looks. And if you didn't already know, "coulis" is just a fancy word for sauce.

Makes 12 to 14 servings

THE GOODS

Tart Crust
1 cup all-purpose flour
3 tablespoons sugar
⅛ teaspoon salt
1 stick unsalted butter, cut into ½ inch pieces
1 egg yolk
1 teaspoon vanilla extract

Tart Filling

1 ¼ cups heavy cream

9 ounces bittersweet chocolate, chopped (I usually use an equal mixture of a hunk of 54% cacao and one that's 65% or above)

2 eggs

1 teaspoon vanilla extract

3 tablespoons bourbon

¼ teaspoon salt

Tart Glaze

2 tablespoons heavy cream

1 ¾ ounces bittersweet or dark chocolate, chopped (I use a chocolate that's above 65% cacao)

1 teaspoon light corn syrup (This is different from high-fructose corn syrup!)

1 tablespoon warm water

1 tablespoon bourbon

¼ teaspoon *fleur de sel* (flaky French sea salt that's great for baking and pretty presentation)

Raspberry Coulis

2 cups fresh raspberries, plus more for serving

2 to 3 tablespoons sugar

1 teaspoon fresh lemon juice

THE BREAKDOWN

1. Preheat the oven to 350°F.
2. In a food processor, blend the flour, sugar, and salt. Add the butter, egg yolk, and vanilla and pulse until the mixture forms a large moist clump.
3. Press the dough into a 9-inch round fluted tart pan with a removable bottom. Press the dough up the sides, press the bottom of the dough four or five times with the tines of a fork, and bake for 10 minutes, then cool.
4. For the filling: Bring the heavy cream to a boil in a medium saucepan, then remove from the heat. Add the chocolate and stir until melted.

5. Whisk the eggs, vanilla, bourbon, and salt in a small bowl and add to the chocolate. Pour the filling into the tart shell and bake for 20 to 25 minutes. Remove from the oven and cool for about an hour.

6. For the glaze: Bring the heavy cream to a boil in a medium saucepan, then remove from the heat and stir in the chocolate. Add the corn syrup, warm water, and bourbon. Gently pour evenly over the tart. Sprinkle the *fleur de sel* over the tart and allow to stand for about an hour.

7. For the raspberry coulis: Heat the raspberries, sugar, and lemon juice in a small saucepan and simmer for about 10 minutes. Strain the seeds out through a small sieve if desired.

8. Carefully remove the tart from the outer part of the pan. Serve with 2 to 3 teaspoons of raspberry coulis and fresh raspberries.

The Facts: 380 calories; 27g fat; 17g saturated fat; 4g protein; 3g fiber

The Cheater's Cookie

These cookies are the ideal treat for cheating and eating. There's a lot going on in these suckers, but they're worth gathering all the ingredients for. They're scrumptious and are chock-full of heart-healthy oats, antioxidant-rich dark chocolate and raisins, healthy fats from walnuts and peanut butter, and the random addition of pretzels for that sweet-salty crunch. Fair warning, the batter makes a mountain of cookies, so these are great for gifts, to bring into the office, or even store in the freezer for when you're dying for something sweet.

Makes 60 small cookies

THE GOODS
    3 cups rolled oats
    1 cup all-purpose flour
    1 teaspoon baking soda

2 teaspoons ground cinnamon

¼ teaspoon freshly grated nutmeg

¼ teaspoon salt

2 sticks unsalted butter, softened

1 cup natural peanut butter, chunky or creamy

1 cup sugar

1 cup light brown sugar

2 large eggs

2 teaspoons vanilla (I like a lot of vanilla, so I usually put in 1 full tablespoon)

1 ½ cups (12 ounces) dark or bittersweet chocolate chips

½ cup chopped walnuts

¾ cup raisins

½ cup pretzels broken into small 1-inch pieces

THE BREAKDOWN

1. Preheat the oven to 350°F.
2. In a large bowl, whisk together the oats, flour, baking soda, cinnamon, nutmeg, and salt.
3. In a stand mixer, beat the butter, peanut butter, granulated sugar, and brown sugar on medium speed until well blended. (If you don't have a stand mixer, combine the ingredients in a large bowl and mix by hand—it'll be a good mini workout for you.)
4. Add the eggs and vanilla and beat until completely blended. Turn the mixer speed to medium-low and slowly add the dry ingredients. Beat until blended and add the chocolate chips, walnuts, raisins, and pretzels. If you have time, chill the dough for 2 hours or overnight.
5. With a spoon, drop rounded tablespoons of dough a few inches apart on greased baking sheets (you'll have to work in batches)—12 to 14 cookies should fit on each baking sheet. Bake the cookies for 15 to 17 minutes. Remove the cookies from the baking sheets and cool.

The Facts: 150 calories; 8g fat; 3g saturated fat; 3g protein; Ig fiber

Luscious Raspberry Lemon Muffins

Makes 24 muffins

THE GOODS
1 ½ cups all-purpose flour
1 ½ cup whole wheat flour
4 teaspoons baking powder
½ teaspoon baking soda
1 teaspoon salt
⅔ cup unsalted butter, at room temperature
¾ cup sugar plus 4 tablespoons
2 eggs
1 tablespoon fresh lemon juice
1 cup low-fat milk
2 cups fresh raspberries
Grated zest of 2 lemons

THE BREAKDOWN
1. Preheat the oven to 375° F. Grease two 12-hole muffin pans or line with paper muffin cups.
2. In a large bowl, combine the flours, baking powder, baking soda, and salt and set aside.
3. In a separate bowl, cream the butter with an electric beater. Slowly add the ¾ cup of sugar, beating until smooth. Beat in the eggs.
4. Add the milk and lemon juice to the batter alternately with the flour and dry ingredients. Stir in the raspberries. Spoon into the prepared muffin pans.
5. Combine the remaining 4 tablespoons of sugar with the lemon zest in a small bowl. Sprinkle evenly over the batter.
6. Bake for about 25 minutes, until the muffins are light golden and a toothpick or cake tester comes out clean when inserted in the center. Remove from the oven and cool.

VARIATION: *Don't have raspberries? Swap them out for blueberries or cranberries.

The Facts: 130 calories; 6g fat; 3.5g saturated fat; 3g protein; 1g fiber

Boozy Applesauce

Apparently I like bourbon in my baked goods, because it's back in this incredibly easy, versatile applesauce—which is actually more like a chunky compote. It's deliciously healthy either way and is great to eat alone as a light snack or dessert, to spoon over vanilla ice cream, or even stir into plain yogurt.

Makes 12 to 16 servings

THE GOODS

12 apples, peeled, cored, and chopped
½ cup sugar
1 teaspoon ground cinnamon, or to taste
2 teaspoons vanilla extract
1 tablespoon bourbon

THE BREAKDOWN

1. In a large saucepan, combine the apples, sugar, cinnamon, and vanilla and cook over medium-low heat for 20 to 25 minutes, until the apples are soft and mushy. Stir at least once to make sure the apples don't stick to the bottom of the pan.
2. Add the bourbon and cook for another 5 to 10 minutes.

The Facts: 90 calories; 0g fat; 0g saturated fat; 0g protein; 3g fiber

- **Stop the Presses!**—Wait! We can't be done just yet, can we? What if you really hit a stumbling block, go completely off the reservation, and forget your cheating habits and daily plan? Not to worry or fret, I won't leave you hanging before these pages run out. Again, look back to your Take-Home Tips on the previous pages. If you find it helpful and/or soothing, copy them or rip out the page and keep it on hand, stashed secretly in your wallet or tacked up on your fridge (or somewhere else memorable but a bit more discreet). If you find yourself completely out of sorts and slipping back into old habits for a week or three, don't just continue to let things slide. Bring back the cheater in you and do some or, better yet, all of the following:

◆ Stop making excuses and reread the bold print and primary goals of the Cheater's Diet. You could come up with a zillion excuses—work's been abnormally insane, you haven't done laundry in three weeks, let alone grocery shop, your dog's been sick. Take responsibility, make eating well a priority again, and reestablish the principle goals that you know work so well—as simple as grocery shopping weekly and getting your water intake back up to snuff. Pull this book back out and read back through some key chapters (like Chapter 1 on portions, Chapter 4 on stress eating, or Chapter 5 on managing alcohol and your social life).

◆ Get another set of ears. Chat with your girlfriend, your sister, a coworker, your mom, or even your hairdresser about getting back on track. The second you verbalize it, you commit to doing it.

◆ Hold yourself accountable again. Keep a food and exercise journal for three days or three weeks, whatever it takes for you to get your healthy eating and cheating groove back on. Or grab a buddy and make a set goal to check in with him or her once a week or more, to help keep you motivated and on task. It sounds a little lame, but we've all done it at some point—whether about eating better and losing weight or about getting over an ex.

◆ Give yourself some credit. This stuff isn't easy, but hopefully it becomes more effortless and exciting as the weeks, months, and years go by. You've put a lot of energy and determination into reaching your goals. Don't look back and get bummed out or pissed off if you falter for a week or month. Praise the positive things you've accomplished and are continuing to accomplish, like cooking at home at least three times a week, exercising on a consistent basis three or more times a week, feeding your body quality food, and learning what your body's individual needs are (in terms of portion sizes, alcohol, and much more).

◆ You've got the skills, tactics, and every bit of knowledge and fortitude to catch yourself, get back up, and keep cheating and charging ahead.

Wrapping It Up: Cheating for the Long Haul

Over the course of eight weeks and eight chapters, you've managed to make healthy eating part of your day-to-day routine (without killing yourself), you've discovered the ins and outs of the grocery store and your local greenmarket, you know when and why to go organic and how to shoot back a couple of drinks (without tipping the scale), you're kicking things up in the kitchen (without causing serious injury to yourself or your home), you're relishing eating things you always thought were forbidden, you've got the gym-exercise thing down pat at least three or four times a week (who knows, a 5K or half-marathon could be in your future), and last but not least, you've managed to drop a pant size or more and have successfully shed that extra weight you were formerly hauling around.

The pounds are off, and thanks to your cheating ways, they're going to stay off for good. Over the next few weeks and months, you'll likely continue to see a little or a lot more weight continue to drop off. I'm not known to sugarcoat things—you will most likely stall out here and there for a few weeks, plateauing momentarily while your body and metabolism reset themselves, which is absolutely normal and expected. Try not to get discouraged—patience, persistence, and pleasurable, smart eating are the keys here. Refer back to earlier chapters in the book, like Chapter 4's "Clean, Lean, and Green Blueprint," to jump-start your progress.

How much total weight can you expect to lose if you continue to "cheat it up"? Eventually, your body will reach it's natural "sweet spot," the healthy weight where it feels most comfortable and confident—a totally sustainable weight that doesn't require you to eat nothing but steamed carrots, tofu, and lettuce in order to maintain it (the thought of which sounds utterly painful to me). That numeric sweet spot might be a little more or a little less than you aimed for on the scale. Keep in mind, it's simply a number (I know that's annoying to read). But if you're strutting your stuff in a hot pair of jeans, you feel fantastic, your energy levels are better than ever, your skin and hair are glowing, you're more conscious about what you put into your body, and all else is in check, that's what's most important. You're awesome, you know it, and everyone around you knows it. Take your cheating self and keep rocking out. This book has provided you the tools to do so, and with them, you're confidently and blissfully eating and drinking the best of the best. Sometimes coming back to the basics is our ultimate, most satisfying secret weapon. So go ahead, cheat it up.

BIBLIOGRAPHY

BOOKS

Krause's Food, Nutrition and Diet Therapy, by Kathleen Mahan
What to Eat, by Marion Nestle

WEB REFERENCES

Alcohol and Hangovers
http://pubs.niaaa.nih.gov/publications/arh22-1/54-60.pdf

Bagels and Portion Sizes
http://p2010.nhlbihin.net/portion/portion.cgi?action=question&number=1

Caffeine Content of Food and Drugs
www.cspinet.org/new/cafchart.htm

Carbohydrates—USDA Dietary Recommendations
www.health.gov/DietaryGuidelines/dga2005/document/html/chapter7.htm

Cinnamon and Health
www.betternutrition.com/document/624

Coffee and Beverage Calories and Nutrition
www.starbucks.com/retail/nutrition_beverage_detail.asp

Coffee and Antioxidant Content
www.medicalnewstoday.com/articles/29838.php

Eggs and the Cholesterol Myth
www.incredibleegg.org/health_heart.html

Fair Trade Coffee
www.groundsforchange.com/learn/fairtrade.php

Farmers' Markets and Local Food Marketing
www.ams.usda.gov/AMSv1.0/FARMERSMARKETS

Fats
www.americanheart.org/presenter.jhtml?identifier=4582

Fish—Environmentally Friendly
www.montereybayaquarium.org/cr/cr_seafoodwatch/sfw_health.aspx

Fish—Omega-3 Fatty Acids
www.americanheart.org/presenter.jhtml?identifier=4632

Food Consumption in America
www.usda.gov/factbook/chapter2.htm

Ingredients in Twinkies
http://abcnews.go.com/Nightline/story?id=3080425

Iron Intake Recommendations
www.ods.od.nih.gov/factsheets/iron.asp#h4

Local Food
www.sustainabletable.org/issues/buylocal/

Mercury in Fish
www.fda.gov/Food/FoodSafety/Product-SpecificInformation/Seafood/Foodborne
    PathogensContaminants/Methylmercury/ucm115644.htm
www.wholefoodsmarket.com/nutrition/methylmercury-seafood.php

Omega-3 Fatty Acids
www.umm.edu/altmed/articles/omega-3-000316.htm

Pasture-Raised Animals
www.sustainabletable.org/issues/pasture/

Portion Sizes and Plate Size
http://steinhardt.nyu.edu/nutrition.olde/PDFS/young-nestle.pdf
/www.precisionnutrition.com/wordpress/wp-content/uploads/2009/07/portion-
    size-me.pdf

Potatoes and Nutrition
www.potatoes.com/Nutrition.cfm

Restaurants and Calorie Content
www.rubytuesdays.com/files/Nutrition.pdf
www.unos.com/kiosk/nutritionUnos.html
www.dennys.com/en/cms/Nutrition%2FAllergens/23.html
www.chipotle.com/ChipotleNutrition.pdf
www.brinker.com/gr/Nutritional/Mac_NutritionalInfo.pdf

Sleep and Weight
www.sleepfoundation.org/article/sleep-topics/obesity-and-sleep

Shopper's Guide to Pesticides
www.foodnews.org

Sodium and Potassium Daily Dietary Recommendations
www.health.gov/DietaryGuidelines/dga2005/document/html/chapter8.htm

Splenda and Artificial Sweeteners
www.splenda.com/page.jhtml?id=splenda/products/main.inc

Sugar Alcohols and Artificial Sweeteners
www.ific.org/publications/factsheets/sugaralcoholfs.cfm

Trans Fats
www.fda.gov/Food/LabelingNutrition/ConsumerInformation/ucm078889.htm
www.pueblo.gsa.gov/cic_text/food/reveal-fats/reveal-fats.htm

JOURNAL ARTICLES

"A Potential Role of the Curry Spice Curcumin in Alzheimer's Disease," by John M. Ringman, *Current Alzheimer Research*, 2005

"A Role for Sweet Taste: Calorie Predictive Relations in Energy Regulation by Rats," by Susan E. Swithers, *Behavioral Neuroscience*, 2008

"Association between Reduced Sleep and Weight Gain in Women," by Sanjay R. Patel, *American Journal of Epidemiology*, 2006

"Caffeinated Beverage Intake and the Risk of Heart Disease Mortality in the Elderly: A Prospective Analysis," by James Greenberg, *American Journal of Clinical Nutrition*, February 2007

"Capsaicin Stimulates Uncoupled ATP Hydrolysis by the Sarcoplasmic Reticulum Calcium Pump," by Yasser A. Mahmmoud, *The Journal of Biological Chemistry*, June 2008

"Checking the Food Odometer: Comparing Food Miles for Local Versus Conventional Produce Sales in Iowa Institutions," by Rich Pirog, *Leopold Center for Sustainable Agriculture*, July 2003

"Chefs' Opinions of Restaurant Portion Sizes," by Marge Condrasky, *Obesity*, 2007

"Dietary Intake of Antioxidant Nutrients and the Risk of Incident Alzheimer Disease in a Biracial Community Study," by Martha Clare Morris, *The Journal of the American Medical Association*, June 26, 2002

"Does White Wine Qualify for French Paradox? Comparison of the Cardioprotective Effects of Red and White Wines and Their Constituents: Resveratrol, Tyrosol, and Hydroxytyrosol," by Jocelyn I. Dudley, *Journal of Agricultural and Food Chemistry*, September 27, 2008

"Drinking Water Is Associated with Weight Loss in Overweight Dieting Women Independent of Diet and Activity," by J. Stookey, *Obesity*, November 2008

"Effect of Capsaicin on Substrate Oxidation and Weight Maintenance after Modest Body-weight Loss in Human Subjects," by M. Lejeune, *British Journal of Nutrition*, September 2003

"Effect of Dark Chocolate on Arterial Function in Healthy Individuals: Cocoa Instead of Ambrosia?" by Charalambos Vlachopoulos, *Current Hypertension Reports*, May 2006

"Effect of Strength Training on Resting Metabolic Rate and Physical Activity: Age and Gender Comparisons," by J. Lemmer, *Medicine and Science in Sports and Exercise*, April 2001

"Effects of Green Tea and EGCG on Cardiovascular and Metabolic Health," by Swen Wolfram, *Journal of the American College of Nutrition*, 2007

"Effects of Low Habitual Cocoa Intake on Blood Pressure and Bioactive Nitric Oxide," by Dirk Taubert, *The Journal of the American Medical Association*, July 4, 2007

"Have Americans Increased Fruit and Vegetable Intake?" by Sarah Stark Casagrande, *American Journal of Preventive Medicine*, 2007

"Hangover Headache Help: Expert Tips on Avoiding—or Treating—Morning-After Head Pain," by Daniel J. DeNoon, *WebMD Health News*, December 29, 2006

"High-dose Antioxidant Supplements and Cognitive Function in Community-dwelling Elderly Women," by Francine Grodstein, *The American Journal of Clinical Nutrition*, April 2003

"Lipophilic and Hydrophilic Antioxidant Capacities of Common Foods in the United States," by X Wu, *Journal of Agricultural and Food Chemistry*, 2004

"Phenol Antioxidant Quantity and Quality in Foods: Beers and the Effect of Two Types of Beer on an Animal Model of Atherosclerosis," by Joe Vinson, *Journal of Agricultural and Food Chemistry*, August 2003

"Prevention of Sudden Cardiac Death by n-3 Polyunsaturated Fatty Acids," by A. Leaf, *Journal of Cardiovascular Medicine*, 2007

"Red Wine's Resveratrol May Help Battle Obesity," *The Endocrine Society*, June 2008

"Reductions in Dietary Energy Density Are Associated with Weight Loss in Overweight and Obese Participants in the PREMIER Trial," by Jenny Ledikwe, *The American Journal of Clinical Nutrition*, May 2007

"Regular Consumption of Dark Chocolate Is Associated with Low Serum Concentrations of C-Reactive Protein in a Healthy Italian Population," by Romina di Giuseppe, *The Journal of Nutrition*, October 2008

"Short-term Effect of Eggs on Satiety in Overweight and Obese Subjects," by Jillon Vander Wal, *Journal of the American College of Nutrition*, 2005

"Personal Health: The Sweet Slurp of Excess," by Joan Stephenson, *The American Chemical Society*

"The Contribution of Expanding Portion Sizes to the U.S. Obesity Epidemic," by Lisa R. Young and Marion Nestle, *American Journal of Public Health*, February 2002

"The Effects of Grapefruit on Weight and Insulin Resistance: Relationship to the Metabolic Syndrome," by Ken Fujioka, *Journal of Medicinal Food*, March 2006

"The Role of Dietary n-6 Fatty Acids in the Prevention of Cardiovascular Disease," by W. C. Willett, *Journal of Cardiovascular Medicine*, 2007

"The Underappreciated Role of Muscle in Health and Disease," by Robert R. Wolfe, *The American Journal of Clinical Nutrition*, September 2006

"Weight Loss Is Greater with Consumption of Large Morning Meals and Fat-Free Mass Is Preserved with Large Evening Meals in Women on a Controlled Weight Reduction Regimen," by Nancy L. Keim, *Journal of Nutrition*, January 1997

MAGAZINE ARTICLES

"8 Things You Always Wanted to Know About Dieting," Shape.com

"10 Foods that Fight Inflammation," BetterNutrition.com

"A Little Wine May Boost Heart-healthy Omega-3," *Reuters*, December 17, 2008

"Alcohol Counts," by Sally Squires, WashingtonPost.com

"Americans' Weight Issues Not Going Away," by Lydia Saad, Gallup.com

"Can Nonstick Make You Sick?" by Brian Ross, *ABC News*

"Chocolate, Wine and Tea Improve Brain Performance," *University of Oxford*, December 22, 2008

"Deconstructing the Twinkie," by John Berman, *ABC News*

"Eating Too Quickly May Encourage Weight Gain," by Jane Collingwood, Psych-Central.com, January 21, 2009

"Food Fight: Calorie Labeling in New York Restaurants," by Sharon Palmer, *Today's Dietician*, June 2007

"Is High Fructose Corn Syrup Really Good for You?" by Lisa McLaughlin, Time.com, September 17, 2008

"New Analysis Suggests 'Diet Soda Paradox'–Less Sugar, More Weight," *HSC News*, June 14, 2005, Posted: Tuesday, June 14, 2005

"Nonstick Pans are OK in New Tests," ConsumerReports.org, June 2006

"Online Grocery Shopping: Way to Go?" by Brian Dakss, CBSNews.com, July 28, 2006

"Portion Sizes in Restaurants Larger than Before," Bio-Medicine.org, October 23, 2006

"Pump It Up: Women May Prevent or Delay 'Middle-aged Spread' by Lifting Weights," *Penn Medicine,* March 3, 2006

"Snooze and Lose! Sleep Off the Weight," by Jenny Stamos Kovacs, Newsvine .com, February 6, 2009

"The Claim: Caffeine Causes Dehydration," by Anahad O'Connor, NYTimes .com, March 4, 2008

"The Overflowing American Dinner Plate," by Bill Marsh, NYTimes.com, August 3, 2008

"The Spice of Life," by Jack Turner, *Bon Appetit*, March 2009

"Throwing the Book at Salt," by Kim Severson, NYTimes.com, January 27, 2009

"U.S. Food Consumption Up 16 Percent Since 1970," by Hodan Farah, *Amber Waves*, November 2005

"Water: How Much Should You Drink Every Day?" by Mayo Clinic staff, Mayo-Clinic.com

"Why Are We So Fat?" by Cathy Newman, *National Geographic*, August 2004

OTHER SOURCES

ESHA Nutrition Analysis Software

INDEX

ABOUT THE AUTHOR

Marissa Lippert is a registered dietitian in Manhattan and knows great food when she tastes it. The founder of Nourish, a nutrition counseling and media communications firm, she helps individuals live, eat, and cook more healthfully without giving up delicious food.

After deciding to pursue her passion for health and food, she earned a master's degree in clinical nutrition from New York University.

She writes a monthly column for *Glamour* and Culinate.com and serves on the expert panel for *Woman's Day* and *Health*. In addition, she's a frequent contributor to *The New York Times* and AOL Health and has appeared on Martha Stewart Living Radio, ABC News, FOX News, and New York 1 News.

Marissa lives in Manhattan and is an avid cook, much to her friends' and family's delight. She makes the most of her tiny NYC kitchen, always bringing balance, flavor, and lots of indulgence to the table!